This Book has bee
and studied.

Ken,
Of all the frameworks that I have been
exposed to over the years, I have found
FAP to be the most helpful in establishing
a foundation for helping others. IT has been
a pleasure to work with you so far and
I hope you are finding Personal meaning and
value at Trinity.

No matter how obvious and disruptive the
clinical problems, AlwAys "catch" and
reinforce the CRB-2S, This will take
you Far!

Warmest Regards,

TL

9-3-2010

A Guide to Functional Analytic Psychotherapy

Mavis Tsai · Robert J. Kohlenberg ·
Jonathan W. Kanter · Barbara Kohlenberg ·
William C. Follette · Glenn M. Callaghan

A Guide to Functional Analytic Psychotherapy

Awareness, Courage, Love, and Behaviorism

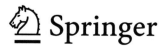 Springer

Mavis Tsai
Private practice and University
 of Washington
Seattle, WA, USA
mavis@u.washington.edu

Robert J. Kohlenberg
University of Washington
Seattle, WA, USA
fap@u.washington.edu

Jonathan W. Kanter
University of Wisconsin-Milwaukee
WI, USA
jkanter@uwm.edu

Barbara Kohlenberg
University of Nevada-Reno, Reno
NV, USA
barbarak@med.unr.edu

William C. Follette
University of Nevada-Reno, Reno
NV, USA
follette@unr.edu

Glenn M. Callaghan
San Jose State University San Jose
CA, USA
glennc@email.sjsu.edu

ISBN: 978-0-387-09786-2   e-ISBN: 978-0-387-09787-9
DOI 10.1007/978-0-387-09787-9

Library of Congress Control Number: 2008938817

Printed on acid-free paper

springer.com

Preface

Our first book, *Functional Analytic Psychotherapy: Creating Intense and Curative Therapeutic Relationships,* was published almost two decades ago. We finished that manuscript a day before our son was born, and as he has grown and flourished, so has FAP. We concluded that book with the statement, "If this book produces just one meaningful, intense, client-therapist relationship that otherwise would have not occurred, then, for us, it was useful." In fact, based on the feedback we have received, countless meaningful interactions have occurred as a result of therapists using FAP principles. Our book has been translated carefully into *Portuguese* (Rachel Kerbauy, Ph.D., Fátima Conte, Ph.D., Mali Delitti, Ph.D., Maria Zilah da Silva Brandão, M.A., Priscila Derdyk, M.A., Regina Christina Wielenska, Ph.D., Roberto Banaco, Ph.D., and Roosevelt Starling, M.A.), *Japanese* (Hiroto Okouchi, Ph.D. Takashi Muto, Ph.D., Akio Matsumoto, M.A., Minoru Takahashi, M.A., Toshihiko Yoshino, Ph.D., Hiroko Sugiwaka, Ph.D., Masanobu Kuwahara, M.A.,Yuriko Jikko, M.A., and Mariko Hirai, M.A.) and *Spanish* (Luis Valero, Ph.D., Sebastian Cobos, B.A., Rafael Ferro, Ph.D., and Modesto Ruiz, M.A.), and we have presented numerous workshops nationally and internationally to enthusiastic audiences. The relevance of FAP rules and methodology appears universal for all therapists who want to create more intense and curative therapeutic relationships. For those who are unfamiliar with FAP's foundations, Chapter 1 of this volume offers an introduction which details the behavioral principles upon which FAP was founded. Although FAP has a long way to go before it meets criteria for an empirically supported treatment, the basic tenets of FAP–the importance of the therapeutic relationship and the use of natural reinforcement to shape client problems when they occur in the therapeutic relationship–are quite robust, and evidence from multiple and diverse areas of research in support of these principles is described in Chapter 2. FAP, when conducted well, requires a thorough and accurate assessment and case conceptualization, the topic addressed in Chapter 3. The heart of FAP methodology is elucidated in Chapter 4 which discusses Therapeutic Technique and the Five Rules. In Chapter 5 we discuss our behavioral account of how the experience of self is created, and why a sense of self is necessary in order for one to engage in mindfulness. The development of intimacy and how it involves risk taking by both client and therapist is the

topic of Chapter 6. In Chapter 7, The Course of Therapy, we describe a typical
FAP treatment from beginning to end. Chapter 8 covers both individual and
group models of FAP supervision, and also offers suggestions for therapist self-
development. Therapists who believe that the world is at a crossroads for
survival and want to go beyond treating their clients' symptoms by bringing
forth their clients' best selves and a commitment to activism will resonate with
the ideas stated in Chapter 9, Values in Therapy and Green FAP.

The behavioral language and concepts used throughout this book help to
give new and more precise insights into clinical phenomena. This terminology
was not developed in the psychotherapy environment, however, and thus can be
cumbersome when used to communicate about clinical experience. In writing
this book we walked a line between the language of behaviorists and that used
by most clinicians, and sought to capitalize on the richness of both. For those
who prefer everyday language, we emphasize therapeutic awareness, courage
and love because these qualities are important in implementing the rules of
FAP. Whatever your orientation, wherever you are in your individual journey
as a therapist, we hope that the ideas and information contained in this book
will inspire you to be more aware, courageous and loving towards your clients
and that they will reinforce you for doing so.

Finally, we want to underscore that therapy is not about just following rules
and adherence measures. Each time you interact with someone, you have the
opportunity to reflect what is special and precious about this person, to heal a
wound, to co-create closeness, possibilities and magic. When you take risks and
speak your truth compassionately, you give to your clients that which is only
yours to give–your unique thoughts, feelings, and experiences. By so doing, you
create relationships that are unforgettable. When you touch the hearts of your
clients, you create a legacy of compassion that can touch generations yet
unborn.

Seattle, WA, USA   Mavis Tsai
                                                              Robert J. Kohlenberg

Acknowledgments

Mavis Tsai

Bob Kohlenberg and I requested Jonathan Kanter, Barbara Kohlenberg, Bill Follette and Glenn Callaghan to be co-authors of this volume because they each have devoted significant time in their careers to thinking, developing, teaching, researching, practicing and writing about FAP. I especially want to thank Jonathan, whose major contributions to this book helped us complete it in a timely manner. Whether his task was to write substantive material or to edit, he was always energetically willing. I also want to thank the additional chapter authors for their thoughtful and hard work. I am indebted to Bob, my devoted partner, who makes life a playground of work and love. Whatever we are collaborating on, he supports, challenges, encourages and brings out the best in me. I am thankful for the support of my cherished friends throughout the long process of writing this book. I want to thank my colleagues near and far whose appreciation of FAP's contributions to their work energizes and sustains me. I would like to acknowledge our Springer Editor Sharon Panulla for recognizing the importance of FAP and assisting us throughout the publication process. Our copy editor Janie Busby Grant did a superb and conscientious job polishing our final manuscript. I am grateful to my clients and students past and present who have shaped who I am as a person, supervisor, teacher and clinician–I love you more than you will ever know.

Robert J. Kohlenberg

I became a radical behaviorist in graduate school long before there was any Skinnerian-informed adult outpatient treatment. I was mistakenly convinced that soon, someone would develop such an approach. I waited, the years went by, and I eventually gave up hope that a radical behaviorally based outpatient therapy would come into being. In the meantime I watched Mavis do magic in the therapy room that seemed to transform everyone she worked with–I wished I could understand and do what she did. Then, in 1980, my daughter Barbara Kohlenberg said, "Dad, I want you to go to an ABA (Association of

Behavior Analysis) meeting with me and attend a workshop by my advisor, Steve Hayes–you've got to see what he is doing." Steve showed that radical behaviorism could inform outpatient therapy and blazed the trail for me to follow. Then, in close collaboration with my precious and inspired partner Mavis, with considerable struggle, time and love, we developed an understanding of how to describe and reproduce the powerful therapeutic results she attained. My dear late friend and colleague Neil Jacobson urged us to write about what we were doing, and FAP was officially born. Early on, my friend and colleague Marsha Linehan helped put FAP on the map by telling her students and associates that they need to understand FAP in order to do good DBT (Dialetical Behavioral Therapy). I want to acknowledge co-authors Jonathan, Barbara, Bill and Glenn as well as my other students (all are chapter contributors) who each made special contributions to sustaining and growing FAP throughout the years. Finally, I want to thank my clients who patiently nurtured the development of my ability to be therapeutically aware, courageous and loving.

Jonathan W. Kanter

I would first like to acknowledge Mavis Tsai and the other co-authors for creating a book-writing process that was consistent with the themes of the book–a process in which both CRB1s and CRB2s occurred for all of us, always lovingly processed in the spirit of producing the best book possible. I would also like to thank Bob Kohlenberg for his years of mentorship and shaping me into my current form as a behavioral scientist and FAP practitioner. My students– Sara Landes, Andrew Busch, Keri Brown, Laura Rusch, Rachel Manos, Cristal Weeks, William Bowe, and David Baruch – also continue to play a large role in the development of my understanding and approach to FAP, and deserve full acknowledgement. Finally, I would like to acknowledge my wife Gwynne Kohl, for her unwavering support and all that she does behind the scenes to facilitate my continued attempt at a productive and meaningful career.

Barbara Kohlenberg

I would first like to thank, with my whole heart, my mother and father, Joan Giacomini and Bob Kohlenberg, for providing me with steady and compassionate love throughout my life. Truly, the love that I put into the world, and in particular how love infuses my clinical work, my friendships, and my family, are very much extensions of the love I have felt all of my life. I also wish to acknowledge my beloved friends, Liz Gifford and Debra Hendrickson, who remind me of the importance of being true to myself in all of my endeavors. My intellectual life has been profoundly shaped by Steve Hayes, who has guided my thinking from graduate school and extending to this very day. I wish to thank

Mavis Tsai, whose love for my father, and whose courage as a clinician, thinker, and friend, has been deeply meaningful for me. My colleagues in the Department of Psychiatry, particularly David Antonuccio and Melissa Piasecki, have been a never ending source of support for me. Of late, my colleague Mark Broadhead has shared both his heart and his intellect with me, and has helped me not feel so alone during a difficult time. I am grateful for my patients, who over the years have allowed me the privilege of hearing the story of their lives, and for allowing me to share their joys and their anguish. My husband, Steve Davis, has shown me so much about love and patience. And finally, to my children, Hannah and Jack, who remind me every day that love is about both feeling and doing, and who have given me the gift of being their mother.

William C. Follette

I would thank all of those who have shaped my thinking, caring and humor. I have no idea who all of you are and how you did it. I can thank Bob Kohlenberg, who has been a mentor and friend through good times and trying times. To all my students, past and present, you may never know how much I continue to learn from you. If one is fortunate, one finds a friend along the way who is there for you when you need someone to laugh with you and sometimes at you, and to accept your friendship and return his in kind. Glenn Callaghan is such a friend. I would like to acknowledge Laura, Mom, Dad, Debbie and those who started this journey with me but were not able to finish.

Glenn M. Callaghan

I want to thank my wonderful wife, partner, and colleague, Dr. Jennifer Gregg for her love, compassion, intellectual guidance, and support. Without her, I would not be the FAP therapist or scholar that I am today. More than that, I would not be the person I am without her. My relationships with Jen, Hope and Jack are the most important ones I will ever have. My deep appreciation goes to Bob Kohlenberg and Mavis Tsai for their offer to be part of this book and their encouragement and understanding in the process of my contributions. I want to thank Bill Follette for being the best colleague and friend I could have imagined finding in this field. I would not be part of this book, a FAP therapist, or really the person I am today without his kindness, patience, and humor over the years. I want to thank all of the FAP clients I have seen for their help in shaping the way I do FAP more effectively with the openness, grace, and bravery they have shown me.

Contents

1 **What is Functional Analytic Psychotherapy?** 1
  Robert J. Kohlenberg, Mavis Tsai, and Jonathan W. Kanter

2 **Lines of Evidence in Support of FAP** 21
  David E. Baruch, Jonathan W. Kanter, Andrew M. Busch,
  Mary D. Plummer, Mavis Tsai, Laura C. Rusch, Sara J. Landes,
  and Gareth I. Holman

3 **Assessment and Case Conceptualization** 37
  Jonathan W. Kanter, Cristal E. Weeks, Jordan T. Bonow,
  Sara J. Landes, Glenn M. Callaghan, and William C. Follette

4 **Therapeutic Technique: The Five Rules** 61
  Mavis Tsai, Robert J. Kohlenberg, Jonathan W. Kanter,
  and Jennifer Waltz

5 **Self and Mindfulness** 103
  Robert J. Kohlenberg, Mavis Tsai, Jonathan W. Kanter,
  and Chauncey R. Parker

6 **Intimacy** 131
  Robert J. Kohlenberg, Barbara Kohlenberg, and Mavis Tsai

7 **The Course of Therapy: Beginning, Middle and End Phases of FAP** . . 145
  Mavis Tsai, Jonathan W. Kanter, Sara J. Landes, Reo W. Newring,
  and Robert J. Kohlenberg

8 **Supervision and Therapist Self-Development** 167
  Mavis Tsai, Glenn M. Callaghan, Robert J. Kohlenberg,
  William C. Follette, and Sabrina M. Darrow

9 **Values in Therapy and Green FAP** 199
  Mavis Tsai, Robert J. Kohlenberg, Madelon Y. Bolling,
  and Christeine Terry

Appendices 213

Index 225

Primary Authors

Mavis Tsai, Ph.D., co-originator of FAP, is a clinical psychologist in independent practice. She is also Director of the FAP Specialty Clinic within the Psychological Services and Training Center at the University of Washington, where she is involved in teaching, supervision and research on treatment development. Her publications and presentations include work on healing Posttraumatic stress disorder interpersonal trauma with FAP, disorders of the self, power issues in marital therapy, incorporating Eastern wisdom into psychotherapy, racism and minority groups, teaching youth to be peace activists, and women's empowerment via reclaiming purpose and passion. She is on the Fulbright Senior Specialists Roster, has presented "Master Clinician" sessions at the Association for Behavior and Cognitive Therapy, and has led numerous workshops nationally and internationally. She is interested in behaviorally informed multi-modal approaches to healing and growth that integrate mind, body, emotions and spirit. e-mail: mavis@u.washington.edu

Robert J. Kohlenberg, Ph.D., ABPP, co-originator of FAP, is a professor of psychology at the University of Washington, where he held the position of Director of Clinical Training from 1997 to 2004. The Washington State Psychological Association honored him with a Distinguished Psychologist Award in 1999. He is on the Fulbright Senior Specialists Roster, and has presented "Master Clinician" and "World Round" sessions at the Association for Behavioral and Cognitive Therapies. He has presented FAP workshops both in the United States and internationally, and has published papers on migraine, Obsessive-compulsive disorder, depression, intimacy of the therapeutic relationship, and a FAP approach to understanding the self. He has attained research grants for FAP treatment development, and his current interests are identifying the elements of effective psychotherapy, the integration of psychotherapies, and the treatment of co-morbidity. e-mail: fap@u.washington.edu

Jonathan W. Kanter, Ph.D., is an assistant professor of psychology, Director of the Depression Treatment Specialty Clinic, and Coordinator of the Psychology Clinic at the University of Wisconsin-Milwaukee. His research focuses on Behavioral Activation, the mechanisms of action in FAP, and stigma related to depression. He has presented numerous workshops on FAP and provides clinical supervision in both FAP and BA. e-mail: jkanter@uwm.edu

Barbara Kohlenberg, Ph.D., is an associate professor at the University of Nevada School of Medicine, Department of Psychiatry and Behavioral Sciences. She has a special interest in combining FAP and Acceptance and Commitment Therapy. She has been principal investigator and a co-investigator on NIH grants focused on treatment development using FAP and ACT, in the areas of addictions, stigma, and burnout. Her interests include FAP, ACT, and the elements of successful psychotherapy. She also is interested in training medical students in interviewing skills for use in medical settings. e-mail: bkohlenberg@medicine.nevada.edu

William C. Follette, Ph.D., is an associate professor of psychology at the University of Nevada, Reno, where he is currently the Director of Clinical Training. He has taught several workshops on FAP and runs a large FAP supervision team at UNR. He has presented a number of panels and symposia at national meetings including the Association for Behavioral and Cognitive Therapies and Association for Behavior Analysis. He has had a grant from NIMH (National Institute of Mental Health) studying FAP as an intervention for those dependent on benzodiazepines. Besides his interests in treatment research and development and clinical behavior analysis, he also conducts research on the acquisition of complex interpersonal skills, depression and functional assessment. e-mail: follette@unr.edu

Glenn M. Callaghan, Ph.D., is a professor of psychology at San Jose State University in California. He has published a variety of articles on FAP ranging from behavioral conceptualizations to research methodology essential to FAP's development to single subject treatment outcome studies. He is co-author of the Functional Analytic Psychotherapy Rating Scale, a coding system used to identify the mechanism of change in FAP. He developed and authored the Functional Idiographic Assessment Template (FIAT) and Functional Assessment of Skills of Interpersonal Therapists (FASIT). His interests in FAP lie with the use of principally-based interpersonal behavior therapies focused on long-standing pervasive repertoire problems such as those seen in recurrent depression, dysthymic disorder, and personality disorders. He is engaged in both psychotherapy and the supervision of FAP therapists, and conducts workshops introducing FAP to new therapists and training FAP skills to intermediate and advanced therapists. e-mail: Glenn.Callaghan@sjsu.edu

Contributing Authors

David E. Baruch Graduate Student, Cardinal Stritch University, Milwaukee, WI, USA, debaruch@gmail.com

Madelon Y. Bolling, Ph.D. Independent Practice; Clinical Instructor, University of Washington, WA, USA, mbolling@u.washington.edu

Jordan T. Bonow Graduate Student, University of Nevada, Reno, NV, USA, jtbonow@yahoo.com

Andrew M. Busch, M.S. Graduate Student, University of Wisconsin-Milwaukee, Milwaukee, WI, USA, ambusch@uwm.edu

Sabrina M. Darrow, M.A. Graduate Student, University of Nevada, Reno, NV, USA, darrow@unr.nevada.edu

Gareth I. Holman Graduate Student, University of Washington, WA, USA, gholman@u.washington.edu

Sara J. Landes, Ph.D. Postdoctoral Fellow, Harborview Medical Center, University of Washington, WA, USA, sjlandes@u.washington.edu

Reo W. Newring, Ph.D. Postdoctoral Psychology Fellow, Behavioral Pediatrics and Family Services Clinic, Boys Town, Great Plains, NE, USA, rwexner@u.washington.edu

Chauncey R. Parker, Ph.D. Independent Practice, Reno, NV, USA, chaunceyparker@gmail.com

Mary D. Plummer, Ph.D. Independent Practice; FAP Clinic Supervisor, University of Washington, WA, USA, marydp@u.washington.edu

Laura C. Rusch, M.S. Graduate Student, University of Wisconsin-Milwaukee, Milwaukee, WI, USA, lrusch@uwm.edu

Christeine Terry Graduate Student, University of Washington, WA, USA, cmt3@u.washington.edu

Jennifer Waltz, Ph.D. Associate Professor of Psychology, University of Montana, Missoula, MT, USA, jennifer.waltz@mso.umt.edu

Cristal E. Weeks, M.S. Graduate Student, University of Wisconsin-Milwaukee, Milwaukee, WI, USA, ceweeks@uwm.edu

Chapter 1
What is Functional Analytic Psychotherapy?

Robert J. Kohlenberg, Mavis Tsai, and Jonathan W. Kanter

As you begin to read this book, we imagine you are intellectually curious and eager to expand your therapeutic skills. You already may have experience using Functional Analytic Psychotherapy (FAP) and want to delve more deeply, or this may be your first exposure. If you are not sure what FAP is, you may be expecting a behaviorally informed dictionary definition, or you may be seeking an answer that speaks more to your intuition. Consistent with the behavioral approach we take in this book, however, we believe there is no absolute, context-free 'best' in terms of definitions, therapeutic interventions or underlying theory. Instead, 'best' always depends on what one is attempting to accomplish. FAP is an idiographic therapy that is experienced differently among those who have learned, practiced, received, researched, taught and/or written about it. Thus, we start with a smörgåsbord of these experiences. We hope at least one will strike a chord in you.

1) *A client*

A female client has been struggling with PTSD symptoms following negative experiences involving trusted healthcare professionals. Consistent with findings from the PTSD literature, she had a pre-existing vulnerability that would account for the unusual intensity and severity of her symptoms. Her history included early abandonment, a lack of care by trusted others, and the death of close family members. The following is an excerpt from an e-mail in which she describes reactions to her therapy session with RJK a few days earlier.

> You've always asked for free association, and this morning I awakened at 6:30 just full of it. So, here goes. Why, I kept asking myself, are you [RJK] being so persistent about this 'perverse' path of whistling in the dark, in which you are at once encouraging my attachment to you (ostensibly), while talking about the end of our therapy and presumably other endings as well? In what kind of uneasy truce, I also wondered, would Freud and the Behaviorists sit at the same table and drink tea? Well, it occurred to me that you are using therapeutic attachment/transference for desensitization/exposure therapy. You are asking me to *be*, again and again, at the edge of my comfort zone, in the space in which one is 'knowingly' attached, trusting you, myself really, to cushion the end, even delight in it. 'Transference-based Exposure Therapy,' huh?

R.J. Kohlenberg (✉)
Department of Psychology, University of Washington, Seattle, WA 98195-1525, USA
e-mail: fap@u.washington.edu

M. Tsai et al., *A Guide to Functional Analytic Psychotherapy*,
DOI 10.1007/978-0-387-09787-9_1, © Springer Science+Business Media, LLC 2009

2) *A graduate student*

FAP pushes me to stretch and to grow and to be theoretically and values-consistent in all aspects of my life. FAP challenges me to see therapy through the client's eyes, to engage in self-introspection and to more accurately analyze myself in my interactions.

3) *A CBT (Cognitive Behavioral Therapy) therapist*

Learning how to 'be' in a therapeutic relationship has been one of the most valuable 'take home' ideas FAP has given me. I now find that much of the time that I am working with a client I am mindful of how 'I am' and focus on the intention to be fully present—and it has been a powerful process, even when it is uncomfortable. I have been impacted in a very profound way, both professionally and personally. I am much more aware of my avoidance patterns. I have become more in touch with my desire to link my personal self and my professional self in a way that is more real, more human and more present. Learning FAP has been a healing and broadening force in my life, and has enriched my life so much. This has been a life-changing experience.

4) *A DBT (Dialectical Behavioral Therapy) therapist*

FAP is about living fully by experiencing emotion, risking as much as our patients, wanting to change the world, wanting to relieve suffering and moving towards love and the capability for love. I just love the blend of creativity, pushing borders, intensity, existential meetings and potent therapeutic technique.

5) *Book co-author*

FAP is an interpersonally-oriented psychotherapy designed to help alleviate client problems that are fundamentally about human relationships. Client suffering may occur in the presence or absence of people. Yet the emotional pain clients feel is about their lack of meaningful connection. What makes FAP unique is the use of basic behavioral assumptions about contingent shaping and the application of reinforcement during a therapy session. At the core of FAP is its hypothesized mechanism of clinical change, through contingent responding by the therapist to client problems live, in-session, while they occur.

6) *Book co-author*

FAP uses behavioral principles to create a sacred space of awareness, courage and love where the therapeutic relationship is the primary vehicle for client healing and transformation. FAP shapes interpersonal effectiveness by nurturing clients' abilities to speak and act compassionately on their truths and gifts, to engage in intimacy and to fully give and receive love.

We originally developed FAP (Kohlenberg & Tsai, 1991) to explain why some of our clients receiving standard CBT exhibited unanticipated and marked transformations in their lives, far beyond the usual expectations of treatment. Each of these remarkable cases involved a naturally occurring and particularly intense, involved and emotional therapist-client relationship. We sought to explain these therapist-client relationships using a radical behavioral analysis (Skinner, 1945, 1953, 1957, 1974) of the psychotherapeutic process that emphasized each individual's unique history.

Certainly the notion that the therapist-client relationship plays a central role in producing change is ubiquitous in the psychotherapy literature and has considerable empirical support (see Chapter 2). Our intent in using radical behavioral concepts to understand this phenomenon was to provide a new perspective on the way in which the therapist-client relationship contributes to therapeutic gains. We used a 'top-down' approach, starting with clinical observations of therapist interventions and their effects, and then using behavioral concepts to explain these effects. We also used a 'bottom-up' approach, applying behavioral concepts, associated theory and laboratory findings to inform, shape and refine therapeutic interventions. FAP as currently practiced reflects over two decades of this iterative process.

One key advantage of the behavioral approach embedded in FAP is that it points to hypothesized mechanisms of change that, in turn, lend themselves to specific and teachable treatment guidelines. Behavioral concepts and definitions enable therapists to implement a broad range of potentially significant therapeutic mechanisms such as 'courage,' 'therapeutic love' and 'creating a sacred space' (see Chapter 4), not typically addressed in cognitive behavioral therapies. Bringing such courage and love into their relationships with clients is a difficult process that takes therapists to the edge of their own comfort zones—often evoking emotional avoidance. We also look to behaviorism to facilitate responsible, ethical risk-taking by therapists that is beneficial for clients.

Basic Behavioral Concepts Underlying FAP

Behaviorism, which is at the core of FAP, is easily misunderstood. For this reason it is appropriate to review some basic behavioral concepts and how they apply to FAP. We refer readers who would like a more detailed description of fundamental behavioral tenets to our first volume (Kohlenberg & Tsai, 1991). In this section we will address three key concepts: behavior as action, the difference between functional analysis and topographical analysis, and reinforcement. Keep in mind that behaviorism is a contextual theory that questions the existence of a fixed, knowable reality and instead adopts pragmatism as its truth criterion (Hayes, Hayes, & Reese, 1988; Roche, 1999). Reality and even the notion of reality in this contextualistic approach to understanding people is a function of the unique experiential histories of those for whom a particular reality is relevant. In other words, one's perception of reality is a product of the context in which such perceiving occurs. Because context plays such a central role in this theory, the most important issue is not if the theory is right in an objective sense but if it is pragmatically useful—does it lead to devising helpful therapeutic interventions, ameliorating human suffering, and facilitating individuals to lead meaningful, productive and fulfilling lives?

Behavior as Action[1]

What is behavior? The way this question typically is answered is at the root of a pervasive misconception about radical behaviorism. All too often behavior is defined in a narrow way that is limited to overt, publicly observable events and does not include thinking or feeling. Behavior (also known as acts), however, actually refers to *anything* a person does. Behavior definitely encompasses observable events such as walking, smoking, laughing, talking and crying. It also includes private acts, such as having a dream, liking a movie, calculating a tip, feeling sad, wishing for a sunny day, thinking, feeling, seeing, hearing, experiencing and knowing. Behavior includes the activity of bodily organs as well, such as the heart beating. Thus every aspect of being human is encompassed by this definition of behavior, as long as the act is expressed as a verb— instead of having memory, people remember; instead of having values, people value; instead of having courage, people act courageously.

Behaviorism is a theory of behavior change, thus if mental entities of interest can be specified as verbs, actions or processes, the appropriate targets of therapy are much clearer. For example, instead of having low self-esteem, people think, believe, attribute, feel and act in ways that they or others label as indicative of low self-esteem. Instead of having problems of the self, people find experiencing an abiding awareness difficult, or become fearful in intimate relationships. Psychoanalyst Schafer (1976) has called for and demonstrated the feasibility of a similar translation of psychoanalytic structures into processes (verbs). Thus translating nouns into verbs also facilitates a common language across different therapeutic systems and assists in psychotherapy integration (Kohlenberg & Tsai, 1994). The following are more examples of behaviors as actions.

> Dreaming, singing, drinking,
> Walking, talking, winking, sailing,
>   wailing, bailing, taking notes, and flailing.
> Wondering and wandering, laundering, and
>   pondering.
> Thinking of an old friend, mixing a fine blend.
> Speaking your truth, drinking French vermouth.
> Running, heaving, sighing, leaving.
> Belching, throwing, blowing, sewing.
> Picking up sticks, getting out of a fix.
> Passing gas, thinking of a glass.
> It's behavior if you can do it
> Doesn't matter if no one knew it.

Having highlighted the importance of verbs, we need to specify a caveat, namely that when you see nouns that appear to be mental entities in this book, we are still talking about process, but are using a short-hand way of conveying meaning, as using only verb language can be unwieldy.

---

[1] This section, including the behavioral poem below, is based in part on Biglan (1995).

Functional Analysis Versus Topographical Analysis

To illustrate what is meant by 'functional analysis' consider the following case study (Haughton & Ayllon, 1965), one of the earliest reported in the behavior therapy literature. The patient depicted in Fig. 1.1 was a long-term resident in a psychiatric ward at a time when both medication and community/social support treatment options were limited. At that point in the history of behavior therapy, medical and psychoanalytic models dominated almost every aspect of treatment. In that context, Drs. Haughton and Ayllon were desperately attempting to demonstrate that contingencies of reinforcement can influence behavior that is almost universally seen as 'pathological.' The researchers sought to discover if the behavior of holding a broom and sweeping the floor could be shaped in this patient through the use of cigarettes as reinforcers. After a few weeks of reinforcement for this behavior, the patient spent most of her time holding the broom (as shown in Fig. 1.1). Two psychoanalytically-oriented therapists, who were not aware of the shaping, were then asked to explain why the patent was acting that way. Dr. A gave the following explanation.

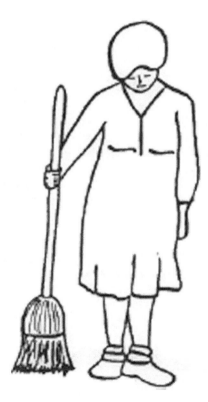

Fig. 1.1 Sketch of patient in reinforced position

The broom represents to this patient some essential perceptual element in her field of consciousness. How it should have become so is uncertain; on Freudian grounds it could be interpreted symbolically, on behavioral grounds it could perhaps be interpreted as a habit which has become essential to her peace of mind. Whatever may be the case, it is certainly a stereotyped form of behavior such as is commonly seen in rather regressed schizophrenics and is rather analogous to the way small children or infants refuse to be parted from some favorite toy, piece of rag, etc.

Dr. B's account was as follows.

Her constant and compulsive pacing holding a broom in the manner she does could be seen as a ritualistic procedure, a magical action. When regression conquers the associative process, primitive and archaic forms of thinking control the behavior. Symbolism is a predominant mode of expression of deep seated unfulfilled desires and instinctual impulses. By magic, she controls others, cosmic powers are at her disposal and inanimate objects become living creatures. Her broom could be then: (1) a child that gives her love and she gives him in return her devotion, (2) a phallic symbol, (3) the scepter of an omnipotent queen. Her rhythmic and prearranged pacing in a certain space are not similar to the compulsions of a neurotic, but because this is a far more irrational, far more controlled behavior. From a primitive thinking, this is a magical procedure in which the patient carries out her wishes, expressed in a way that is far beyond our solid, rational and conventional way of thinking and acting.

What was wrong with the explanations given by Drs. A and B? We would argue that they were not based on functional analysis. They made the mistake of assuming that one could infer causality by merely looking at the topography (the formal appearance) of the behavior. As behaviorists we seek to avoid such inferences and instead attempt to discover the causal factors that account for the behavior. It is not that the accounts given by Dr. A and Dr. B could never be correct. Rather, there are numerous possible causes for the patient's behavior. Without a functional analysis, it is impossible to know which explanation is appropriate for this particular 'symptom' of this particular patient at this particular time. Behaviorists believe that behavior independent of context has no meaning. Causes, according to behaviorists, are environmental stimuli that influence behavior in specific contexts. A functional analysis is an attempt to identify these stimuli and how they historically acquired their influence on behavior.

There are primarily three types of stimuli of concern in functional analysis.

1) *Reinforcing* stimuli are stimuli that follow a behavior, thereby making it more or less likely to occur in the future. Reinforcing stimuli in essence are consequences that affect the future probability or strength of a particular behavior. For example, a glass of water reinforces the behavior of a thirsty person asking for a glass of water. In FAP, reinforcement is the most important function to understand, and the key to FAP is understanding how therapists naturally reinforce client behavior.

2) *Discriminative* stimuli are stimuli that reliably precede a behavior and predict that reinforcement may occur. Discriminative stimuli may be complex. In the above example, an actual glass of water (or a nearby glass and available water) and a person who is able to hear the request are aspects of the

discriminative stimulus for the behavior of asking for a glass of water. In other words, discriminative stimuli are circumstances under which certain behaviors are reinforced and thus are more likely to occur. Behavior that occurs due to the presence of a discriminative stimulus and whose strength is affected by its consequences, or reinforcement, is commonly known as voluntary behavior, and technically termed 'operant' behavior. Operant behavior involves both discriminative and reinforcing stimuli. One would not ask for a glass of water if based on past experience there were no chance of obtaining it (reinforcing stimuli) and no one to hear the request (discriminative stimuli).

3) *Eliciting* stimuli, like discriminative stimuli, also precede behavior. They cause a different type of behavior, however, and reinforcement is not necessary. Eliciting stimuli elicit involuntary or reflexive behavior, technically called 'respondent' behavior. Respondent behavior is the type that enters into the Pavlovian conditioning paradigm, such as salivating in response to food on the tongue. Many 'gut' emotional reactions can be considered respondent behavior.

Functional analysis answers the question 'What is a behavior's function?' by identifying the reinforcing, discriminative, and eliciting stimuli of which behavior is a function. FAP is primarily (but by no means only) concerned with reinforcement, and thus it is discussed in detail below. For now, the crucial point is that reinforcement is a historical process. One asks for water, not because reinforcement will occur and the water will be received in that instance, but because asking the question has been reliably reinforced with water *in the past*.

Functional analysis requires understanding each client's unique history, and this understanding allows us to define topographically similar behaviors according to different functions. For example, consider the behavior of drinking alcohol excessively at a party. For one individual, this could represent negative reinforcement, if in the past alcohol has eased social anxiety and made the individual less nervous. For another individual, this could represent positive reinforcement, if in the past alcohol consumption has led to fun times. Of course, it is often the case that multiple functions are involved, especially with complex behavior. The important point for now is that as behaviorists, we define behavior according to its function. To say that the individual has an alcohol drinking problem is not sufficient. This is simply a description of the topography of the behavior—what it looks like. We prefer descriptions such as the problem functions to alleviate anxiety, to gain benefits from lowered social inhibition, or that the problem has multiple functions. As discussed earlier, keep in mind that behaviorism is a contextual system. Thus, functional analysis is preferred not because it is 'right' or 'better' in an absolute or objective sense but only to the extent that it is pragmatic and leads to useful therapeutic interventions.

A functional analysis can be conducted in many ways. The ideal method involves performing an experiment that carefully controls and manipulates different variables—in essence the creation of a real history in the laboratory—while measuring the frequency of the behavior in question in order to clearly identify which variables function as reinforcers. With rare exceptions (e.g. Kanter et al., 2006), such experimental functional analyses are difficult to do during outpatient psychotherapy. In fact, because functions are determined by history, the therapist rarely has direct access to this history. Instead the therapist simply asks questions to discern, as accurately as possible, the potential functions of a behavior (see Chapter 3 for a detailed discussion of assessment). The FAP therapist also closely observes how the client responds to the therapist, which is an important source of information to aid functional analysis.

Reinforcement

In radical behavioral theory, reinforcement is seen as ubiquitous in our daily lives. The term 'reinforcement' is used here in its precise, generic sense, referring to all consequences or contingencies that affect (increase or decrease) the strength of behavior, including positive and negative reinforcement and punishment. The strengthening or weakening of behavior occurs at an unconscious level, such that awareness or feelings are not required. Although individuals often experience pleasure when being positively reinforced or displeasure when negatively reinforced or punished, this awareness is not a necessary part of the reinforcement process and should not be confused with it.

Reinforcement is the ultimate and fundamental cause of action. Complete radical behavioral explanations necessarily involve identifying reinforcement history. For example, a client may say he yelled at his spouse because he was angry. As a behavioral explanation this is incomplete, however, and requires information about past contingencies which account for both the actions of getting angry and yelling. That is, not every spouse gets angry under those circumstances, nor even if angry, do all spouses yell. A complete explanation addresses these issues in addition to the individual's internal states and current situation.

Even though complete explanations always refer to history and are preferred, it may be sufficient or useful at times to view clients' problems as resulting from more proximal discriminative stimuli (influences) in the current environment, including one's private thoughts and emotions.

Three aspects of reinforcement particularly relevant to the psychotherapy situation are natural versus contrived reinforcers, within-session contingencies and shaping.

Natural versus contrived reinforcers. Unfortunately, simply saying 'good' or offering a tangible reward to a client for behaving as the therapist wants are typical images that come to mind when the term 'reinforcement' is mentioned. These images are not only technically erroneous but exemplify contrived reinforcement. The distinction between natural and contrived reinforcement is especially important in the change process (Ferster, 1967; Skinner, 1982). Reinforcement almost always occurs naturally and is rarely the result of someone 'trying' to reinforce another. Natural reinforcers are typical and reliable in daily life, whereas contrived ones generally are not. For example, giving a child candy for putting on a coat is contrived, whereas getting chilled for being coatless is a natural reinforcer. Similarly, fining a client a nickel for not making eye contact is contrived, while the spontaneous wandering of the therapist's attention when the client is looking away is natural.

Contrived reinforcers can be highly effective in the treatment of clients who are restricted in movement and/or who live in controllable environments such as schools, hospitals or prisons. In these settings, contrived reinforcers can be used consistently and not just in the context of a brief therapeutic interaction. Contrived reinforcement can fall short, however, when the changed behavior is expected to generalize into daily life. Consider for example a client for whom expressing anger is a problem, and he or she actually expresses anger during a therapy session about the therapist's inflexibility regarding payment terms. If the therapist responds by smiling and saying, 'I'm glad you expressed your anger toward me,' this is likely to be contrived reinforcement as such a consequence is unlikely to occur in the natural environment. Clients who learn to express anger because it was followed by smiles would not be prepared to express anger appropriately during daily life. A natural reinforcer probably would have consisted of the therapist taking the client seriously, discussing and perhaps altering the payment policy. Any changes produced by these consequences would be more likely to carry over into daily life.

Unfortunately, the deliberate use of reinforcers can lead them to become contrived or 'phony' and to lose their effectiveness (Ferster, 1972). This problem was alluded to by Wachtel (1977), who observed that behavior therapists were often overly exuberant in their use of praise, thereby diminishing its effectiveness. Furthermore, deliberate use of consequences can be viewed as manipulative or aversive by clients and induce efforts on their part to reduce or alter therapeutic change efforts—what Skinner (1953) would call 'counter-control.'

The use of reinforcement in psychotherapy thus presents a major dilemma. On the one hand, natural reinforcement that is contingent on the goal behavior is the primary change agent available in the therapeutic situation. On the other hand, if the therapist attempts to purposely 'use' the extant natural reinforcers, they may lose their effectiveness, induce counter-control and produce a manipulative treatment. The dilemma is obviated, however, when the therapy is structured so that the genuine reactions of the therapist to client behavior naturally reinforce improvements as they happen. More specifically, because the dominant aspect of psychotherapy is interactional, the immediate natural reinforcement of client improvements is most likely when the client-therapist relationship naturally evokes the client's presenting problems. The following is an example of such a relationship.

A male client has just demonstrated an in-session improvement—after avoiding talking about his grief over the death of his mother for months, he has broken down and begun crying about her death. Up to this point, the client's marriage has been disrupted, partly because his avoidance of expressing grief was achieved by being more emotionally distant from his wife. At this moment, the FAP therapist should ask oneself a series of questions such as, 'How am I feeling toward this client at this particular moment?', 'Am I feeling close, intimate, connected, supportive, or am I feeling distant, bored, disconnected?', 'Would expressing my own reaction to the client right now enhance our relationship and bring us closer, or would it scare him and punish him for showing his feelings?', 'How likely is it that my reaction in this moment would be typical of his wife? Would she feel the same as I do?' Given appropriate answers to these questions, the FAP therapist might amplify his or her feelings to the client by saying, 'You showing me your feelings right now makes me feel as close to you as I ever have. It connects me to you in a deep way.' This constitutes natural reinforcement. The therapist might later encourage the client to let his wife see these feelings as well.

In essence, FAP provides a simple set of guidelines (the five rules discussed in Chapter 4) specifying when and how to apply natural reinforcement in the therapeutic relationship.

Within-session contingencies. A well known feature of reinforcement is that the closer in time and place a consequence is to the behavior, the greater the effect of that consequence. It follows, then, that treatment effects will be stronger if clients' problem behaviors and improvements occur during the session, where they are closest in time and place to the available reinforcement. For example, if a female client states that she has difficulty trusting others, the therapy will be much more powerful if her distrust actually manifests itself in the therapeutic relationship where the therapist can react immediately, rather than just talking about such incidents that occur in between sessions. Significant therapeutic change results from the contingencies that occur during the therapy session within the client-therapist relationship.

Shaping. The concept of shaping implies that there is a large response class of client behaviors for the therapist to reinforce. It is the behavioral equivalent of saying 'Clients will do their best to improve and therapists just need to recognize when this happens.' Shaping is contextual in that it takes into account a client's learning history and the behaviors present and absent from the client's repertoire. Thus, the same behavior may be considered a problem for one client but an improvement for another. For instance, take the case of a male client who pounds on his armrest and yells at the therapist, 'You just don't understand me!' If this behavior came from a client who entered therapy unable to express feelings, it would constitute an improvement, and the therapist's openness to this outburst would be important. Of course, if outbursts like this were typical, the therapist might suggest an alternative way to express feelings of displeasure that does not involve aggressive physical demonstrations.

A Behavioral View of Psychotherapy

What occurs during outpatient psychotherapy sessions? Essentially, a client and a therapist sit in an office and talk to each other. The client is there due to daily life problems, voluntarily attending on a regular basis and pays for the therapist's time. The therapist does not observe the client outside of the weekly fifty-minute therapy sessions or control events in the client's day-to-day environment. Nevertheless, the process is intended to help the client outside of the office in his or her daily life.

In light of the above, an interesting theoretical question facing every psychotherapist is, 'What does the therapist do in-session that helps the client with problems occurring outside the session?' The therapist's world views and theories of behavior have marked implications for the methods and form of psychotherapeutic practice employed. Putting on a behaviorist hat, we would argue that the answer lies in functional analysis. Everything a therapist can do to help clients involves the presentation of the three types of stimuli discussed above (reinforcing, discriminative and eliciting stimuli), each defined by their functions or the effects they have on clients.

Each and every action of a therapist can have one or more of the above three functions at the same time. Consider a therapist asking, 'What are you feeling right now?' This question could have a discriminative function, in effect saying, 'It is now appropriate to describe your feelings.' The client's response to this question is the occurrence of an operant. It is also possible, however, that the question might be aversive to the client and thus punish the behavior that immediately preceded it. For example, imagine the client was crying immediately before the therapist asked the question, but does not know exactly why he or she was crying and hates not having answers. In this case the therapist's question may punish the emotional expression of crying and make it less likely to occur in the future. This weakening of the client's prior behavior is the result of the reinforcing function (punishment in this case). The eliciting function of the question might cause the client to turn red, sweat, get anxious or induce other private bodily states. Specifically why the client reacts in these ways can be found in his or her history.

Application of functional analysis to outpatient psychotherapy may seem like a strange idea. It has become quite clear, however, that functional analysis is extremely beneficial in other areas of psychology. Indeed, by applying basic functional analytic principles to effect behavior change in controlled and institutional settings, such as classrooms and inpatient units, applied functional analysts have had an immense impact on the field. Such analysts have created a range of successful treatments for many populations defined by severe behavioral disruptions and physical and cognitive impairments.

For many years, despite ongoing success in settings such as those mentioned above, functional analysts (with the notable exception of Hayes (1987)) did not attempt to apply the fundamental principle of reinforcement to the adult, outpatient psychotherapy context. Factors that delayed the birth of FAP have been described elsewhere in detail (Kohlenberg, Tsai, & Dougher, 1993; Kohlenberg, Bolling, Kanter, & Parker, 2002; Kohlenberg, Tsai, & Kohlenberg, 1996). Here, we simply note that one reason for the reluctance to apply principles of reinforcement in therapy may have been distaste for arbitrary or contrived reinforcement, which many non-behaviorists erroneously assume to be the only form of reinforcement. For example, it is difficult for therapists to see the relevance of reinforcers often used in basic research (e.g., food pellets or water), or those used in applied work in controlled settings (e.g., play privileges or tokens to purchase cigarettes) to their work with adult, outpatient clients. FAP, we believe, elegantly solves this problem, and harnesses the power of reinforcement to create genuine and life-changing therapy experiences.

FAP's 'Here and Now' Therapeutic Focus

FAP is based on the assumptions that, (1) the only way a therapist helps the client is through the discriminative, reinforcing and eliciting functions of what the therapist does, and (2) these stimulus functions will have their strongest effects on client behavior occurring during the session. Thus the most important characteristic of a problem suitable for FAP is that it can occur during the therapy session. Client improvements also must take place during the session and be naturally reinforced by the therapist's actions and reactions. Implementing this 'here and now' approach is the core of FAP.

Clinically Relevant Behavior

Central to the implementation of FAP's 'here and now' approach is the concept of clinically relevant behavior (CRB). The FAP therapist needs to distinguish between three types of clinically relevant client behavior that can occur during the session; these CRBs are of central importance to the therapy process.

CRB1s: Client problems that occur in-session. CRB1s are in-session occurrences of client repertoires that have been specified as problems according to the client's goals for therapy and the case conceptualization. There should be a correspondence between specific CRB1s and particular daily life problems. Understanding CRB1s requires an appreciation of behavior in terms of broad response classes that include varying behavioral topographies; some occur in-session in relation to the therapy process and the therapist, while some occur out of session in relation to work, friends, family, significant others and so forth. In successful FAP, CRB1s should decrease in frequency over the course of therapy. Typically, CRB1s are under the control of aversive stimuli and consist of avoidance (including emotional avoidance), but CRB1s are by no means restricted to problematic avoidance repertoires. The following behaviors are actual instances of presenting clinical problems.

- A woman who has no friends and 'does not know how to make friends' avoids eye contact, answers questions by talking at length in an unfocused and tangential manner, has one 'crisis' after another, demands to be taken care of, gets angry at the therapist for not having all the answers and frequently complains that the world 'shits' on her and that she gets an unfair deal.
- A man who avoids entering into love relationships always decides ahead of time what he is going to talk about during the therapy hour, watches the clock so he can end precisely on time, states that he can only come to therapy every other week because of tight finances (he makes $70,000 a year) and cancels the next session after making an important self-disclosure.
- A self-described 'hermit' who would like to develop a close relationship and who has been in therapy for three years continues to muse periodically that his therapist is 'only in this for the money' and is secretly contemptuous of him.
- A woman who has a pattern of getting into relationships with unattainable men develops a crush on her therapist.
- A woman who has a history of people leaving her because they 'get tired' of her introduces new and involved topics at the end of the hour, frequently threatens to kill herself and shows up drunk at her therapist's house in the middle of the night.
- A man suffering from speech anxiety 'freezes up' and is unable to talk to his therapist during the session.
- A depressed man who feels controlled by his wife shows up session after session with nothing to contribute to the therapy agenda and passively accepts whatever the therapist suggests.
- A man who must always be the life of the party spends most of each session telling entertaining stories to the therapist, at first feeling satisfied after each session but eventually feeling that his therapy is not progressing.
- A woman who erroneously believes her husband is cheating on her feels that the therapist likes his other clients more than her.

CRB2s: Client improvements that occur in-session. CRB2s are in-session improvements in CRB1 repertoires and should increase in frequency over the course of successful FAP. During the early stages of treatment CRB2 behaviors are rare or of low strength when an instance of the clinical problem, CRB1, occurs. For example, consider a client whose problem is withdrawal and accompanying feelings of low self-esteem when 'people don't pay attention' to him during conversations and in other social situations. This client may show similar withdrawal behaviors when the therapist does not attend to what he is saying or interrupts him. Possible CRB2s for this situation include repertoires of assertive behavior that would have directed the therapist back to what the client was saying, or the ability to discern the therapist's waning interest before the therapist actually proceeded to the point of interrupting him.

Consider another case, of a client who has been sexually abused as a child by her father and is troubled by constant anxiety and insomnia. In addition, she avoids intimate relationships and is not open, trusting or vulnerable. Therapeutic goals would be to reduce generalized avoidance and increase the CRB2s of: (1) contacting feelings such as pain, anger and grief, (2) learning to ask for what she wants (i.e., that her needs are important and deserve attention), (3) learning to accept caring from her therapist through a sensation of softening her heart, feeling her breath and breathing more deeply.

CRB3s: Client interpretations of behavior. Thus far we have emphasized that functional analysis, the process of attempting to understand behavior in terms of histories of reinforcement and other stimulus functions, is crucial to FAP. Such analysis is a critical component of FAP because this functional talk will help the therapist more effectively describe behavior in terms that will lead to useful FAP interventions. Identifying the nature of the reinforcers that have historically shaped and maintained a behavior should enable the therapist to identify and engage in specific reinforcing responses to change that behavior.

Another vital component of FAP is the process through which clients learn to view the world through such functional lenses. In this sense, any attempt by a client to describe the causes of his or her behavior in therapy is an opportunity for the FAP therapist to shape more functional, and hopefully more helpful, talk. To highlight the importance of this issue, clients' talk about their own behavior and the causes of it is labeled CRB3. CRB3s include 'reason giving' and 'interpretations.'

Most client talk in therapy is not particularly functional. While the best CRB3s involve the observation and description of one's own behavior and associated reinforcing, discriminative and eliciting stimuli, any 'causal' talk may be seen as CRB3 because it represents an opportunity to shape something important to FAP in the therapy session. For example, a client may say, 'I yelled at my child because I am a terrible person.' This statement certainly identifies a cause for a behavior, but not a particularly useful cause. This should be considered an opportunity to shape more functional talk. The therapist may help the client identify the discriminative stimuli that occasioned the behavior (e.g., the child was not listening and they were late for daycare), and the reinforcing conditions that strengthened the behavior over time (e.g., yelling works, at least in the short term, to quiet the child). The therapist and the client may also discuss other historical factors relevant to the situation, such as the client never having had the opportunity to learn alternative responses. Notice that improved functional talk may not only help the client feel better about himself or herself, but also may lead to useful interventions in terms of both discriminative stimuli (e.g., leave earlier for daycare) and reinforcement (e.g., praise the child when behaving properly).

CRB3s are especially important to FAP when they relate to CRB1s and CRB2s, because CRB3s should help with the generalization of CRB2s from therapy to outside life. Consider a female client who, after an intense therapeutic interaction says, 'Wow, it blows my mind that I can get so upset in here and you tolerate it. My dad would have run screaming.' Although the client did not use terms like reinforcement or punishment, she is clearly contrasting a reinforcing response from the therapist (in reaction to her emotional display) with a punishing response from her father. The therapist could then ask, 'But what about your husband? Will he tolerate it?' The client might then consider that he would. This type of therapy experience, in which reinforcement is experienced in the therapy room and then identified via CRB3 to the outside world, should lead the client to try out the CRB2 more readily.

Take another example, of a woman in her early forties who had not been sexually intimate with anyone for over 15 years. After three years in FAP, she became the lover of a man she met through her church. Her CRB3 was, 'The reason I'm in this intimate situation is because you [the therapist] were there for me. It's such a phenomenal change. If not for you, I wouldn't be in this situation. With you it was the first safe place I had to talk about what I feel, to find reasons why it's desirable to be sexual. There was a period of time that I was more overtly attracted to you and you were accepting of my feelings. I learned in here that it was better to be whole and feel my sexuality than to be armored and empty, and I practiced learning how to be direct with you.' This kind of statement can help increase the transfer of client gains in the therapy situation to daily life. In this case, the behavior to be generalized helped her to form an intimate relationship and increase the ensuing daily life positive reinforcement.

One final point about CRB3s relates to the fact that many therapeutic systems assume that the important behavior in therapy is talking (it is commonly called 'talk' therapy, after all!). In FAP, the label CRB3 acknowledges the fact that a tremendous amount of talk occurs in therapy, and therefore we want it to be the kind of talk that is most helpful (functional talk). The ultimate goal in FAP, however, is not to shape CRB3 repertoires, but to shape CRB2s, and CRB3s are only useful to the degree they facilitate this. Therapists sometimes confuse CRB3 repertoires with the behavior to which they refer. A client stating that she withdraws whenever she becomes dependent in a relationship (CRB3) is very different from actually withdrawing during the session because she is becoming dependent on the therapist (CRB1). Unfortunately, some therapists focus on those verbal repertoires that describe a problem behavior occurring in daily life and fail to observe the problem behaviors (CRB1s) or improvements (CRB2s) as they occur. In FAP, when CRB2 occurs, the best response might be to lean forward, maintain close eye contact, and allow oneself to feel and express whatever comes naturally. This interaction then can be talked about after the moment passes.

A Behavioral Cosmology

FAP calls for the therapist to learn behavioral philosophy and to be able to speak like a behaviorist. Some may judge this approach cold and distancing, but that is untrue. In fact, the philosophy at its core fosters deep emotional connections, empathy and love. We end this chapter with a behavioral cosmology—a metaphor that extends behaviorism to account for the interconnectedness of all life and which can lead to a mindful awareness of one's 'here and now' experience. In FAP, attention to the 'here and now' experience of the client is fundamental, and one of the best ways to do this is to 'experience' (the verb). Needless to say, what clients 'experience' is often the most productive focus of therapy, and if ignored, can be counter-therapeutic. In order to best attend to clients' experience, therapists first need to be in touch with their own experience. We began this chapter with personal accounts of FAP experience, before describing how behaviorism attempts to account for everything that people do, leading to the 'here and now' emphasis in psychotherapy. We conclude with how behaviorism leads to a 'here and now' experience for the therapist, one that can facilitate the emotional and empathic connections essential to FAP.

A behavioral explanation of who we are and how we think, feel and perceive is a verbal description of our history, in particular the contingencies of reinforcement that account for the emergence of our behavioral repertoires. Contingencies of reinforcement differentially strengthen and weaken specific repertories of operant behavior. In addition, another type of contingency also has shaped important aspects of who we are. These are the contingencies of survival that determined whether our ancestors survived or died. Our ancestors' genetic material, physical structure and behavioral tendencies were shaped by these contingencies of survival. Operant behavior is one tendency shaped in this way. Contingencies of reinforcement, from this perspective, work to produce operant behavior because our ancestors whose adaptive behavioral patterns were strengthened by certain life-sustaining consequences survived. For example, our ancestors learned how to retrace their steps to watering holes because they were reinforced by finding water. They passed on to us the tendency to have behavior strengthened by reinforcing contingencies.

One technique through which we can connect with and identify our present moment experience is by attempting to become aware (see Chapter 5 for the behavioral meanings of 'aware') of the contingencies of reinforcement that have shaped who we are. The following is an account of one author's (RJK) experience of the present moment in the form of a metaphor.

> I am here, at this moment, in front of my computer. When I pause, I can experience myself as standing at the front edge of a flowing stream of experiences that extends into the past. My imagery is that I am standing at the front of a slow moving river that has brought me to this instant. As I look back over my shoulder, I can see myself getting up this morning, and my interactions with Mavis, my racquetball partner, my students, my son and my dog that filled the passage of time, leading me to this point. In order to account for these 'getting to this instant' actions and interactions, I can look even further back in the stream, before I got up, and see that I have learned to get up early enough to get to my office on time, to prepare for a class or a therapy session, because when I did so there were consequences. Just as right now, I am reinforced by words appearing on the monitor as I type and make progress on this manuscript, one that marks a milestone in my life. My interactions today are a tiny fraction of the multitude of experiences I've had—with Mavis, my children, my friends, my siblings, my

students, my clients, my parents and my grandparents. Unlike the feelings I am experiencing now (e.g., alertness, contemplation, engagement, excitement), as I look back in the stream I realize that I was usually unaware of these contingencies or consequences of my past actions. These contingencies, regardless of my awareness of them, changed the synapses in my brain and are responsible for what I do, feel, notice, think and sense in this moment. The stream of time and all the contingencies I have been exposed to include the event most responsible for my current behavior (working on this manuscript), namely an inspiring conference I attended. Specifically, the interactions or contingencies that occurred with my colleagues, students and daughter at that conference are the stimuli for my current writing. Yet, each of these people at that past moment had their own streams of experiences trailing off behind them that, in turn, influenced what they did during that meeting. In a sense, there was a confluence of streams during that meeting, and I undoubtedly was affected by many of the experiences in their streams that entered into their interactions. Of course, each of their streams was influenced by confluences with other streams that had occurred earlier in their days, their weeks, and ultimately, their lives.

Experiential Exercise

Let us conduct a brief exercise similar to the one described above. Choose a time to do this that is convenient for you. First close your eyes, and focus your attention on your breathing. Breathe naturally, focusing on the sensations of inhaling and exhaling. It's normal to become distracted at this stage, and if you do so, simply gently return to the task of noticing your breath. After about ten breaths, try to use imagery to conceptualize your experience. One useful image is of a stream as described in the example above. Imagine that you are at the front of a stream of past experiences. If you look back a little at this stream you can see yourself at some point a few hours ago (waking up, having lunch, driving your car, etc.). Then glance back further in the stream over the past few days, weeks or months and see yourself having a particularly pleasant, intimate or involved interaction with a specific person. Try to recall the details—what he or she looked like, what you said to each other, how you felt being with this person. Now, imagine that person also has a stream extending behind him or her, and your interaction with each other involves a confluence of both of your streams. At that moment rivulets from each of your streams join together and then return. Sense how what happened between the two of you was influenced not only by your history but the other's history as well. After you have experienced this image, pause and read the next step.

Look further back in time from that significant interaction, far back down your stream. As you go back, see yourself as a young adult, a teenager, an adolescent, a child, a toddler taking your first steps. Spend a moment acknowledging some of the most important people and events that have shaped who you are. Then focus on a specific image, or just the notion that you were an infant, with a stream of preceding experiences that shaped you (regardless of your awareness of those experiences). Try to look back further, see yourself as a fetus in the womb, and then go back in time to the point at which the joining of sperm and egg formed an embryo. The sperm and the egg had their own streams of past experience that account for the genetic material of each. Finally, let yourself feel a sense of interconnectedness to others and to the pulse of the universe as you gradually open your eyes.

The exercise above halted at the joining of sperm and egg. However, according to Skinner, the complete metaphor would include reversing oneself down the evolutionary chain to the slime that formed at the edges of primordial soup, and then, the geophysical events that led to amino acid formation and so forth. From this behaviorally informed metaphor of our histories of contingencies of reinforcement and survival, there is a cosmic unity and interconnectedness between all of us and to the material world origins we have in common.

The above experience is eloquently described in this quotation from an 1854 speech attributed to Chief Seattle:

> Every shining pine needle, every sandy shore, every mist in the dark woods, every meadow, every humming insect... all are holy in the memory and experience of my people. We know the sap which courses through the trees as we know the blood that courses through our veins. We are part of the earth and it is part of us... The rocky crests, the dew in the meadow, the body heat of the pony, and man all belong to the same family. The shining water that moves in the streams and rivers is not just water, but the blood of our ancestors... Each glossy reflection in the clear waters of the lakes tells of events and memories in the life of my people. The water's murmur is the voice of my father's father... The wind that gave our grandfather his first breath also received his last sigh... All things are connected like the blood that unites us all. Man did not weave the web of life, he is merely a strand in it. Whatever he does to the web, he does to himself...

From a behavioral perspective, such profound contact with the present moment is crucial, in that it should lead to increased awareness and contact with immediate contingencies and an enhanced ability to be more naturally reinforcing to your clients and others who come into contact with you and your stream of experience.

References

Biglan, A. (1995). *Changing cultural practices: A contextualist framework for intervention research*. Reno, NV: Context Press.

Chief Seattle (1854). Retrieved January 31, 2008, from http://www.cs.rice.edu/~ssiyer/minstrels/poems/184.html

Ferster, C. B. (1967). Arbitrary and natural reinforcement. *The Psychological Record, 22*, 1–16.

Ferster, C. B. (1972). Clinical reinforcement. *Seminars in Psychiatry, 4*(2), 101–111.

Haughton, E., & Ayllon, T. (1965). Production and elimination of symptomatic behavior. In L. Ullman, & L. Krasner (Eds.), *Case studies in behavior modification* (pp. 94–98) New York: Holt Rinehart.

Hayes, S. C. (1987). A contextual approach to therapeutic change. In N. Jacobson (Ed.), *Psychotherapists in clinical practice: Cognitive and behavioral perspectives* (pp. 327–387). New York: Guilford.

Hayes, S. C., Hayes, L. J., & Reese, H. W. (1988). Finding the philosophical core: A review of Stephen C. Pepper's world hypotheses: A study in evidence. *Journal of the Experimental Analysis of Behavior, 50*(1), 97–111.

Kanter, J. W., Landes, S. J., Busch, A. M., Rusch, L. C., Brown, K. R., Baruch, D. E., et al. (2006). The effect of contingent reinforcement on target variables in outpatient psychotherapy for depression: A successful and unsuccessful case using functional analytic psychotherapy. *Journal of Applied Behavior Analysis, 39*(4), 463–467.

Kohlenberg, R. J., Bolling, M. Y., Kanter, J. W., & Parker, C. R. (2002). Clinical behavior analysis: Where it went wrong, how it was made good again, and why its future is so bright. *The Behavior Analyst Today, 3*(3), 248–254.

Kohlenberg, R. J., & Tsai, M. (1991). *Functional analytic psychotherapy: Creating intense and curative therapeutic relationships.* New York: Plenum Press.

Kohlenberg, R. J., & Tsai, M. (1994). Functional analytic psychotherapy: A radical behavioral approach to treatment and integration. *Journal of Psychotherapy Integration, 4*(3), 175–201.

Kohlenberg, R. J., Tsai, M., & Dougher, M. J. (1993). The dimensions of clinical behavior analysis. *Behavior Analyst, 16*(2), 271–282.

Kohlenberg, R. J., Tsai, M., & Kohlenberg, B. S. (1996). Functional analysis in behavior therapy. In M. Hersen, R. M. Eisler, & P. M. Miller (Eds.), *Progress in behavior modification* (pp. 1–24). Newbury Park, CA: Sage Publications.

Roche, B. (1999). 'New wave' analysis. *The Psychologist, 12*(10), 498–499.

Schafer, R. (1976). *A new language for psychoanalysis.* New Haven, CT: Yale University Press.

Skinner, B. F. (1945). The operational analysis of psychological terms. *Psychological Record, 52*, 270–276.

Skinner, B. F. (1953). *Science and human behavior.* New York: McMillian.

Skinner, B. F. (1957). *Verbal behavior.* New York: Appleton-Century-Croft.

Skinner, B. F. (1974). *About behaviorism.* New York: Knopf.

Skinner, B. F. (1982). Contrived reinforcement. *The Behavior Analyst, 5*, 3–8.

Wachtel, P. L. (1977). *Psychoanalysis and behavior therapy: Toward an integration.* New York: Basic Books.

Chapter 2
Lines of Evidence in Support of FAP

David E. Baruch, Jonathan W. Kanter, Andrew M. Busch, Mary D. Plummer,
Mavis Tsai, Laura C. Rusch, Sara J. Landes, and Gareth I. Holman

What empirical evidence supports FAP? On the one hand, FAP is based on a handful of basic behavioral principles that were theoretically and empirically derived from decades of laboratory experimentation. On the other, FAP has yet to be tested in a randomized controlled trial. Our belief is that the basic tenets of FAP—namely the importance of the therapeutic relationship and the use of natural reinforcement to shape client problems when they occur naturally in the therapeutic relationship—are robust, and lines of evidence in support of these principles converge from multiple and diverse areas of research. In this chapter we review these lines of evidence. It should be clear from the outset, however, that this review by no means seeks to justify the paucity of direct empirical evidence in support of FAP. Rather, we believe that the findings of this review strongly suggest that additional empirical research specifically investigating the efficacy of FAP is warranted, as it was developed from a solid foundation of principles and evidence and represents a convergence of some of the most robust findings in psychological research.

While FAP is a therapy based on behavior analytic principles, at its heart it is an interpersonal therapy. FAP is based on the assumption that both the causes of, and treatment for, psychopathology are intimately related to interpersonal relationships. This assumption has substantial support in the literature with respect to depressive disorders. It is well established that interpersonal problems, troubled relationships, and lack of social support predict the onset (Stice, Ragan, & Randall, 2004), course (Lara, Leader, & Klein, 1997; Miller et al., 1992), duration (Brown & Moran, 1994) and relapse of depression (Hooley & Teasdale, 1989). Conversely, the presence of social support has protective effects (Peirce, Frone, Russell, Cooper, & Mudar, 2000) and predicts recovery from depression (Lara et al., 1997; Sherboume, Hays, & Wells, 1995). While several alternative therapies focus on the therapeutic relationship and associated processes, FAP utilizes basic learning principles to harness the therapist-client relationship, focusing on the establishment of a more effective

D.E. Baruch (✉)
Graduate Student, Cardinal Stritch University, Milwaukee, WI, USA
e-mail: debaruch@gmail.com

M. Tsai et al., *A Guide to Functional Analytic Psychotherapy*,
DOI 10.1007/978-0-387-09787-9_2, © Springer Science+Business Media, LLC 2009

interpersonal repertoire in order to effect generalization of these new skills to relationships in clients' lives.

Case studies involving FAP as a stand alone treatment have included jealousy (López, 2003), anxiety disorder without agoraphobia (Bermúdez, Ferro, & Calvillo, 2002), chronic pain (Vandenberghe, Ferro, & Furtado da Cruz, 2003), posttraumatic stress disorder (Kohlenberg & Tsai, 1998), aggressive-defiant patterns in a child (Gosch & Vandenberghe, 2004), obsessive-compulsive disorder (Kohlenberg & Vandenberghe, 2007; Vandenberghe, 2007), and depression (Ferro, Valero, & Vives, 2006). Several case studies of other interventions incorporating FAP have also been published. These include case studies using FAP and Acceptance and Commitment Therapy (ACT; Hayes, Strosahl, & Wilson, 1999) in the areas of fibromyalgia (Queiroz & Vandenberghe, 2006), anorgasmia (Oliveira-Nasser, & Vandenberghe, 2005), and exhibitionism (Paul, Marx, & Orsillo, 1999). A Dialectical Behavioral Therapy (DBT)-FAP combination has also been used in the case of an individual diagnosed with a personality disorder NOS (not otherwise specified) (Wagner, 2005). These reports provide anecdotal evidence and clinical guidance, and suggest the breadth of presenting problems for which FAP and FAP enhancements may be appropriate. This abundance of case literature begs the question—what is the empirical basis of FAP?

Our goal in this chapter is to highlight the converging lines of evidence from multiple disciplines that support key FAP principles. Concurrently, we note the ways in which FAP theory contributes to each of these literatures, and in doing so informs therapists about the promotion of client change using a unique and powerful methodology. To this end, we seek to address not only areas of convergence but also highlight where FAP diverges in either interpretation of findings or their implications for therapy.

The Therapeutic Alliance

FAP is based on the notion that the therapeutic relationship is an important factor in psychotherapy—hardly a controversial notion. Nevertheless, FAP makes the argument that to harness fully the relationship as a mechanism of change, it must be conceptualized in a manner that makes specific the so-called 'non-specific' relationship factor. That is, what are the specific factors that make the therapist-client interaction curative? Before clarifying this position further, we first review the supporting evidence for the relevance of the relationship to psychotherapy.

The concept of therapeutic alliance can be traced back to the earliest writings of Freud (1912/1958), who first addressed the importance of friendly or affectionate feelings between the patient and the therapist as a foundation for any future therapeutic gains. The alliance concept also draws heavily on Rogers' (1957) assertion that therapeutic empathy, unconditional positive regard and genuineness constitute necessary and sufficient conditions for successful psychotherapy. In the past 25 years, interest in the therapeutic alliance as an essential element in the therapy process has burgeoned, such that contemporary psychotherapy researchers broadly define it as the collaborative and affective bond between therapist and client and their ability to agree on treatment goals and tasks (Martin, Garske, & Davis, 2000).

Evidence for the importance of the therapeutic alliance emerges from two primary sources. First, although researchers from different theoretical orientations have assessed the therapeutic alliance in different ways using an assortment of measures, they consistently have found that the strength of the alliance is predictive of outcome (Barber, Connolly, Crits-Christoph, Gladis, & Siqueland, 2000; Horvath, 2001; Martin et al., 2000). Second, researchers unable to find a consistent difference in the effectiveness of psychotherapies across orientations (e.g., Lambert & Bergin, 1994) have conceptualized the therapeutic alliance as a common factor across different therapies. Indeed, some researchers have even begun to argue that the quality of the alliance is more important than the type of treatment in predicting positive therapeutic outcomes (e.g., Safran & Muran, 1995), such that the therapeutic alliance has been referred to as the 'quintessential integrative variable' of therapy (Wolfe & Goldfried, 1988).

Although it is clear from the therapeutic alliance literature that the strength of the alliance is related to treatment outcome, there is evidence that many therapists fail to focus on the therapeutic relationship in-session. Coding all therapist turns at speech during the session, Goldfried and colleagues (Castonguay, Hayes, Goldfried, & DeRubeis, 1995; Goldfried, Castonguay, Hayes, Drozd, & Shapiro, 1997; Goldfried, Raue, & Castonguay, 1998) showed that CBT (Cognitive Behavior Therapy) therapists do not frequently focus on the therapy relationship in-session, yet an increased focus was found during significant, high-impact sessions when master therapists conducted therapy. Similarly, Kanter, Schildcrout and Kohlenberg (2005) have shown that therapists in several studies of CBT for depression rarely focus on the therapeutic relationship for an extended period of session time.

Perhaps the limited focus on the therapeutic relationship may be explained by the lack of consensus as to what therapists must do to secure a strong relationship, how much and what type of attention to pay directly to the therapeutic relationship, the mechanism underlying the relationship or its curative effect. A FAP analysis sheds light on these issues by, (1) behaviorally specifying the 'active ingredients' of the therapeutic relationship that will ultimately facilitate client change, and (2) functionally assessing client behaviors for their clinical relevance in alliance building, rather than looking solely at the form or topography of a behavior. In other words, use of the term 'therapeutic alliance' tends to focus primarily on what the behavior looks like, rather than the function it serves. In contrast, a FAP conceptualization of in-session behavior would focus on how a particular behavior functions for the client, not whether it looks like alliance-type behavior.

To investigate further the above point, imagine a behavior that appears topographically to be associated with alliance building in-session, but may in fact function as compliance. Consider for example an unassertive male client who dutifully completes his homework but feels that he is not 'getting anything' out of it. What looks like alliance behavior in this case is actually a CRB1, an in-session example of a problematic behavior such that he is not expressing a relevant feeling he is experiencing. If this client were to state his doubts about the validity of the homework, topographically it may look like alliance disrupting behavior, but functionally it is an improvement, and will lead to a strengthening of the therapeutic alliance if the client's concerns are taken seriously by the therapist. On the other hand, if compliant behavior is assessed to be a CRB2 (e.g., in the case of a client whose difficulty in meeting others' expectations interferes with his relationships), then it would be interpreted by a FAP therapist to be alliance building behavior. Thus a FAP perspective allows the explanation and prediction of the means by which an alliance can be enhanced and even harnessed as the result of general contingent reinforcement by the therapist of client CRB2s (Follette, Naugle, & Callaghan, 1996).

In sum, rather than making general statements about the predictive relationship between the therapeutic alliance and therapy outcome, FAP specifies what the therapist needs to do to build alliance and to utilize it as a context for change (Kohlenberg, Yeater, & Kohlenberg, 1998). Specifically, FAP makes three overarching assumptions, namely that (1) clients' CRBs are evoked by the therapeutic context, (2) CRBs can be shaped through application of contingencies in the therapeutic relationship, and (3) these contingencies involve natural reinforcement. The next three sections will review research findings corroborating these assumptions.

Principles of FAP

CRBs are Evoked by the Therapeutic Context

FAP again adopts an uncontroversial position by claiming that clients' problematic interpersonal patterns (CRB1s) will emerge in the therapeutic context. Perhaps millions of pages of psychotherapy theory have been written about this topic, with the theoretical and empirical literature addressing the theory of transference perhaps the penultimate example. Although the term transference hails from a different theoretical perspective, research on it nonetheless is relevant to FAP, as it provides support for the claim that CRB1s may be evoked by the therapeutic context.

Until recently, transference remained a largely theoretical construct and underwent little empirical examination (Connolly et al., 1996). In fact, the ratio of theoretical to empirical articles on transference has been reported to be approximately 500 to 1 (Ogrodniczuk, Piper, Joyce, & McCallum, 1999). Nevertheless, transference has been found to occur in a diverse set of daily social relationships (Andersen & Baum, 1994; Andersen & Cole, 1990; Andersen, Glassman, Chen, &

Cole, 1995) and in the context of the therapy relationship (Connolly et al., 1996; Crits-Christoph, Demorest, & Connolly, 1990; Luborsky, McLellan, Woody, O'Brian, & Auerbach, 1985). Thus there is ample evidence supporting the claim that transference reactions occur in therapy. While this research is relevant to FAP, in that it corroborates the occurrence of CRBs, FAP and psychodynamic theory diverge with respect to the most effective response to transference reactions and CRBs (see *reinforcement contingencies and transference interpretations* sections below).

CRBs can be Shaped Through Application of Contingencies in the Therapeutic Relationship

Is it important to contingently reinforce live, in-session behavior? A fundamental premise of FAP is that the closer in time and place client behavior is to the therapist's intervention (i.e., contingent reinforcement), the stronger the effect of the intervention. In other words, a 'delayed' or far-removed therapist response is expected to be less beneficial than reinforcement of live behavior. For example, some therapists may argue that they reinforce client improvements when they provide praise (e.g., saying 'Good job' in response to a client who reported being assertive in interactions with her employer during the preceding week). FAP contends that such use of reinforcement would be more effective if provided at the same time and in the same place as the behavior it is intended to reinforce (the client being assertive with her employer in the workplace). This belief underlies the focus on similar classes of behavior (CRB2) emerging in the context of therapy that can be immediately reinforced.

What research supports this well-accepted maxim? On one hand, literally thousands of studies have used immediate reinforcement to establish and maintain behavior. Indeed, nothing less than a review of the history of research on learning theory, from cats in Thorndike's puzzle boxes, rats in T-mazes, pigeons in Skinner boxes, to humans in sound attenuation chambers, is required to describe all the evidence (e.g., Catania, 1998). Essentially, the animal literature strongly supports the notion that delay of reinforcement adversely affects subsequent learning, although the relationship between delay and learning is complex and mediated by several factors (Renner, 1964; Tarpy & Sawabini, 1974). In general, studies involving human subjects have generated similar results (Greenspoon & Foreman, 1956; Saltzman, 1951; Bilodeau & Ryan, 1960). The delay effect—that reinforcement becomes less effective as the delay between a response and reinforcement increases—is most clearly demonstrated in humans with complex tasks (Hockman & Lipsitt, 1961) and when intervening behavior occurs between a response and reinforcement (Atkinson, 1969).

The human delay literature, while supportive of the above claim, is difficult to generalize to the psychotherapy situation. This is primarily because the lengths of delay studied in research preparations (up to 12 seconds) are much too small to be relevant to the question of whether immediate responses to in-session behavior are preferable to feedback about behavior that occurred outside of session, perhaps as long as a week ago. Nevertheless, immediate contingent responding has been found to enhance treatment for hair-pulling clients (Rapp, Miltenberger, & Long, 1998; Stricker, Miltenberger, Garlinghouse, Deaver, & Anderson, 2001; Stricker, Miltenberger, & Garlinghouse, 2003).

Does contingent reinforcement run counter to 'unconditional' positive regard? Reinforcement contingencies and their immediacy may be important in certain experimental situations or with discrete problems such as hair pulling, but are such issues relevant to adult, clinical populations dealing with abstract problems of intimacy, loneliness, anger, heartbreak, and so on? Perhaps these concerns require something more sophisticated than simple contingencies of reinforcement. As we will explain next, FAP theory suggests otherwise, and research on Rogerian, 'non-directive' therapy highlights how contingent reinforcement is relevant to psychotherapy.

FAP's emphasis on the therapeutic relationship and natural responding may lead some to mistake it for a variant of Carl Roger's client-centered, humanistic style of therapy (see Rogers, 1957). While both approaches believe in the power of the therapeutic relationship to produce change, FAP theory diverges significantly with respect to the claim from Rogerian theory that change may occur solely through non-directive or non-contingent therapist behavior. We would argue that a question to ask is whether non-directive or unconditional positive regard really is non-contingent. People may be reinforced readily without awareness (Frank, 1961; Krasner, 1958), and thus a client may feel unconditional positive regard while being unaware of a contingent process. Two studies speak directly to this conditioning phenomenon. In one experiment (Greenspoon, 1955) subjects were asked to list as many nouns as they could. As they did so, an experimenter responded with subtle sounds of approval ('mmm-hm') or disapproval ('huh-uh') to each term. They found that despite being unaware of the contingency, subjects increased their frequency of nouns when they were followed by 'mmm-hm' and decreased them when followed by 'huh-uh. ' Such research has led Frank (1961) to conclude, 'This much, at least, seems safely established: One person can influence the verbalizations of another through very subtle cues, which may be so slight that they never come to the center of awareness' (p. 108).

The crucial point emerging from the above discussion is that therapists may be contingently reinforcing client behavior without being conscious of doing so. If that is the case, then therapist responses such as 'mmm-hm' that signal clients to continue speaking may contingently reinforce a favored class of behavior (i.e., improvements) inadvertently. Accordingly, therapy that might 'feel' like unconditional positive regard or non-directive may in fact be contingent. Investigating this possibility, Truax (1966) conducted a process analysis of Carl Rogers himself providing therapy (e.g., non-directive therapy comprised of emphatic understanding, acceptance and unconditional positive regard).

Consistent with FAP, results revealed that despite consciously attempting to respond non-contingently, improvement in therapy was associated with differential, albeit inadvertent, reinforcement of client improvements. Such findings suggest that, while many therapists may not realize it, they are *constantly* shaping their clients' behavior through verbal and non-verbal reinforcement contingencies, punishment and extinction.

Rogerian theory asserts that unconditional positive regard and empathy are both necessary and sufficient for full recovery. FAP agrees that such an approach is necessary (e.g., a focus on natural reinforcement), however, a non-directive approach is seen not only as rare, but also insufficient. Recognizing the inevitable impact of therapists' behavior on clients, FAP encourages therapists to harness the therapeutic relationship to shape naturally and contingently more effective interpersonal client behavior.

How do transference interpretations differ from contingent responding? In light of findings that transference change has been found to mediate treatment outcome (O'Connor, Edelstein, Berry, & Weiss, 1994), several researchers have examined the transference interpretation as a mechanism of change in relationship-focused treatments (Leichsenring & Leibing, 2007). Transference interpretation occurs when the therapist explains the client's transference in order to provide insight into unconscious conflicts underlying current problematic patterns of behavior. In short, findings suggest that higher levels of transference interpretations are actually associated with poorer outcome in clients with low levels of interpersonal functioning, particularly when the interpretation revolves around the therapeutic relationship (Connolly et al., 1999; Ogrodniczuk et al., 1999).

FAP predicts that any response to in-session problematic interpersonal behavior that fails to take context or function into consideration would miss opportunities to reinforce CRB2s or inadvertently reinforce CRB1s. This may be an explanation for the poor treatment results following large numbers of transference interpretations. For example, in many cases a psychodynamic therapist would ignore noncompliant behavior from a client. For a historically passive client who has trouble asserting needs, however, noncompliance may actually be functioning as a CRB2. Thus, while in practice there may be considerable overlap between psychodynamic and FAP treatment approaches, theoretical differences lead to important clinical implications in terms of responses to problematic interpersonal behavior evoked by the therapeutic relationship.

The Importance of Natural Reinforcement

Will contingent responding undermine intrinsic motivation? In FAP an overriding emphasis is placed on the notion that CRB2s should be reinforced naturally, typically through interpersonal verbal exchanges. Yet an often cited criticism of behaviorism is that when a person's behavior is reinforced the person begins to emit the behavior specifically to obtain external rewards (external motivation) which impairs the development of self-determinism (Deci, Koestner, & Ryan, 1999; Kohn, 1993). Applying this criticism to FAP leads to the suggestion that perhaps the reinforcement of interpersonal behaviors by FAP therapists extrinsically links motivation for these new behaviors to the therapist, thus limiting the generalization of the gains to other relationships and in fact reducing intrinsic motivation to learn new interpersonal behaviors. Does this critique hold?

Intrinsic motivation generally is defined as behavior believed to be motivated by the activity itself, as opposed to behaviors extrinsically motivated by external rewards such as prizes, rewards, or approval (Cameron, Banko, & Pierce, 2001). Recent findings suggest, however, that it is an oversimplification to mark all forms of external motivation as inherently harmful. Researchers have begun to identify settings and conditions in which external motivation actually may provide important benefits (Dickinson, 1989; Cameron et al., 2001). Nevertheless, the distinction between extrinsic and intrinsic motivation maps roughly to the distinction promoted by FAP between contrived and natural reinforcement respectively. For example, while a meta-analysis conducted by Cameron et al. (2001) revealed that verbal reinforcement may support intrinsic motivation, FAP focuses on whether the reinforcement was delivered in a contrived or natural manner.

Take for example a client in which a CRB2 is taking a risk by stating an opinion in front of the therapist. A response of 'Good job sharing an opinion with me,' would most likely be a contrived reinforcer (e.g., approval from therapist). FAP theory suggests that a more naturally reinforcing response by the therapist, such as taking the opinion seriously, would not only reinforce the CRB2, but would do so in a way that would facilitate generalization to other relationships. In this way, FAP utilizes reinforcement contingencies in order to shape improved interpersonal functioning and support intrinsic motivation.

How can one contingently reinforce and utilize interpersonal expectancy effects? The effects of natural contingent reinforcement in therapy may often be mistaken for common 'non-specific' factors. Research examining the interpersonal expectancy effect helps clarify this issue. In general, interpersonal expectancy effects are the result of one person's expectations on another person's behavior. In a meta-analytic review of research investigating interpersonal expectancy effects, Harris and Rosenthal (1985) provided a list of empirically supported teacher behaviors that have been shown to result in expectancy-confirming responses in students. This list included:

- Creating a less negative atmosphere (e.g., not behaving in a cold manner)
- Maintaining closer physical distances
- Providing more input by introducing more material or more difficult material
- Creating a warmer atmosphere
- Exhibiting less off-task behavior
- Having longer and more frequent interactions

- Asking more questions
- Encouraging more
- Engaging in more eye contact
- Smiling more
- Praising more
- Accepting the student's ideas by modifying, acknowledging, summarizing or applying what he or she has said
- Providing more corrective feedback
- Nodding more
- Waiting longer for responses

This list suggests that the behaviors and cues involved may be quite subtle and operate outside the conscious awareness of both the teacher and the subject.

From a FAP perspective, the above list is a perfect example of natural reinforcers in action, the type of natural reactions people display in everyday interactions that shape and maintain such interactions. It also is noteworthy that items on this list represent some of the most ubiquitous 'non-specific factors' of therapists across a wide spectrum of therapeutic modalities. As discussed earlier, these are undoubtedly the kinds of responses that Carl Rogers himself contingently, and non-consciously, deployed when attempting to be unconditional. Although these subtle cues influence client behavior in all therapy modalities, FAP is unique in that it explicates these subtle interactions and challenges therapists to deliberately and strategically harness them to shape improved interpersonal functioning.

Can contingent, natural reinforcement promote generalization? FAP maintains that interpersonal behaviors naturally shaped in-session will be more beneficial for clients than simply providing rules on how to be more effective. Specifically, FAP distinguishes itself from other psychotherapeutic approaches in terms of its focus on contingency-shaped behavior rather than rule-governed behavior. Compared to contingency-shaped behavior, which is behavior learned through direct contact with reinforcement (i.e., learning to solve a puzzle through trial and error), rule-governed behavior is behavior controlled by verbal descriptions of reinforcement (i.e., following instructions as to how to solve a puzzle) (Hayes, Zettle, & Rosenfarb, 1989; Skinner, 1953, 1957). Thus rule-governed behavior allows for behavioral change to occur without direct shaping. From a behavioral perspective, most psychotherapeutic approaches can be seen as providing rules to clients for how to behave more effectively.

Clients commonly expect their therapists to provide them with more, new or better rules that will lead to symptom reduction. Therapy based on rule specification, however, may obstruct clients' progress in dynamic and evocative contexts (e.g., interpersonal relationships) where the same behavior may be punished by one person and reinforced by another. In this situation, exquisite sensitivity to contingencies, rather than rule-governed behavior, is required. Behavioral research supports this assertion. For example, a large body of evidence suggests that when a person's behavior is contingency-shaped, the individual is better able to adapt to changing contingencies than when that behavior is rule-governed (e.g. Catania, Mathews, & Shimoff, 1982; Rosenfarb, Bunker, Morris & Cush, 1993; Shimoff, Catanina, & Mathews, 1981).

FAP's focus on natural reinforcement helps therapists avoid the promotion of rule-governed behavior in clients. For this reason, FAP therapists are not provided with formal instructions on how to respond to a CRB but are instead instructed to respond 'naturally.' Natural responding entails the notion that there are an infinite number of responses that all function to reduce CRB1s and increase CRB2s. To accomplish this, FAP therapists must draw on their own private reactions to their clients (thoughts, emotions, physiological responses) and naturally respond to each CRB accordingly. Thus when clients engage in improved behavior (CRB2s)—particularly behavior that breaks the rules they typically adhere to—FAP emphasizes the interpersonal effect of therapist behavior and revealing reactions to clients in the moment. In this way, natural and contingent therapist responses may not only shape improved client functioning but do so in a way that promotes generalization and client adaptability.

Existing Research on FAP Principles

A final line of evidence in support of FAP and FAP's proposed mechanism of action comes from research on FAP itself. The efficacy of FAP as a stand alone treatment has been supported by a single-subject investigation (Callaghan, Summers, & Weidman, 2003; described below). The incremental effectiveness of adding FAP to CBT has been demonstrated both via single-subject (Gaynor & Lawrence, 2002; Kanter et al., 2006) and group design studies (Kohlenberg, Kanter, Bolling, Parker, & Tsai, 2002).

In a non-randomized trial of FAP-enhanced cognitive therapy (termed FECT) for depression, Kohlenberg and colleagues (2002) compared client outcome in 20 subjects treated with CT (Cognitive Therapy) to 28 clients treated by the same therapists following training in FECT. Results revealed that FECT was incrementally more efficacious than CBT, such that 79% of the FECT participants responded (experienced a larger than 50% decrease in depression symptomatology) compared with 60% of the CT participants. Furthermore, FECT participants experienced significant improvements in their interpersonal functioning compared to CT participants. Subsequent process analyses (Kanter et al., 2005) illustrated that rates of FAP interventions (e.g., increased focus on CRBs) increased almost threefold during FECT and that these interventions related to weekly client reports of progress in therapy.

Finally, in the only randomized-controlled study incorporating FAP, Gifford and colleagues (2008) compared a combination of ACT (Acceptance and Commitment Therapy) and FAP to Nicotine Replacement Therapy (e.g. Rigotti, 2002) in a smoking cessation trial. There were no differences between conditions at post-treatment, however participants in the ACT and FAP condition experienced significantly better outcomes at one-year follow-up. Thus to date the majority of research assessing FAP has focused on the enhancement of other treatments through the addition of FAP interventions. Given this fact, a vital question is whether there is empirical support for FAP's proposed mechanism of change.

Recent investigations examining the mechanism of FAP have been undertaken in a manner consistent with FAP's underlying functional philosophy through the employment of functional analytic research methodologies. Given the flexibility of FAP and the overarching notion that (due to FAP's intense focus on function) application of its mechanism may look very different for different therapists and clients, the first goal of this research was specification of the FAP mechanism. This process involved a specification, in functional terms, that would allow for varying topographies of technique. The mechanism defined for this research was *therapist contingent responding with natural reinforcement to CRBs*. Thus such research aims not to provide empirical support for FAP as a treatment package via a randomized controlled trial, but rather to isolate and identify FAP's purported mechanism of action and demonstrate the effects of this mechanism on the behavior of individual clients.

The first requirement of this research was a reliable and valid measure that would allow for the reliable identification of in-session problems (CRB1s), improvements (CRB2s), and contingent therapist responses. Callaghan et al. (2003) created and applied such a measure, the Functional Analytic Psychotherapy Rating Scale (FAPRS), designed to measure turn-by-turn client and therapist behavior in FAP. To employ the FAPRS, a coder utilizes detailed case conceptualizations to identify instances of CRBs (e.g., CRB1s or CRB2s) while also coding therapist contingent responses to CRBs. Several more codes were used to distinguish FAP and 'traditional' therapist responses, discussion about the therapeutic relationship vs. contingent responding, and so forth (refer to Callaghan, Ruckstuhl, & Busch, 2005 for a full description). A key advantage of this turn-by-turn methodology is that it analyzes the FAP process on the level of the therapist-client interaction (i.e., on a moment-to-moment basis). In this way, the research on FAP's mechanism of change occurs at a level that can directly inform the clinical work of the FAP therapist.

Callaghan and colleagues (2003) used the FAPRS to code segments of therapist-client interactions for the treatment of a personality disordered client with histrionic and narcissistic features. Not only were CRBs identified (supporting the belief in FAP that general interpersonal problems may present themselves in the therapeutic context), but therapist contingent responding to CRBs was identified as well. Crucially, findings also indicated that CRB1s decreased and CRB2s increased over the course of FAP.

Kanter and colleagues (2006) provided single subject data on two subjects who received CBT and then FAP in a within-subject A/A + B design. Results were mixed. Subject 1 demonstrated slight decreases in his targeted behaviors (e.g., communication skills) but dropped out of the study before completion. Subject 2 demonstrated immediate improvements in her targeted behaviors (e.g., attention seeking, being vulnerable) upon introduction of FAP. Busch and colleagues (in press) applied the FAPRS coding system to Subject 2, replicating previous findings that therapist responding successfully shaped client in-session behavior. Importantly, both out-of-session client behaviors (collected via client diary cards) and in-session behaviors (CRBs) improved following the phase shift. Thus, results garnered using the FAPRS have provided support for the mechanism of change (contingent responding).

Conclusion

This chapter has reviewed several converging lines of evidence in support of FAP principles, including the therapeutic alliance, transference, transference interpretations, 'unconditional' positive regard, immediate reinforcement (delay to reinforcement), intrinsic versus extrinsic motivation, interpersonal expectancy effects, and rule-governed behavior. Each of these research areas is uncontroversial and relatively robust. Thus, although not directly providing support for FAP and FAP techniques, these lines of evidence together describe a compelling picture of what a treatment based on such evidence might look like. We believe FAP is just such a treatment.

Research directly examining FAP is, admittedly, in its infancy. Nevertheless, data exist to support both the incremental validity of FAP when combined with other interventions and the proposed mechanism of change in FAP—namely therapist contingent responding with natural reinforcement to CRBs. Combined with the above reviewed converging lines of evidence in support of the principles of FAP, the rationale for FAP appears strong. It remains to be demonstrated, however, that FAP can outperform existing treatments in standard randomized clinical trials. We hope this chapter may inspire researchers to conduct such trials.

References

Andersen, S. M., & Baum, A. B. (1994). Transference in interpersonal relations: Inferences and affect based on significant-other representations. *Journal of Personality, 62*, 460–497.

Andersen, S. M., & Cole, S. W. (1990). 'Do I know you?': The role of significant others in general social perception. *Journal of Personality and Social Psychology, 59*, 384–399.

Andersen, S. M., Glassman, N. S., Chen, S., & Cole, S. W. (1995). Transference in social perception: The role of chronic accessibility in significant-other representations. *Journal of Personality and Social Psychology, 69*, 41–57.

Atkinson, R. C. (1969). Information delay in human learning. *Journal of Verbal Learning and Verbal Behavior, 8*, 507–511.

Barber, J. P, Connolly, M. B., Crits-Christoph, P. Gladis, L., & Siqueland, L. (2000). Alliance predicts patients' outcome beyond in-treatment change in symptoms. *Journal of Consulting and Clinical Psychology, 6*, 1027–1032.

Bermúdez, M. A. L., Ferro G. R., & Calvillo, M. (2002). Una aplicacion de la Psicoterapia Analitica Funcional en un trastorno de angustia sin agorafobia. [An application of

Functional Analytic Psychotherapy in a case of anxiety disorder without agoraphobia.] *Análisis y Modificación de Conducta, 28*, 553–583.

Bilodeau, E. A., & Ryan, F. J. (1960). A test for interaction of delay of knowledge of results and two types of interpolated activity. *Journal of Experimental Psychology 59*, 414–419.

Brown, G. W., & Moran, P. (1994). Clinical and psychosocial origins of chronic depressive episodes: I. A community survey. *British Journal of Psychiatry, 165*, 447–456.

Busch, A. M., Kanter, J. W., Callaghan, G. M., Baruch, D. E., Weeks, C. E, & Berlin, K. S. (in press). A micro-process analysis of Functional Analytic Psychotherapy's mechanism of change. *Behavior Therapy*.

Callaghan, G. M., Ruckstuhl, L. E., & Busch, A. M. (2005). Manual for the Functional Analytic Psychotherapy Rating Scale III. Unpublished manual.

Callaghan, G. M., Summers, C. J., & Weidman, M. (2003). The treatment of histrionic and narcissistic personality disorder behaviors: A single-subject demonstration of clinical effectiveness using Functional Analytic Psychotherapy. *Journal of Contemporary Psychotherapy, 33*, 321–339.

Cameron, J., Banko, K. M., & Pierce, W. D. (2001). Pervasive negative effects of rewards on intrinsic motivation: The myth continues. *Behavior Analyst, 24*, 1–44.

Castonguay, L. G., Hayes, A. M., Goldfried, M. R., & DeRubeis, R. J. (1995). The focus of therapist interventions in cognitive therapy for depression. *Cognitive Therapy and Research, 19*, 485–503.

Catania, A. (1998). *The taxonomy of verbal behavior*. New York: Plenum Press.

Catania, A. C., Matthews, A. A., & Shimoff, E. (1982). Instructed versus shaped human verbal behavior: Interactions with nonverbal responding. *Journal of the Experimental Analysis of Behavior, 38*, 233–248.

Connolly, M. B., Crits-Christoph, P., Demorest, A., Azarian, K., Muenz, L., & Chittams, J. (1996). Varieties of transference patterns in psychotherapy. *Journal of Consulting and Clinical Psychology, 64*, 1213–1221.

Connolly, M. B., Crits-Christoph, P. Shappell, J., Barber, J. P., Luborsky, L., & Shaffer, C. (1999). Relation of transference interpretations to outcome in the early sessions of brief supportive-expressive psychotherapy. *Psychotherapy Research, 9*, 485–495.

Crits-Christoph, P., Demorest, A., & Connolly, M. B. (1990). Quantitative assessment of interpersonal themes over the course of a psychotherapy. *Psychotherapy, 27*, 513–521.

Deci, E. L., Koestner, R., & Ryan, R. M. (1999). A meta-analytic review of experiments examining the effects of extrinsic rewards on intrinsic motivation. *Psychological Bulletin, 125*, 627–668.

Dickinson, A. (1989). The detrimental effects of extrinsic reinforcement on "intrinsic motivation." *Behavior Analyst, 12*, 1–15.

Ferro, R., Valero, L., & Vives, M. C. (2006). Application of Functional Analytic Psychotherapy: Clinical analysis of a patient with depressive disorder. *The Behavior Analyst Today, 7*, 1–18.

Follette, W. C., Naugle, A. E., & Callaghan, G. M. (1996). A radical behavioral understanding of the therapeutic relationship in effecting change. *Behavior Therapy, 27*, 623–641.

Frank, J. D. (1961). *Persuasion and healing: A comparative study of psychotherapy*. Baltimore, MD: Johns Hopkins Press.

Freud, S. (1912/1958). The dynamics of transference. In J. Starchey (Ed., & Trans.), *The standard edition of the complete psychological works of Sigmund Freud* (Vol. 12, pp. 99–108). London: Hogarth Press. (Original work published 1912)

Gaynor, S. T., & Lawrence, P. (2002). Complementing CBT for depressed adolescents with Learning through In Vivo Experience (LIVE): Conceptual analysis, treatment description, and feasibility study. *Behavioural & Cognitive Psychotherapy, 79*–101.

Gifford, E. V., Kohlenberg, B. S., Hayes, S. H., Pierson, H., Piasecki, M. M., Antonuccio, D. O., Palm, K. M. (2008). Applying acceptance and the therapeutic relationship to smoking cessation: A randomized controlled trial. Unpublished Paper, University of Nevada, Reno, NV.

Goldfried, M. R., Castonguay, L. G., Hayes, A. M., Drozd, J. F., & Shapiro, D. A. (1997). A comparative analysis of the therapeutic focus in cognitive-behavioral and psychodynamicinterpersonal sessions. *Journal of Consulting and Clinical Psychology, 65,* 740–748.

Goldfried, M. R., Raue, P. J., & Castonguay, L. G. (1998). The therapeutic focus in significant sessions of master therapists: A comparison of cognitive-behavioral and psychodynamic-interpersonal interventions. *Journal of Consulting and Clinical Psychology, 66,* 803–810.

Gosch, C. S., & Vandenberghe, L. (2004). Análise do comportamento e a relação terapeuta-criança no tratamento de um padrão desafiador-agressivo. [Behavior analysis and the therapist-child relationship in the treatment of an aggressive-defiant pattern]. *Revista brasileira de terapia comportamental e cognitiva, 6,* 173–183.

Greenspoon, J. (1955). The reinforcing effect of two spoken sounds on the frequency of two responses. *American Journal of Psychology, 68,* 409–416.

Greenspoon, J., & Foreman, S. (1956). Effect of delay of knowledge of results on learning a motor task. *Journal of Experimental Psychology, 51,* 226–228.

Harris, M. J., & Rosenthal, R. (1985). The mediation of interpersonal expectancy effects: 31 meta-analyses. *Psychological Bulletin, 97,* 363–386.

Hayes, S. C., Strosahl, K. D., & Wilson, K. G. (1999). *Acceptance and commitment therapy: An experiential approach to behavior change.* New York: Guilford Press.

Hayes, S. C., Zettle, R. D., & Rosenfarb, I. (1989). Rule-following. In S. C. Hayes (Ed.), *Rule-governed behavior: Cognition, contingencies, and instructional control* (pp. 191–220). New York: Plenum Press.

Hockman, C. H., & Lipsitt, L. P. (1961). Delay-of-reward gradients in discrimination learning with children for two levels of difficulty. *Journal of Comparative and Physiological Psychology, 54,* 24–27.

Hooley, J. M., & Teasdale, J. D. (1989). Predictors of relapse in unipolar depressives: Expressed emotion, marital distress, and perceived criticism. *Journal of Abnormal Psychology, 98,* 229–235.

Horvath, A. O. (2001). The alliance. *Psychotherapy: Theory, Research, Practice, Training, 38,* 365–372.

Kanter, J. W., Schildcrout, J. S., & Kohlenberg, R. J. (2005). In vivo processes in cognitive therapy for depression: Frequency and benefits. *Psychotherapy Research, 15,* 366–373.

Kanter, J. W., Landes, S. J., Busch, A. M., Rusch, L. C., Brown, K. R., Baruch, D. E., et al. (2006). The effect of contingent reinforcement on target variables in outpatient psychotherapy for depression: A successful and unsuccessful case using Functional Analytic Psychotherapy. *Journal of Applied Behavior Analysis, 39,* 463–467.

Kohlenberg, B. S., Yeater, E. A., & Kohlenberg, R. J. (1998). Functional analytic psychotherapy, the therapeutic alliance, and brief psychotherapy. In J. D. Safran & J. C. Muran (Eds.), *The therapeutic alliance in brief psychotherapy* (pp. 63–93). Washington, DC: APA Press.

Kohlenberg, R. J., Kanter, J. W., Bolling, M. Y., Parker, C., & Tsai, M. (2002). Enhancing cognitive therapy for depression with functional analytic psychotherapy: Treatment guidelines and empirical findings. *Cognitive and Behavioral Practice, 9,* 213–229.

Kohlenberg, R. J., & Tsai, M. (1998). Healing interpersonal trauma with the intimacy of the therapeutic relationship. In V. M. Follette, J. I. Ruzek, & F. R. Abueg (Eds.), *Cognitive-behavioral therapies for trauma* (pp. 305–320). New York: Guilford.

Kohlenberg, R. J., & Vandenberghe, L. (2007). Treatment resistant OCD, inflated responsibility, and the therapeutic relationship: Two case examples. *Psychology and Psychotherapy: Theory Research and Practice, 80,* 455–465.

Kohn, A. (1993). *Punished by rewards: The trouble with gold stars, incentive plans, A's, praise, and other bribes.* Boston, MA: Houghton Mifflin Co.

Krasner, L. (1958). Studies of the conditioning of verbal behavior. *Psychological Bulletin, 55,* 148–170.

Lambert, M. J., & Bergin, A. E. (1994). The effectiveness of psychotherapy. In A. E. Bergin & S. L. Garfield (Eds.), *Handbook of psychotherapy and behavior change* (4th ed., pp. 143–189). Oxford: John Wiley & Sons.

Lara, M. E., Leader, J., & Klein, D. N. (1997). The association between social support and course of depression: Is it confounded with personality? *Journal of Abnormal Psychology, 106*, 478–482.

Leichsenring, F., & Leibing, E. (2007). Psychodynamic psychotherapy: A systematic review of techniques, indications and empirical evidence. *Psychology and Psychotherapy: Theory, Research and Practice, 80*, 217–228.

López, F. J. C. (2003). Jealousy: A case of application of Functional Analytic Psychotherapy. *Psychology in Spain, 7*, 86–98.

Luborsky, L., McLellan, A. T., Woody, G. E., O'Brian, C., & Auerbach, A. (1985). Therapist's success and its determinants. *Archives of General Psychiatry, 42*, 602–611.

Martin, D. J., Garske, J. P., & Davis, M. K. (2000). Relation of the therapeutic alliance with outcome and other variables: A meta-analytic review. *Journal of Consulting and Clinical Psychology, 68*, 438–450.

Miller, I. W., Keitner. G. I., Whisman, M. A., Ryan, C. E., Epstein, N. B., & Bishop, D. S. (1992). Depressed patients with dysfunctional families: Description and course of illness. *Journal of Abnormal Psychology, 101*, 637–646.

O'Connor, L. E., Edelstein, S., Berry, J. W., & Weiss, J. (1994). Changes in the patient's level of insight in brief psychotherapy: Two pilot studies. *Psychotherapy: Theory, Research, Practice, Training, 31*, 533–544.

Ogrodniczuk, J. S., Piper, W. E., Joyce, A. S., & McCallum, M. (1999). Transference interpretations in short-term dynamic psychotherapy. *Journal of Nervous and Mental Disease, 187*, 572–579.

Oliveira-Nasser, K. C. F., & Vandenberghe, L. (2005). Anorgasmia e esquiva experiencial, um estudo de caso. [Anorgasmia and experiential avoidance, a case study]. *Psicologia Clínica, 17*, 162–176.

Paul, R. H., Marx, B. P., & Orsillo, S. M. (1999). Acceptance-based psychotherapy in the treatment of an adjudicated exhibitionist: A case example. *Behavior Therapy, 30*, 149–162.

Peirce, R. S., Frone, M. R., Russell, M., Cooper, M. L., & Mudar, P. (2000). A longitudinal model of social contact, social support, depression and alcohol use. *Health Psychology, 19*, 28–38.

Queiroz, M. A. M., & Vandenberghe, L. (2006). Psicoterapia no tratamento da fibromialgia: Mesclando FAP e ACT. [Psychotherapy in the treatment of fibromialgia: Interweaving FAP and ACT.]. In H. J. Guilhardi & N. Aguire (Eds.), *Sobre Comportamento e Cognição* (pp. 238–248). Santo André: ESETec.

Rapp, J. T., Miltenberger, R. G., & Long, E. S. (1998). Augmenting simplified habit reversal with an awareness enhancement device: Preliminary findings. *Journal of Applied Behavior Analysis, 31*, 665–668.

Renner, K. E. (1964). Delay of reinforcement: A historical review. *Psychological Bulletin, 61*, 341–361.

Rigotti, N. A. (2002). Treatment of tobacco use and dependence. *New England Journal of Medicine, 346*, 506–512.

Rogers, C. R. (1957). The necessary and sufficient conditions of therapeutic personality change. *Journal of Consulting Psychology, 21*, 95–103.

Rosenfarb, I. S., Burker, E. J., Morris, S. A., & Cush, D. T. (1993). Effects of changing contingencies on the behavior of depressed and nondepressed individuals. *Journal of Abnormal Psychology, 102*, 642–646.

Safran, J. D., & Muran, J. C. (1995). Resolving therapeutic alliance ruptures: Diversity and integration. *In Session: Psychotherapy in Practice, 1*, 81–92.

Saltzman, I. J. (1951). Delay of reward and human verbal learning. *Journal of Experimental Psychology, 41*, 437–439.

Sherboume, C. D., Hays, R. D., & Wells, K. B. (1995). Personal and psychosocial risk factors for physical and mental health outcomes and course of depression among depressed patients. *Journal of Consulting and Clinical Psychology*, *63*, 345–355.

Shimoff, E., Catania, A. C., & Matthews, B. A. (1981). Uninstructed human responding: Sensitivity of low-rate performance to schedule contingencies. *Journal of the Experimental Analysis of Behavior*, *36*, 207–220.

Skinner, B. F. (1953). *Science and human behavior*. New York: Mcmillian.

Skinner, B. F. (1957). *Verbal behavior*. New York: Appleton-Century-Croft.

Stice, E., Ragan, J., & Randall, P. (2004). Prospective relations between social support and depression: Differential direction of effects for parent and peer support? *Journal of Abnormal Psychology*, *113*, 155–159.

Stricker, J. M., Miltenberger, R. G., & Garlinghouse, M. (2003). Augmenting stimulus intensity with an awareness enhancement device in the treatment of finger sucking. *Education & Treatment of Children*, *26*, 22–29.

Stricker, J. M., Miltenberger, R. G., Garlinghouse, M. A., Deaver, C. M., & Anderson, C. A. (2001). Evaluation of an awareness enhancement device for the treatment of thumb sucking in children. *Journal of Applied Behavior Analysis*, *34*, 77–80.

Tarpy, R. M., & Sawabini, F. L. (1974). Reinforcement delay: A selective review of the last decade. *Psychological Bulletin*, *81*, 984–997.

Truax, C. B. (1966). Reinforcement and nonreinforcement in Rogerian psychotherapy. *Journal of Abnormal Psychology*, *71*, 1–9.

Vandenberghe, L. (2007). Functional analytic psychotherapy and the treatment of obsessive compulsive disorder. *Counseling Psychology Quarterly*, *20*, 105–114.

Vandenberghe, L., Ferro, C. L. B., & Furtado da Cruz, A. C. (2003). FAP-enhanced group therapy for chronic pain. *The Behavior Analyst Today*, *4*, 369–375.

Wagner, A. W. (2005). A behavioral approach to the case of Ms. S. *Journal of Psychotherapy Integration*, *15*, 101–114.

Wolfe, B., & Goldfried, M. (1988). Research on psychotherapy integration: Recommendations and conclusions from an NIMH workshop. *Journal of Consulting and Clinical Psychology*, *56*, 448–451.

Chapter 3
Assessment and Case Conceptualization

Jonathan W. Kanter, Cristal E. Weeks, Jordan T. Bonow, Sara J. Landes,
Glenn M. Callaghan, and William C. Follette

Assessment is significant only if it affects what one does in therapy (Hayes,
Nelson, & Jarret, 1987). Assessment in FAP focuses on clinically relevant
behaviors (CRBs) and related variables throughout the course of therapy,
informing therapists' responses to client behavior in the moment. Of all therapies that attempt to address the interpersonal functioning of outpatient adults,
FAP embodies the strongest behavior analytic approach. FAP therapists seek
to functionally define CRBs, recognize basic behavioral principles, appreciate
the distinctiveness of each case and idiographically define the targets of treatment for a particular client. FAP case conceptualizations are dynamic, changing both with the client's behavior and the therapist's understanding of it.
Definitions of CRBs take into account the client's history, presenting problems
and in-session behavior.

Although much of this chapter is written in the language of functional
analysis, such language need not be used with clients. Alternative client-friendly
language (including phrases such as "opening your heart," "speaking your
truth") is described in many of the examples presented in this book, despite
the fact that such terms would make many functional analysts' heads spin. This
is because FAP therapists use language that is functional, contextual and
pragmatic. We seek to use terminology that makes sense to our clients, that
enhances the intimacy of the therapeutic relationship, that fosters growth and
deep, meaningful change. A treatment that allows for the flexible, functional
use of language is a truly functional treatment—in contrast, a treatment that
dogmatically insists on using functional terminology is topographically functional but not *functionally* functional. The flexible language used with clients in
FAP overlays a functional analysis of client behavior. That analysis is focus of
this chapter.

J.W. Kanter (✉)
Department of Psychology, University of Wisconsin-Milwaukee, Milwaukee, WI
53201, USA
e-mail: jkanter@uwm.edu

M. Tsai et al., *A Guide to Functional Analytic Psychotherapy*,
DOI 10.1007/978-0-387-09787-9_3, © Springer Science+Business Media, LLC 2009

The Context of Assessment

As is the case for many other treatment approaches, a DSM (Diagnostic and Statistical Manual)-based diagnostic assessment is not considered a sufficient assessment strategy in FAP. A syndromal diagnosis suggests the application of specific, empirically supported treatment packages but does not inform specific interventions within a package—this requires additional assessment and conceptualization. Prominent psychologists such as David Barlow (Barlow, Allen, & Choate, 2004), Gerald Rosen and Gerald Davison (2003) have recently called for empirically supported principles that link directly with specific intervention strategies. Assessment and case conceptualization in FAP is sympathetic to this aim, as while diagnostic assessment remains a component of this process, it ultimately is designed to inform directly the case conceptualization and targeted therapist interventions.

FAP does not prescribe a single means of assessing target variables. FAP practitioners work in a range of settings with a variety of clients, and an intrinsic component of FAP is that assessment strategies are tailored to the unique needs of each situation. Indeed, some FAP therapists working in private practice are now known specifically, and are sought out for their intense focus on intimate interpersonal relationships. In such cases a full ranging assessment is not necessary; instead the client and therapist may proceed quickly to identification of CRBs related to the client's specific interpersonal issues. FAP therapists also work in a range of other settings, including residential facilities for clients with developmental disabilities, community and university-based clinics, and prisons. In these settings a broader range of target problems may be seen and assessment will likely be more elaborate and extensive, tailored to the specific population and context. This chapter will focus on assessment strategies for relatively high functioning individuals, as typically seen in private practice and outpatient clinics. Targeted behaviors in these settings tend to involve interpersonal difficulties and associated mood, anxiety and personality disorders.

Assessment in FAP is inextricably linked to treatment and is part of the initial relationship-building process between client and therapist. During therapy the therapist and client *together* determine what behaviors are causing the client difficulty in his or her daily life; the collaborative nature of the assessment process is one reason FAP is an intense intervention. In concert with FAP as a whole, the assessment process allows the therapist to be a genuine human being, and functions not only to produce an assessment outcome, but also to express interest, concern and genuine care toward the client.

An Overview of Functional Idiographic Assessment

Assessments in FAP are functional and idiographic. When conducting such an assessment, it is crucial to draw a distinction between function and topography. The topography of a stimulus or behavior is simply what it looks like. When we describe what people do, we are usually referring to the topography or form of their behavior (e.g., describing a person as 'laughing', or scolding a noisy child as 'punishment'). In FAP a topographical analysis is less clinically useful than a description of function.

The function of a stimulus is related to its effect on behavior (i.e., whether it increases it, decreases it, or sets the occasion for its emission). If the child continues to make noise in the future, the scolding may have acted not as a 'punishment' but a 'reward' (such that attention from the parent served as a reinforcer for the behavior). Similarly, the function of a behavior is defined by the effect the behavior has on the environment. If the behavior is considered in the context of its antecedents (the conditions that *precede* the behavior) and consequences (what *follows* the behavior), this conceptualization becomes clearer. Often a person may display the same topographical behavior in different contexts, and the behavior may function very differently in each of those contexts. For example, laughing at a comedy club may function to express joy, whereas laughing at a funeral may function as avoidance of negative emotion.

It is also important to note that the function of a stimulus or behavior may not be as intended. An individual who expresses too much (or too little) emotion while seeking to connect with others may actually drive them away, or attempts at delivering compliments may be taken the wrong way. Offering money to people after they do charity work may make them less likely to volunteer again. Behavior both within and outside sessions can function quite differently from what the client intends. This gap between intended and actual effect is often a source of confusion and distress for clients—and the same can be true of therapists! Thus it is essential for therapists to continually reassess whether their actions are functioning to reinforce and punish client behaviors as expected (refer to Rule 4 in Chapter 4).

The key aim of behavioral assessment is the identification of functional relationships between antecedents, behaviors and consequences. This process, however, can be very difficult. One behavior may serve as an antecedent stimulus for the emission of another behavior, which in turn may provide a consequence for the first behavior and an antecedent for the emission of a third behavior. It is also vital to recognize that thoughts and feelings, in addition to external stimuli, can act as cues to engage in specific behaviors. There exists some misconception about the role of thoughts and feelings in a behaviorally based treatment. Thoughts and feelings are not only accorded a role in the radical behavioral perspective, but are considered to be important factors in the assessment of behavior. Thoughts and feelings are viewed simply as covert behaviors, and therefore are subject to the same analysis as overt behaviors and similarly can act as cues. Thus when conducting a functional assessment, it is vital to examine the function of any thoughts or feelings that may be occurring immediately before or after a behavior.

An important caveat to the above statements is that the focus in FAP is not on the accuracy of a thought or feeling (as in Cognitive Therapy) but instead on what function it may provide. Consider a client who ruminates while at social functions, experiencing thoughts such as, "I don't have anything interesting to say, no one will want to talk to me..." A cognitive therapist may address the specific thoughts that the client is having by asking the client to test these thoughts against reality (i.e., am I really not interesting? Do others really not want to talk to me?). In contrast, a FAP therapist may find that while the client is ruminating he or she is avoiding taking any interpersonal risks such as starting a conversation with others, or meeting someone new. This implies that the function of the client's rumination is negative reinforcement or avoidance, and suggests specific treatment techniques to address the function of the behavior, regardless of the contents of the ruminative thoughts.

Assessing functional relationships between variables often requires repeated observations over time. Discussion of a client's interpersonal interactions in daily life (e.g., gaining information about the client's behavior, the situation) is an integral component of nearly every therapeutic treatment. This process provides the opportunity for a therapist to observe a client's behavior and the variables influencing it by proxy. During these conversations client problem behaviors readily become evident to the therapist; however their function may not be as clear. It particularly is difficult to identify correctly the functions of clients' behaviors if they provide inaccurate or incomplete reports. It may seem obvious that an adolescent client who often tells jokes to classmates is doing so to receive social approval, until it is revealed that telling jokes helps him or her avoid completing schoolwork.

Fortunately, therapists can observe directly how clients interact in-session. In FAP it is assumed that the same functional processes that occur in a client's daily life often will occur also in the room with the therapist, although possibly in a different topographical form. Thus the therapist is considered an inextricable part of these interactions. A major source of information for the functional assessment emerges from observing how the client reacts to the therapist's behavior in a variety of circumstances. Over time, the therapist will be able to develop hypotheses about the functions of various behaviors and stimuli. These hypotheses can be tested during a functional analysis. In FAP a functional assessment becomes a functional analysis when the therapist systematically manipulates antecedent and consequential variables during interactions with clients, observes the predicted changes in behavior as they occur, and compares these changes to previous levels of responding. For example, a therapist might purposefully change his or her tone of voice and rate of speech when responding to a reserved client's emotional expressions in order to determine the most reinforcing way to respond to such disclosures.

While basic behavioral research has narrowed the function of behaviors to discrete categories, the key aim of functional assessment in FAP is not to find a specific technical label for the client's behavior, but to identify the internal and environmental cues that are acting to evoke and maintain the client's maladaptive behaviors. The therapist attempts to organize instances of client ineffective behavior into functional response classes (e.g., avoidance of intimacy) defined by similar events (e.g., partner's attempts at intimacy) that evoke and maintain (e.g., through negative reinforcement) those responses. In essence, the therapist simply seeks to identify the discriminative stimuli and reinforcing stimuli that functionally define the target behaviors.

The key to understanding the concept of functional class is the recognition that there are many different ways of accomplishing the same goal. If different behaviors have the same effect, they are said to be members of the same functional class. It becomes both important and difficult to identify a functional class, however, when vastly different topographies of behaviors with the same function occur in-session. When this situation occurs it can be very difficult for the client and therapist to recognize that a single functional class may account for the emergence or persistence of interpersonal difficulties. For example, a number of seemingly unrelated client behaviors (e.g., arguing with the therapist, missing sessions, suicidal ideation) might actually be of the same functional class (e.g., preventing increased intimacy in the therapeutic relationship, where intimacy is aversive to the client). Identification of these behaviors as of the same functional class likely will lead to dramatically different, and more effective, responses by the therapist.

The process of functional identification is inherently conducted idiographically (i.e., on an individual basis). This flexibility is one point of differentiation between FAP and other manualized therapies. This does not, however, mean that a therapist will never have two clients with the same target behavior classes. Indeed, several common interpersonal behaviors are frequently seen in different clients. If a FAP therapist consistently formulates the same case conceptualization for every client, caution and outside consultation is advised. Such similarities are not assumed in FAP but are discerned through assessment. FAP is not prescriptive with respect to how to formulate a case conceptualization. Rather, the emphasis is placed on the therapist composing a working case conceptualization that will guide him or her in choosing how to respond when clinically relevant behaviors or improvements occur.

The functional assessment process should result in the recognition of patterns of functional classes that can be used to organize client CRBs, and lead to the formation of a case conceptualization. The assessment process is quite complex, but the product is actually very simple; one possible format for FAP conceptualization can be found in Appendix A. A case conceptualization is a (brief) summary of relevant historical variables, behaviors outside-of-session (Os) that are daily life problems (O1s) or daily life goals (O2s), variables maintaining those problems in the client's environment, the client's assets and strengths, CRB1s, CRB2s, planned interventions, and a listing of T1s (therapist problematic behaviors) and T2s (therapist target behaviors). All of these components of the case conceptualization are described in further detail below, with T1s and T2s elaborated on in Chapter 8, Supervision and Therapist Self Development.

Further information can be added to the case conceptualization if other treatment modalities are being used in concert with FAP, such as the incorporation of problematic beliefs when using FAP Enhanced Cognitive Therapy

(Kohlenberg, Kanter, Bolling, Parker, & Tsai, 2002; Kohlenberg, Kanter, & Tsai, in press) or socio-political behaviors (SPs) that are seen as problems (SP1s), and improvements (SP2s) if one is modifying FAP for such issues (Terry, Bolling, Ruiz, & Brown, in press).

A FAP therapist seeks to change client behavior through an in-session focus, thus the variables listed in the case conceptualization should be as specific and as operationalized as possible. The more clearly the threshold for CRB1s and 2s is defined, the easier it will be for the therapist to identify and respond to these behaviors. Furthermore, the case conceptualization should be a dynamic tool, the main purpose of which is the accurate identification of functional classes, hence allowing for appropriate responding by the therapist. It is even possible that the same topographical behavior is of more than one functional class. When uncovering the functions of certain behaviors, more than one theme may emerge. This does not mean that one theme is wrong or another is right, but rather that one behavior may serve different functions in different situations. Clients often have a limited repertoire of behaviors, and thus a single behavior that results in different consequences is common.

Assessment Over the Course of Therapy

Assessment is sometimes seen as a precursor to therapy, but in a functional treatment such as FAP, assessment is ongoing and flexible. It is an interactive and iterative process of revising hypotheses about the client's behavior and its function. The assessment and case conceptualization process continues throughout the course of therapy; changes will occur within and external to the initially identified functional classes. Subsequent to the initiation of the therapy process, several sessions may be needed in order to collaboratively determine treatment goals and pinpoint specific target behaviors or response classes. For example, a client may report different treatment goals at different sessions. Only after several weeks may the therapist come to understand that the actual target can best be defined as indecisiveness about goals, and it may take several more weeks for the client to become aware of this pattern and agree that changing it should be a treatment target.

After older behaviors are refined and new target behaviors are discovered, repeated assessment is necessary, typically a less intensive process later in therapy. With each new alteration in target behaviors the case conceptualization similarly changes, evolving in step with the client's changing interpersonal repertoire and responding to life events encountered during therapy. CRB2s that were not initially part of the client's repertoire may have to be shaped over the course of therapy. In this situation relatively gross approximations to an ideal CRB2 may be considered a CRB2 and reinforced early in therapy, but would not be con-sidered a CRB2 at a later point after a more adaptive behavior has become part of the client's repertoire. More specifically, the operational definition of a CRB will be modified over the course of therapy based on the client's progress. For example, a client who does not assert her needs early in therapy may say, "It's very warm in here today." The therapist may view this statement as an early approximation of assertiveness and respond by offering to turn up the air conditioning and discussing alternative methods of asserting her needs. Later in therapy the same client may not be reinforced for such a vague statement. The therapist instead may respond by prompting a more specific request. It is also common for new CRB classes to manifest themselves as clients expand their repertoires. For example a client who overcomes a deficit in making intimate disclosures may begin to make excessive demands of a new romantic partner.

Other changes during the course of therapy also need to be monitored closely. The beginning phase of the therapy relationship may evoke a different class of CRB than an already established relationship occurring in the middle of therapy, and similarly the termination phase may also evoke different CRB. A client's fear of abandonment may evoke inappropriate behaviors in many of their relationships, but this fear may not be elicited until therapy termination is approaching, and thus only could be approached as a target behavior in this context. Furthermore, client goals legitimately may change over the course of therapy as environmental situations change, O1s/CRB1s are successfully addressed and O2s/CRB2s become part of the client's repertoire. For example, after overcoming a fear of talking to new people, a client may begin to focus on improving a newly formed romantic relationship. Targets then may change from a lack of verbal behavior to personal disclosures that will improve intimacy.

Tactics in Practical Case Formulation

The general considerations described above form the conceptual principles that drive ongoing case conceptualization. In practical terms, FAP relies on the rapid establishment of an intense, important relationship with the client. Thus the prolonged information gathering assessment period existent in traditional therapy is not generally practical. FAP recognizes that there are many paths to goal accomplishment, and this applies to both clients and therapists. Some therapists are able to begin therapy with relatively little formal assessment by forming loosely held hypotheses that are readily changed with the addition of new information, while others are more methodical in their data gathering strategies. Regardless of the approach, the assessment must occur in a manner that enhances the therapeutic relationship. As noted earlier, FAP does not dictate the means by which to formulate case conceptualizations, but rather emphasizes the development of a working case conceptualization that will guide the therapist's responses to CRBs. The goal of assessment is thus a case conceptualization that delineates the client's relevant life history, behaviors outside-of-session and CRBs. There are a number of useful strategies for informally assessing these variables.

Life History

Some clients, if not the majority, will feel understood maximally if they can relate a narrative (often presented chronologically) revealing their beliefs about their path to the present situation. While the relation of this story may not be necessary for the therapist to operate successfully, it can enable one to learn the client's preferred language and yield useful information as to how best to indicate understanding and to approach change. In some cases the details of such a narrative directly can be useful in case formulation, such as when clients describe repeated instances of a specific problem behavior class (e.g., making excessive demands in relationships). Other more savvy clients even may be able to describe the variables that influence their behaviors (e.g., commonalities among anxiety-inducing situations that lead to avoidance). In these cases, the client will aid the therapist in identifying CRB classes.

When gathering this information, it is important to keep in mind that the variables that maintain a behavior may not be the same as the variables that shaped a behavior initially (e.g., sarcastic comments that originally served to gain attention and laughter from peers are later maintained by distancing the client from others). In addition, behavior may be maintained by schedules of reinforcement or punishment in which consequences were presented previously at high levels but are currently at lower levels, or vice versa (e.g., a client who as a child was physically abused repeatedly by his father). Such histories often manifest verbal rules that are elicited in current situations and guide behavior. These rules can override cues in the environment for more socially appropriate behavior, resulting in weak present environmental control and, often in maladaptive behavior. Furthermore, it is relatively common for clients to be unable to report accurately their behavior and its controlling variables. Their misinterpretation of situations may in itself be a target of therapy.

Ultimately, while FAP is a behavioral therapy aimed at achieving current behavior change, assessment of historical variables (including distant childhood histories) can play a role in fully conceptualizing a client's target behaviors and their function. In FAP, however, the therapist focuses on past events and relationships only in order to understand current behavior and relationships; insight into the past is not an end goal in FAP.

Consistent with the above discussion, Appendix B incorporates a "Preliminary Client Information" questionnaire, a tool for therapy that can be mailed or emailed to the client prior to the first session. This questionnaire asks for a detailed life events summary, a description of strengths and assets, therapy goals, and any other factors or events that may be important for the therapist to know. The information provided in this manner may be discussed during the first several sessions of therapy.

A number of questions can be used to prompt clients to provide relevant historical information, however it is the function of the question that is crucial. Asking a question that does not serve a therapeutic purpose (e.g., relationship building or assessment) is actually a waste of an opportunity to ask one that does. It is up to the therapist to decide if a question is likely to function as desired. This can be difficult to determine at the beginning of therapy, and thus the following are stock questions FAP therapists often use in assessing a client's life history.

- What would you say is your biggest problem in relationships?
- When did your difficulty forming and maintaining relationships begin?
- Have you had any important relationships in the past?
- Are there times in your life when your difficulties in relationships were better or worse?

Goals and Values

Functional assessment often appears a tedious, technical process. In FAP this is not the case. One means of dignifying the assessment process is to begin with a discussion of the client's verbal statements of goals and values.[1] Most therapies begin with a discussion of client goals, namely what the client wants from treatment and from life. FAP takes this aspect of assessment very seriously, as the goal of FAP is not symptom reduction but to help clients move toward these goals and lead productive, meaningful and fulfilling lives. Everything in assessment hinges on an appreciation of these life goals.

When conducted at the beginning of therapy, the process of identifying and clarifying a client's reported values will aid the therapeutic process in three ways. First, eliciting discussions about the client's hopes and dreams will begin to build the therapeutic relationship, as it allows the therapist to reinforce the client's attempts at the change process. Second, values clarification will help identify what stimuli function as natural reinforcers for a client. This will enable the therapist to respond to the client's behavior changes more meaningfully (i.e., by functionally reinforcing CRB2s). Additionally, behaviors that are in line with a client's values are more likely to be automatically reinforcing, such that a client will 'feel good' when exhibiting behaviors that support what is valued. A client's clarified values will act as an establishing or motivating operation by strengthening the behavior in the client's repertoire. Any additional reinforcement contingencies that have been arranged will act as 'icing on the cake' to further strengthen the behavior over time. Third, and most important, ascertaining a client's values will provide an overall direction for therapy. Discussion of values provides context for the client's goals and provides the therapist with useful information about what target behaviors would be best to focus on.

---

[1]From a technical behavioral perspective, values are much more than simple statements of client goals. A complete discussion of values should focus on overt and verbal behavior in addition to the variables controlling that behavior (Leigland, 2005).

There are many methods for clarifying client's values. One is to prompt the client with questions about his or her life, goals and dreams. These can include:

- What do you see as your ideal self?
- If money were no object, what would you do with your life?
- If you could wave a magic wand and change whatever you wanted, what would your life look like?
- Who do you admire, and what do you admire about them?

Another method is to have the client engage in self-monitoring. This can be done informally by asking clients what they enjoy doing, or a more involved approach would be to ask clients to collect data regarding their daily activities. A third process that can be used to help a client identify his or her values is to lead the client through experiential exercises, such as the funeral exercise used in Acceptance and Commitment Therapy (ACT; Hayes, Strosahl, & Wilson, 1999). In this exercise clients are asked to imagine eulogies, both probable and desired, that would be spoken at their funerals. This process may enable the client to ascertain what really matters to him or her.

The "Life Snapshot" (Appendix C) is another means of assessing and exploring an individual's values. The Life Snapshot asks clients first to rate how important various values are to them, and then to rate how satisfied they are with their behavior with respect to that value. In essence, it can be seen as an elaboration (albeit one more flexible and inclusive of additional FAP-related values) of the Valued Living Questionnaire (VLQ) used in Acceptance and Commitment Therapy (Wilson & Groom, 2002). Each of these questionnaires is a rapid means of assessing client values and progress on important life dimensions, both at the beginning of treatment and throughout the therapeutic process.

Finally, a mission statement is a helpful tool that can act to remind clients of their values and guide them in engaging in more adaptive, value-driven behaviors (see Chapter 9). A mission statement can take many forms, whether describing where the client sees himself or herself in the future, simply listing a client's values, or even poetry about goals the client wishes to reach. The statement acts as a 'rule' for clients to live by, such that before they engage in a behavior they can consider their mission statement and choose a behavior that is in line with their 'mission.'

Behavior Outside of Session (Os)

Another important area of assessment is client behaviors outside-of-session (Os), both problematic (O1s) and positive (O2s). Early in therapy, investigation of such behaviors will provide information for the initial case conceptualization. As therapy progresses, assessment of client behavior outside-of-session can be used as an indicator of the generalization of the behavioral repertoires shaped by the therapist in-session.

Clinically Relevant Behaviors (CRBs)

CRBs most often are assessed directly during therapy sessions. As noted earlier, given the premise that the therapeutic relationship will evoke the client's daily life behaviors, it is assumed that the therapist's reactions mirror the reactions of the client's friends, family and significant others. If the therapist has a strong reaction to a behavior, especially if it occurs more than once, then that behavior may well be a CRB. To test this theory the therapist should ask questions that will help confirm whether or not the behavior is in fact a CRB, and also assess the function of that behavior in the moment. When engaging in such a process, it is crucial that therapists are skilled in the accurate identification of their own emotional responses. They must be mindful of and focused on the therapeutic relationship throughout the entire session in order to be able to identify and address these CRB interactions. In addition, therapists need to be aware of idiosyncrasies in their own histories that might lead to non-generalizable emotional reactions. In other words, the therapist needs to be sure that his or her own response to the client is functionally similar to the way in which important individuals in the client's life might react.

A therapist does not need to assess CRBs covertly; indeed, it is often helpful to ask the client directly about behaviors to determine if they are important. Examples of such questions include:

- How are you feeling right now?
- What just occurred between us to make you feel that way?
- What are you hoping from your relationship with me?
- What frustrates you about me?
- I notice you look upset. What just happened between us?

In-to-Out Parallels. Potential CRBs determined through direct interaction with the client should be discussed to determine if functionally similar Os occur in their daily life, and if targeting these Os is consistent with the client's goals for therapy. This may be seen as an 'in-to-out' assessment process in which therapists consider their own moment-to-moment responses to the client, and how they feel interacting with the client throughout the session, in order to speculate about and identify Os based on the in-vivo occurrence of CRB. This process demonstrates that FAP does not attempt to fool the client into behaving more effectively, as FAP techniques should be described explicitly and behavior change should entail a collaboration between the client and therapist, with the purpose of reaching the client's goals. For example, a therapist might say:

> I am having a reaction to what you just did. I'm wondering if you are aware of other people who have reacted similarly. I'm trying to determine if my reaction is unique to me or not, or if it would be helpful for us to talk about it in more detail.

Out-to-In Parallels. Assessment of CRBs also can occur as an 'out-to-in' process, beginning with a discussion of the occurrence of Os with a client. In this method Os (based on the client's goals) are first identified, and then in-session instantiations of these Os (CRBs) can be speculated, assessed and discussed with the client. Examples include:

- Does that ever happen in here?
- Does what happens between you and your partner ever occur between
- us in here?
- Is that the same as when you and I had that disagreement and you got really quiet?
- Do I make you feel that way as well?
- Do you see me as similar to your husband in any of these ways?

'In-to-out' and 'out-to-in' parallels specifically relate in-session behavior to out-of-session behavior, and thus in addition to serving an assessment function they also act to aid generalization (refer to rule 5 in Chapter 4). Indeed, the processes of assessing Os/CRBs and providing functional descriptions of Os/CRBs are inextricably linked, such that the FAP therapist is continually refining an understanding of the client's behavior through attempts to assess and functionally describe it.

Assessment of Antecedents, Behavioral Repertoires and Consequences

As underscored throughout this chapter, FAP assessment focuses on identifying functionally-defined response classes, individual instances of which will be both Os and CRBs. Producing a functional definition requires an analysis of the antecedents and consequences of the behavior, in addition to the behavioral repertoire itself.

Antecedents. For each class of problems, the therapist first assesses whether there is a problem such that the client fails to identify when a particular type of behavior should be emitted. Does he/she recognize or discriminate the appropriate situations (antecedents) when a class of behaviors would lead to a predictable outcome if emitted? For a client with problems expressing intimacy, the first logical assessment issue is whether he or she recognizes the appropriate occasions to do so. Regardless of how well one expresses intimacy, timing is fundamentally important. For instance, what could have been a promising relationship could be halted in its tracks if one declares, "I want you to be the mother of my children," on the first date. Before therapy can establish the target of building a repertoire for expressing intimacy, the therapist needs to assess whether the client can recognize appropriate occasions to use such behavior; if not, teaching of such discrimination first must occur.

Response repertoires. Next, assessment targets the adequacy of, or problems within the response repertoire itself. This can be difficult, as it requires therapists to appreciate the difference between function and topography discussed earlier. In some cases a therapist initially may decide that a client does not have an adequate repertoire of a certain kind, simply because the client adopts different behaviors from those the therapist would use to achieve the same ends. For example, therapists often are quick to identify problems with emotional expression. This is in fact a common clinical problem, but can be diagnosed inappropriately. Therapists (and often their friends) usually discuss feelings easily...If the client does not do so using the same terms and cues with which the therapist is familiar, it is easy to assume that there is a clinical problem. The real assessment issue, however, is whether the behaviors the client uses to express affect are effective with the people in his or her actual or desired environment. Thus it is vital that the therapist be aware of the effects of behaviors the client emits to achieve a particular goal, particularly those that may be different from the therapist's, but that are effective across a sufficiently broad social group.

Even taking into account the above caution, response repertoires for major classes of social interactions very often are a clinical problem. While the ultimate criterion for judging the adequacy of a functional class of behaviors is whether they achieve the desired goal for the client, there are common ways in which these repertoires fail to function adequately. A client may manifest a behavioral 'deficit' such that he or she does not emit any or sufficient behavior under the right conditions to attain the desired level of reinforcement. A client may fail to (or too subtly) request change from others. At this point presume that the repertoire for asking for change in others was never learned appropriately, such that individuals in the client's life do not recognize that he or she is requesting change.

A client also can have difficulty with respect to emitting behavioral 'excesses'. A client can be too self-centered, request too much attention or assurance, demand too much compliance or dominate conversations. Each of these or other excesses inhibits the flow of social interactions and development of intimacy. At a very simplistic level many clinical problems can be conceptualized as either excesses or deficits. Either of these states can interfere with the client receiving the desired social reinforcement.

Another level of complexity familiar to most clinicians is the conceptualization of some behavioral problems in terms of common interpersonal functions, such as 'avoidance' of certain classes of consequences. Earlier in this chapter examples of an avoidance response class were given, including missing sessions, anger, suicidal talk and excessive compliments. All of these behaviors could function to avoid growing intimacy. Avoidance behaviors when emitted avert or prevent certain consequences. A related behavioral repertoire that is often dysfunctional is 'escape' responses, which act to terminate some present state. Sometimes an escape response is subtle, such as when a client says, "Oh, I forgot to mention that I have to leave session early today to pick up my child." Other times the topography can be very different, such as when a client refuses to talk or becomes angry with the therapist in the same way he or she does with a spouse when attempting to disengage from a situation. Exactly what consequences a client is escaping or avoiding is not always obvious.

Consequences. The final factor to assess is whether interpersonal behaviors are under appropriate consequential control. The assessment question is: when a useful behavior is emitted, is it appropriately reinforced by the environment such that it is likely to be emitted again in the same or similar circumstances? Sometimes other significant figures in the environment do not reinforce behavior appropriately, and the client may want to decide to emit this behavior anyway, or to expand his or her social circle to include more reinforcing others.

Structured Case Formulation Using the Functional Idiographic Assessment Template (FIAT)

If the generally unstructured assessment method described above is personally unappealing, a semi-structured initial assessment process is also available to FAP therapists, based on the Functional Idiographic Assessment Template (FIAT; Callaghan, 2006). As has been emphasized earlier, assessment is individually tailored to each client. That said, common deficits often interfere with clients effectively relating to others. The FIAT, a structured interview, is derived from one suggested means of organizing a case conceptualization, based on frequently recurring therapy targets. The FIAT is an attempt to define recurrent problem areas and provides a structure for interpreting the complex social interactions that are often the targets of therapy.

Although the FIAT is not firmly established as the definitive approach to identifying Os/CRBs and determining a case conceptualization, it is one means to do so. The FIAT is a continually evolving system. Therapists seeking additional training in the FIAT may contact Dr. Glenn Callaghan (refer to the FAP website: www.faptherapy.com for contact details). Here the FIAT is briefly summarized, and one means of incorporating it into FAP is described.

To begin the FIAT assessment and interview process, the therapist should ask the client to complete the FIAT Questionnaire (FIAT-Q; Callaghan, 2006, and available at www.faptherapy.com) prior to the first therapy session. The FIAT-Q is a 117 item self-report questionnaire that provides a preliminary self-report assessment of the five FIAT classes (assertion of needs, bidirectional communication, conflict, disclosure and interpersonal closeness, emotional experience and expression; see below for a more detailed description of each class). The completion of the FIAT-Q before the commencement of therapy can help guide the discussion of client goals and background information that occurs in the first session. Further, as illustrated in Chapter 4, the therapist can make immediate therapeutic use of the FIAT-Q as an aid for identifying potential CRBs.

Ideally, the therapist reviews the FIAT-Q in order to focus the FIAT interview, which can be done in the first or second session. There are no specific guidelines, normative standards or cutoff scores established for the FIAT-Q. As such, the therapist should use the information generated from the FIAT-Q flexibly. For example, the therapist may find that according to the FIAT-Q a certain class of behavior does not appear to be causing the client difficulty. Knowing this, the therapist does not need to discuss that class in depth, although a brief review may be helpful in ascertaining the accuracy of FIAT-Q responding. In this way, the therapist can choose to focus only on the classes identified by the FIAT-Q if there appears to be a clear distinction in the severity of problems across classes. Alternately, the therapist can scan the FIAT-Q responses for extreme scores and review those items with the client.

The FIAT consists of a pre-defined interview and format for broad classes of interpersonal behaviors using structured questions similar to those described earlier. The five broad classes defined by the FIAT often yield useful case conceptualizations. Each class requires an analysis of antecedents, behavioral repertoire and consequences through client and therapist assessment questions. These questions ask clients to recall specific instantiations of problem behaviors in their daily lives, or use the therapist's observations of the behaviors as they occur in-vivo. Information gathered through these assessment questions is designed to parlay directly into a case conceptualization and inform the course of treatment.

As detailed in the FIAT manual, a sample list of questions is provided for the therapist to use with the client both during the initial assessment period and throughout therapy. These questions primarily focus on out-of-session behaviors, and the client's responses to these questions typically inform the conceptualization of O1s and O2s that may become a focus of treatment. Therapist assessment questions are designed for the therapist alone to consider after having interacted with the client. These questions help determine the presence of in-vivo client issues during the assessment period and over the course of therapy. When answering these questions the therapist must identify the extent to which the behaviors occurred in-session, and their own responses as elicited by the client's behavior.

The first class of problems defined in the FIAT, Class A, is composed of problems relating to the assertion of needs. This can entail a failure to specify, request or recognize an interpersonal need. Client assessment questions for this class include:

- Do you feel like other people are able to meet needs that you have?
- Are your needs met when you have them, or are they met later on?
- Are you able to make requests from others to meet your needs?

Therapist assessment questions for this class include:

- Does the client have problems getting his or her needs met?
- Are there times when the client has trouble getting his or her needs met in-session?
- Is the client able to make requests from the therapist?

Class B encapsulates a wide range of problems with bi-directional communication. These can include failure to notice or describe one's impact on another person, being insensitive to interpersonal consequences, not discriminating needs of others, providing punishing feedback to others, misreading signals, long-winded discussions, or escaping or avoiding some important classes of communication. Client assessment questions for this class include:

- Are you able to notice the impact that you have on others, that is, how others perceive you or feel about you when you are interacting?
- How would you describe this impact?
- Are you aware or do you notice when other people are giving you feedback about your behavior?

Therapist assessment questions for this class include:

- Can the client discriminate when he or she affects the therapist during session?
- Does the client value the feedback of the therapist?
- Is the importance that the client places on the therapist consistent with the nature or development of the therapeutic relationship?

Class C incorporates problems with conflict. Again, there are many possible sources of difficulty at each antecedent, behavior, or consequence component of the analysis. The client may discriminate conflict when it is not intended (i.e., being overly defensive), have an aggressive or passive repertoire, or may find reasonable problem-solving aversive or indicative of a larger problem than the other person in a conversation. Client assessment questions for this class include:

- Are you able to notice that you have emotional experiences as they are happening?
- Can you distinguish different types of emotional experiences from each other?
- Do you hint to people about what you are feeling when you are experiencing an emotion?

Therapist assessment questions for this class include:

- Does the client have problems expressing his or her emotions?
- Is the client able to identify when he or she has emotional experiences?
- Does the client identify the therapist as someone to share his or her emotions with?

Class D includes problems with disclosure and interpersonal closeness. Excesses or deficits are prominent features of this class, in addition to problems discriminating appropriate occasions for disclosure. Clients may be unable or unsure as to how to label the feelings they want to disclose, or they may misunderstand the meaning of disclosure from others. Client assessment questions for this class include:

- Have you had a best friend, or people that you would say you are close with?
- Do you currently have any close relationships, people you are friends with, with whom you can talk about how you are doing?
- Do you value or feel that close relationships are important to you?

Therapist assessment questions for this class include:

- Does the client evidence a desire or need for a close therapeutic relationship?
- Does the client self-disclose to the therapist during the therapy session?
- Does the client recognize that the therapist is a participating member in the interaction?

Class E incorporates problems with emotional experiencing and expression. Problems relevant to this class include difficulties discriminating context in order to label appropriately an emotion, or even being aware that such expression is expected or appropriate. The ability to label and report emotion appropriately requires a very complicated learning history, including an environment that supports and teaches emotional discrimination. Recent treatment developments such as ACT (Hayes et al., 1999) target emotional avoidance as a significant impediment to initiating behavioral change. FAP also provides a safe place in which clients can experience complex emotions, while engendering a relationship in which people can learn to label correctly those emotions. Client assessment questions for this class include:

- Is it normal for conflict to occur between you and other people you are in relationships with?
- Are you aware when conflict is going on between you and another person?
- Do you tend to give in to others easily if there is conflict, accepting their position or view, even though you may not agree with it?

Therapist assessment questions for this class include:

- Does the client engage in any type of conflictual interactions with the therapist in-session?
- Is the client aware that conflict is occurring when it happens in-session?
- Does the client recognize that conflict can occur between him or her and the therapist?

The FIAT does have specific difficulties. Even in the abbreviated discussion of the FIAT classes above, it is clear that the classes can and do overlap. These classes encompass a broad range of client behaviors, but they are not exhaustive nor are they the only approach to partitioning clinical problems. The reader should recognize the importance of the strategy used to identify the problem behavior in the richness of the context in which it occurs. A case conceptualization cannot be formed without considering the circumstance in which a problem does or should occur, the quality of the response given the goal of the client (and the appropriateness of the goal), and the events that occur after the response that make the behavior more or less likely to occur again in similar circumstances. At the time of writing there are neither normative nor reliability data available for the FIAT. Various researchers are attempting to resolve these issues. Nonetheless, many FAP therapists find the FIAT extremely useful in its current form.

Case Example:[2] Identifying FIAT Classes

Thirty-year-old Gary sought therapy to help him form better relationships with others and to develop the skills to enable him to enter and maintain an intimate relationship. He stated that he desired stability in his life, but was unable to describe why he was unable to maintain good relationships. Gary reported features of both Narcissistic and Histrionic Personality Disorders. For example, he reported feeling uncomfortable in situations in which he was not receiving a great deal of attention. Furthermore, Gary's style of interaction was provocative and his emotions shifted quickly, making it difficult for others to know what he was feeling. He often exaggerated or even inaccurately reported his feelings, such that others found it difficult to respond to him. He also had unreasonable expectations of others and appeared to expect others to comply automatically with his expectations. Gary lacked empathy and failed to recognize the feelings of others as reasonable, and displayed arrogant behaviors towards others. Clearly these problems prevented Gary from meeting his interpersonal goals, but he lacked an understanding of the relationship between his behaviors and his problems. At time of intake Gary asked, "Am I doomed to go through life single?"

Using the FIAT, four classes were identified. Class E, difficulties identifying and responding to emotional experience, was the primary class of problem behaviors for both in-session problems (CRB1s) and outside-of-session problem behaviors (O1s). Specifically, Gary engaged in inaccurate identification and labeling of his emotional experiences. For example, he reported or expressed anger when he felt sad, or laughed when describing painful topics. He also had a restricted range of emotional expression that tended toward extreme reactions, and he amplified his feelings in order to produce an effect on others. In addition, his mood often changed quickly, making it difficult for the therapist and others to identify his emotions. The targets for improved behavior (CRB2s) for this class were to develop the client's skills to accurately identify and label his emotional experiences, to express these feelings clearly to the therapist (and then to others outside-of-session), and to exhibit a broader repertoire of emotional expression with the therapist and others.

The second group of targeted client problems was Class A—problems identifying and asserting needs or values. Gary had difficulties clearly identifying and requesting what he needed from others. Instead, he often would say that decisions made by others were fine, but then engage in behaviors attempting to change those decisions to better reflect what he would like to have happen, without clearly requesting such changes. These expressions of dissatisfaction often were sarcastic, and he would deny that he wanted things done differently. He reported that he often expected others to know his wishes without having

---

[2]All identifying information has been altered for clients presented in this book in order to protect their confidentiality.

expressed them. For Gary, improvements with respect to this class occurred when he clearly identified what he wanted from others and then made a direct request. If he were questioned about wanting something different from the therapist or others, an improvement consisted of Gary acknowledging this, even if he were unclear about his desires.

Class B, problems with identification and response to feedback and impact on others, was another important targeted class of responding. Gary was largely insensitive to the impact he had on others, engaged in excessive self-focused talk, and often left listeners feeling uninvolved in social interactions with him. He reported the he usually already knew what others would say and displayed a lack of interest in what the other person actually said. Gary was both unaware of his aversive impact on others and unclear about how to engage in more effective ways of responding. Improvements for Gary consisted of demonstrating his awareness and attempting to notice his impact on others. The goal was not to create a hypersensitivity to his impact, but to recognize when his impact may be one that distances others, and to engage in a different response if he so chose.

The final class of problems was Class D and concerned Gary's difficulties in self disclosing or developing and maintaining a pro-social repertoire. This set of problems included his engaging in a restricted range of over-practiced responses with the therapist and others. This process tended to make the client appear superficial and less interested in a social interaction, even when this was not the case. Gary also assumed that he knew what others were thinking about him instead of asking them. Improvements in this area included more spontaneous interactions, asking others their thoughts, and being interested in what others had to say.

A more detailed account of Gary's FAP treatment and outcome can be found in Callaghan, Summers, and Weidman (2003).

Client Self-Monitoring During Treatment

The primary goal of assessment is to determine which behaviors are problematic for the client, and how they should be targeted through treatment. Depending on the client, behavior or setting, this is not always feasible. It is highly recommended, however, that the client be asked to track behaviors outside-of-session on a daily basis to monitor progress. The tracking of behavior outside-of-session allows the therapist to observe how the client is functioning in daily life and to determine if treatment is generalizing. Behaviors may be tracked using a simple diary card format.

Toward the conclusion of the initial assessment the therapist should spend time with the client collaboratively determining which response classes will be tracked. The response class should be given a simple name using the client's preferred vocabulary for the problem, and two or three representative exemplars of each response class should be listed on the diary card. The exemplars should not be topographically similar but of course should serve the same function in the client's daily life. This can facilitate the client tracking the response class functionally, rather than becoming stuck by tracking only a specific topographical example of the class and hence providing a skewed view of his or her behavioral progress.

The defining and tracking of response classes must be determined idiographically based on each client's insight, motivation and level of functioning. The goal is to create as close to a frequency count of the target or problem behavior as possible. Some response classes may best be tracked in terms of the desired target behavior that should occur more often (e.g., sharing of emotions, asserting one's needs), while others may be tracked in terms of the problem behavior that should decrease in frequency (e.g., excessive flirting, arguing).

It also may be necessary to track not just occurrences of the target or problem behavior, but opportunities for the behavior to occur. For example, for one client a tracked target behavior may be the response repertoire 'insensitively arguing with my ex-wife.' If the client has ceased communicating with his ex-wife, however, this decreased opportunity will confound the monitoring (i.e., will appear as decreased arguing). Similarly, a client may be working on being more assertive with others, but lacks the opportunity to do so. Monitoring the number of opportunities can help track avoidance of engaging in a behavior. It also may be useful to track 'urges' to engage in a problem behavior, in addition to actual occurrences of the problem behavior. 'Urges' and opportunities may in fact be similar. These idiosyncratic issues need to be resolved on a class-by-class and client-by-client basis. If possible, group case supervision is crucial during the initial weeks of therapy to help the therapist determine the most effective way to monitor particular response classes for a specific client.

For some clients, especially clients with a personality disorder or with pervasive interpersonal difficulties, OIs and CRB1s are very frequent in their interpersonal repertoire. For example, a client Tom had an interpersonal style that was subtle and aversive to his therapist. The therapist found it difficult to pinpoint distinct behaviors that were CRB1s. Through group consultation about the case conceptualization, the CRB1 was identified as the client's 'smooth style' of interacting with others. For clients with such frequent or pervasive CRB1s, it is better to have the client track occurrences of the CRB2 instead of the CRB1.

Assessment of the Therapist

Much of this chapter has focused on the client. The therapist, however, plays a crucial role in FAP. Therapists brings their own history and experience to any assessment or therapy session, hence coloring the interpretation of a client's behavior. Such background experiences can influence what therapists notice, how they interact with a new client, and the particular ways they respond to various clinical behaviors the client emits. Observers, including therapists, never can be unbiased in how they interpret behavior. It is a constant struggle to separate one's own history when reacting to certain client characteristics and behaviors in order to judge how others would react in similar circumstances.[3] To assist in this endeavor it is recommended that two key areas directly related to the therapist be assessed during FAP.

Therapist Stimulus Functions

FAP therapists should seek to become aware of their own stimulus properties that can affect a client's clinical presentation, particularly in terms of their ability to evoke client CRBs. An extremely attractive therapist of either gender can produce a very different behavioral repertoire in a client, compared with a therapist with different physical characteristics. Sometimes such stimulus features can be helpful, but on other occasions they may interfere. The key point is that all behavior can be understood only in the context in which it occurs. In one circumstance a behavior may indicate anxiety, whereas in another it may indicate attraction. The assessment process requires openness, in terms of understanding behaviors as possibly having very different functions in different circumstances.

FAP therapists also reinforce CRBs. The above discussion has focused on the assessment of Os/CRBs, but equally important to FAP is the assessment of how clients respond to interactions with the therapist. Technically, the therapist needs to be aware of his or her evoking, eliciting and reinforcing/punishing functions for the client and assess the client's reactions throughout each session. For instance, a therapist who makes statements such as "I'm glad that you told me that," or "I feel closer to you now that you've shared that with me," may assume that these statements are reinforcing to the client. The nature of reinforcement, however, is such that the only true way to know if a consequence is an effective reinforcer is if the behavior increases or maintains its frequency over time. In the moment, this effect is unknown, but it can be assessed by specifically asking clients how they feel following an interaction, or even asking if they would be more likely to emit that response again in the future. The therapist must still keep track of behavior frequency over time, but the client's responses can help guide therapist consequences in the present.

Using both the client's responses to such questions, in addition to information from the change in frequency of behaviors over time, the therapist can hypothesize what types of interactions are more or less reinforcing to a client.

[3]As discussed by Turk and Salovey (1988), there is a growing awareness that clinicians' judgments are prone to a variety of heuristic errors or personal rules of thumb that are used to make judgments in uncertain circumstances.

They can also judge how best to effectively respond to the client's behaviors—yet another aspect of FAP that is idiographic to each client and helps separate it from other manualized therapies. This process works in lieu of the formal reinforcer assessments in traditional functional analysis, as a formal assessment would be too arbitrary for outpatient psychotherapy.

T1s (Therapist Problem Behaviors) and T2s (Therapist Target Behaviors)

Therapist assessment also includes an appraisal of therapist behaviors (as described further in Chapter 8) that may be relevant to, and interact with the client's CRBs. A brief list of T1s (e.g., avoiding client anger, making jokes when anxious) and T2s (e.g., staying present while client expresses anger, staying mindful when anxious) both in general as well as specific to the client can be included in the client's case conceptualization. Many FAP therapists find it helpful to have a list of their personal T1s and T2s available to help them to remain mindful of their own target behaviors while interacting with clients. Another informative method of assessing T1s and T2s is the supervision process. Having a colleague assist in identifying strengths and weaknesses increases the likelihood that a therapist will use and build his or her own repertoires for responding to clients in maximally effective ways. This is discussed in detail in Chapter 8, Supervision and Therapist Self Development.

Possible Roadblocks to Assessment

At the conclusion of this chapter it is important to highlight several factors that can prevent effective employment of the strategies and techniques discussed above. One common roadblock is that throughout assessment (and therapy) clients may not recognize a therapeutic interaction as being similar to how they engage with others in their daily life. As such, when a therapist explores this possibility they may either deny such similarities exist or simply be unable to recognize them. This can be a function of the client's lack of insight into his or her own behavior. The therapist's response should be to explore the response, searching for similar interactions the client may have had with others, and asking many of the questions described above. Using this process the therapist will often discover that the in-session interaction was similar to outside interactions, in addition facilitating a therapeutically potent interaction in the moment.

Another difficulty arises when working with a client who states no interpersonal goals and yet is interpersonally ineffective, as assessed by client report (e.g., describing situations or telling stories) and/or by observation in-session. The assumed mechanism of change in FAP is therapist contingent responding to client behavior in-session; this assumes that the behavior that emerges in-session is interpersonal behavior. Therefore, the therapist and client need to work together to determine goals that ensure FAP is the appropriate treatment. One means of addressing this issue is to revisit the FAP rationale (see Chapter 4), by discussing with the client the key premise that problematic behavior in the client's daily life is likely to occur in the therapy session with the therapist. This process can allow the client and therapist to work on the issue in-session. The therapist may emphasize that "this is how FAP is done" and "how therapy will work." A second way to address the issue is to view the client's indecisiveness (i.e., if the client is indecisive) as a CRB1 and address it within therapy. A third means of addressing the issue is obtain an agreement from the client to do 'exploratory' FAP in order to create new goals using many of the 'in-to-out' techniques described above. This may work well if the therapist simultaneously revisits the FAP rationale with the client. When potential roadblocks to assessment are addressed with sensitivity, the path to an effective FAP treatment is enhanced.

References

Barlow, D. H., Allen, L. B., & Choate, M. L. (2004). Toward a unified treatment for emotional disorders. *Behavior Therapy, 35*(2), 205–230.

Callaghan, G. M. (2006). The Functional Idiographic Assessment Template (FIAT) system. *The Behavior Analyst Today, 7*, 357–398.

Callaghan, G. M., Summers, C. J., & Weidman, M. (2003). The treatment of histrionic and narcissistic personality disorder behaviors: A single-subject demonstration of clinical improvement using Functional Analytic Psychotherapy. *Journal of Contemporary Psychotherapy, 33*(4), 321–339.

Hayes, S. C., Nelson, R. O., & Jarrett, R. B. (1987). The treatment utility of assessment: A functional approach to evaluating assessment quality. *American Psychologist, 42*(11), 963–974.

Hayes, S. C., Strosahl, K. D., & Wilson, K. D. (1999). *Acceptance and commitment therapy: An experiential approach to behavior change*. New York: Guilford Press.

Kohlenberg, R. J., Kanter, J. W., Bolling, M. Y., Parker, C., & Tsai, M. (2002). Enhancing cognitive therapy for depression with functional analytic psychotherapy: Treatment guidelines and empirical findings. *Cognitive and Behavioral Practice, 9*(3), 213–229.

Kohlenberg, R.J., Kanter, J., & Tsai, M. (in press). FAP and cognitive behavior therapy. In J. Kanter, R. J. Kohlenberg, & M. Tsai (Eds.), *The practice of FAP*. New York: Springer.

Leigland, S. (2005). Variables of which values are a function. *Behavior Analyst, 28*(2), 133–142.

Rosen, G. M., & Davison, G. C. (2003). Psychology should list empirically supported principles of change (ESPs) and not credential trademarked therapies or other treatment packages. *Behavior Modification, 27*(3), 300–312.

Terry, C., Bolling, M., Ruiz, M., & Brown, K. (in press). Confronting power and privilege in therapy. In J. Kanter, R.J. Kohlenberg, & M. Tsai (Eds.), *The practice of FAP*. New York: Springer.

Turk, D. C., & Salovey, P. (Eds.). (1988). *Reasoning, inference, and judgment in clinical psychology*. New York: Free Press.

Wilson, K. G., & Groom, J. (2002). *The Valued Living Questionnaire*. Available from Kelly Wilson at Department of Psychology, University of Mississippi.

Chapter 4
Therapeutic Technique: The Five Rules

Mavis Tsai, Robert J. Kohlenberg, Jonathan W. Kanter, and Jennifer Waltz

> *Psychotherapy is effective and successful when...it is human involvement and struggle. It is the willingness of the therapist to extend himself or herself for the purpose of nurturing the patient's growth—willingness to go out on a limb, to truly involve oneself at an emotional level in the relationship, to actually struggle with the patient and with oneself. In short, the essential ingredient of successful deep and meaningful psychotherapy is love.*
>
> (Peck, 1978, p. 173)

The five rules described in this chapter are intended to provide a jumpstart for the reader in using FAP. Used appropriately, they can bring about what Peck considers the essential ingredients of successful therapy—involvement, struggle, willingness to go out on a limb, and love. Rather than the rigid, stern quality associated with the common usage of the term 'rule', the rules proposed here are based on Skinner's conception of verbal behavior (1957, p. 339), using the elaboration by Zettle and Hayes (1982). Within this context, these FAP rules are suggestions for therapist behavior that result in reinforcing effects for the therapist—more of a 'try it, you'll like it' approach than 'you'd better do it.'As such, they lend themselves to integration with other therapeutic approaches and accommodate individual differences across therapists. Although the rules are clearly delineated here for instructional purposes, in practice they join together and therapist interventions typically encompass several rules simultaneously. For those who prefer non-technical language, a non-behavioral equivalent is provided in parentheses adjacent to each rule. These rules and the clinically relevant behaviors (CRBs) described in previous chapters are revisited frequently throughout the remainder of the book.

Psychotherapy is a complex interaction involving multi-determined behavior, and thus these suggestions for therapeutic technique are not intended to be complete nor to exclude the use of procedures not described here. Indeed, other therapy methods can be complemented and enhanced by applying FAP rules. The implementation of FAP rules can shift the focus of treatment to CRBs.

M. Tsai (✉)
3245 Fairview Avenue East, Suite 301, Seattle, WA 98102, USA
e-mail: mavis@u.washington.edu

M. Tsai et al., *A Guide to Functional Analytic Psychotherapy*,
DOI 10.1007/978-0-387-09787-9_4, © Springer Science+Business Media, LLC 2009

Whether this shift in focus is momentary or dominates the therapy, FAP rules can facilitate therapists in taking advantage of therapeutic opportunities that otherwise may go unnoticed.

Rule 1: Watch for CRBs (Be Aware)

This rule forms the core of FAP and its adoption can lead to a more intense and interpersonally-oriented treatment. The more accurately therapists can detect and respond therapeutically to CRBs, the more likely it is that the therapy will be fascinating and profound. As behaviorists, we do not believe that 'watching,' a private event, will directly intensify and improve treatment. 'Watching' or 'being aware,' however, initiates the process and eventually can have a marked effect on how therapists 'see' their clients, the case conceptualization, and the focus and nature of the intervention.

To illustrate the above point, consider a question asked by a client of RJK: "Will you call my doctor and ask her to renew my Xanax prescription?" We have presented this request at numerous workshops and asked experienced therapists how they would respond. Most frequently, they say that "The client is too dependent and should be told to do it herself," or that they have "a policy of not calling their clients' physicians for such purposes." In contrast, if the therapists were attuned to CRBs, they might have asked themselves whether the behavior was a CRB1 or a CRB2. That is, for this particular client, is the question a here-and-now occurrence of the same type of problem in her daily life (CRB1), or does it represent an improvement on what she typically does in the outside world (CRB2)? The answer is, of course, that it depends on the nature of the client's daily life problem. If the client does not typically ask for what she wants and is fearful of doing so, then this is a courageous CRB2 and should be reinforced. If the client is overly dependent, however, and has difficulties in life because she is constantly requesting others do for her what she could do for herself, then it is a CRB1 and the therapist should help the client make the call on her own. On a deeper level (that is, involving a broader response class), the client's daily life problems might entail a lack of trust in others to take her needs seriously, and hence a reluctance to risk possible interpersonal rejection by asking for favors. In this case, the request is thus a significant CRB2 related to forming and maintaining intimate relationships (see Chapter 6).

Therapists can sharpen their ability to detect CRBs in a number of ways, including by being aware of therapeutic situations that frequently evoke CRBs, using their own reactions as a barometer, focusing on possible CRBs based on the FIAT-Q (Functional Idiographic Assessment Template Questionnaire, see Chapter 3) responses, and detecting hidden meaning in verbal behavior.

Being Aware of Therapeutic Situations that Frequently Evoke CRBs

Situations that often evoke CRBs include the time structure of therapy (i.e., 45–50 minute hour), fees, therapist characteristics (e.g., age, gender, race and physical attractiveness), silences or lapses in the conversation, client expression of affect, the client feeling good or doing well, positive feedback and expressions of appreciation and caring by the therapist, feeling close to the therapist, therapist vacations, 'mistakes' or unintentional therapist behavior, unusual events (e.g., the client seeing the therapist with a partner outside of therapy, the therapist becoming pregnant or leaving town for an emergency), and therapy termination. When these circumstances occur it is important that therapists be even more aware of possible client CRBs and hence probe more deeply for client reactions (see Kohlenberg & Tsai, 1991, p. 63–68, for a detailed discussion of situations that can evoke CRBs).

Using One's Own Reactions as a Barometer

A therapist's personal reactions to a client can be a valuable sensor for CRBs. Questions one can ask oneself include: "What are the ways your client has a negative impact on you? Does your attention wander because he drones on and on? Is she avoidant of your questions? Does he frustrate you because he procrastinates with respect to his homework assignments? Does she say one thing and do another? Is he mean or unreasonable with you? Is she late with her payments? Is he critical of your every intervention? Does she shut down when you are warm? Does he pull away when the two of you have had a close interaction? Does she seem to have no interest or curiosity about you as a person?"

A key issue is knowing when one's own responses to a client are representative of how others in the client's life might respond. In other words, one's own reactions are an accurate guide to client CRBs to the extent that these responses are similar to the responses of those in the client's life. It is important, therefore, when using one's own reactions as a guide, to have some understanding of the other important people in the client's life and how they might respond. Overtly, this may involve nothing more than asking, "I'm having [x] reaction to you right now—how would your [significant other] react?" This approach, however, also requires a continued effort over time to truly and deeply understand the consequences that have shaped and maintained the client's behavior in the outside world.

It also is imperative that therapists continually engage in the personal work necessary to address their own deficits (T1s), promote their target behaviors (T2s), and ensure that any negative reactions to their clients are not based on personal issues. Being in touch with oneself will help with recognizing when one is being avoidant versus responsive to clients. At a minimum, ongoing peer consultation ensures that any negative reactions towards clients are representative of how others in the client's daily life might respond. As therapists take advantage of therapeutic opportunities to evoke and reinforce CRB2s, their positive reactions are by definition a barometer of client improvement.

Identification of Possible CRBs Based on FIAT-Q Responses

Table 4.1 has been constructed by adapting the FIAT-Q (Callaghan, 2006), presented as a FAP assessment tool in Chapter 3, to an in-vivo table of CRBs. These CRBs are based on the five response classes: assertion of needs, bi-directional

Table 4.1 Possible CRB1s based on FIAT-Q responses

Class A: Assertion of needs (identification and expression)

The term 'needs' is used to stand for anything that one wants or values, including the need to state who one is, opinions, ideas, convictions, passions, longings, desires, dreams, requests for social support, or other needs that are more practical.

- Difficulty identifying needs or type of help or support wanted from therapist
- Difficulty expressing needs
- Difficulty getting needs met from therapist
- Expresses needs too subtly or indirectly
- Pushes therapist away with neediness
- Too demanding when asking to have needs met
- Giving as a way to let therapist know what is needed in return
- Extremely independent, feels too vulnerable when receiving help
- Inability to tolerate therapist saying no to requests
- Other:

Class B: Bi-directional communication (impact and feedback)

This class of behaviors involves how clients impact or affect other people, how they give and respond to feedback. 'Feedback' refers to the responses and reactions to their behavior or the behavior of others. It is the information from others that lets individuals know how they are doing. It may be verbal (expressed in words) or nonverbal (e.g., facial expressions).

- Difficulty receiving positive feedback (appreciations, compliments)
- Difficulty receiving negative feedback (criticism)
- Difficulty providing positive feedback (appreciations, compliments)
- Difficulty providing negative feedback (constructive criticism)
- Unreasonable expectations of self (perfectionism, sense of failure)
- Unreasonable expectations of therapist
- Hyper-sensitive or overly aware of impact on therapist
- Little awareness of impact on therapist
- Inaccurate assessment of impact on therapist
- Difficulty in tracking or following what the client is saying
- Too tangential when talking
- Talks too much or too long without checking impact
- Too quiet
- Too much eye contact

Table 4.1 (continued)

- Too little eye contact
- Body language does not match verbal content
- Other:

Class C: Conflict
The ability to identify and then deal with interpersonal conflict will determine the long-term success of relationships. Here, 'conflict' refers to having disagreement or an uncomfortable interaction.

- Difficulty tolerating conflict or disagreement
- Conflict avoidant
- Engages in conflict as way to avoid closeness
- Expresses too much anger
- Unwilling to compromise
- Difficulty expressing negative feelings
- Ineffective at resolving conflict
- Apologizes too often
- Assumes everything is his/her fault
- Blames therapist for problems
- Creates unnecessary conflict
- Expresses anger indirectly—e.g., by being passive aggressive
- Unwilling to forgive therapist
- Other:

Class D: Disclosure and interpersonal closeness
One's feelings about interpersonal closeness, and how one self-discloses or talks about one's experiences with others, are response classes implicated in intimacy. Interpersonal closeness simply refers to being 'connected to' or 'close with' another person. Interpersonally close relationships are those that involve telling others how one feels, being understood by another person, and appreciating others and their needs.

- Fear of closeness or attachment
- Difficulty expressing closeness and caring
- Difficulty receiving closeness and caring
- Reluctance to take emotional risks, list:
- Reluctance to self disclose
- Reluctance to let true self be seen or heard
- Difficulty conversing
- Downplays the importance of what he/she shares
- Talks too much about self
- Does not listen well
- Asks for too much support
- Feels need to be secretive
- Too intrusively asks therapist about personal experiences
- Not aware of therapist's needs (e.g., going overtime in-session, not giving therapist openings to talk)
- Talks too much and too tangentially
- Difficulty trusting
- Trusts too easily, too soon
- Other:

Class E: Emotional experience and expression
The term 'emotional experience' refers to all types of emotions or feelings, not just 'negative' feelings such as sadness, anxiety, loneliness, but also love, pride, joy, humor, etc. Feelings may occur in the moment as event or interaction is experienced, or they may occur afterwards, as when an experience is being remembered.

Table 4.1 (continued)

- Difficulty identifying feelings
- Unaware of feelings as they are happening
- Intentionally hides feelings
- Flat or distant emotional expression
- Appears ominous or scary
- Difficulty crying
- Difficulty feeling and/or expressing sorrow, sadness, grief
- Difficulty feeling and/or expressing anxiety, fear
- Difficulty feeling and/or expressing joy, pride, humor (circle that which applies)
- Engages in negative self talk when feeling emotions
- Expresses feelings in an overly intense manner
- Overly focused on feelings, unable to control their expression
- Talks about feelings too much
- Feelings are too labile and intense
- Unable to have perspective on feelings, overwhelmed by them and cannot detach
- Annoys or puts off therapist by the way feelings are expressed
- Avoidant of or suppresses certain feelings. Describe avoided feelings and methods of avoidance:
- Other:

impact, conflict, disclosure and interpersonal closeness, and emotional experience and expression. The items in this table alert therapists to the specific in-vivo behaviors that may indicate possible CRB1s. It may be helpful to show this chart to clients and collaboratively check off the items that may be an issue for them in-session and regularly discuss how they are progressing.

Detecting Hidden Meaning in Verbal Behavior

A FAP verbal behavior classification system based on Skinner's (1957) approach can be helpful in detecting CRBs. This section provides only a brief summary; refer to Kohlenberg and Tsai (1991) for a detailed description. This system essentially focuses on two types of verbal behavior that differ from each other in their causes, 'tacts' and 'mands' It should be noted that Hayes, Barnes-Holmes and Roche (2001) have elaborated and refined the theory of verbal behavior and the meaning of these terms. In the service of using verbal behavior notions to aid in the detection of CRBs, in this section Skinner's terminology is retained in a manner consistent with Barnes-Holmes, Barnes-Holmes & Cullinan (2000).

Tacts. A tact is defined as a verbal response that is under the precise control of discriminative stimuli, and that is reinforced by generalized secondary reinforcers. For example, if a black dog runs in front of your two-year-old daughter at the park and she responds by saying "black dog", she would be 'tacting' because the form of her response ("black dog") is controlled by the prior stimulus, and is reinforced by a conditioned generalized reinforcer ("yes, that's a black dog"). The contingency or reinforcer can be broad or general (e.g., "uh-huh," "right") to indicate she was understood, but the prior discriminative stimulus (Sd) must be specific.

The concept of tact is similar to that of label or name, however it is not a symbolic representation of a particular stimulus. From a behavioral view, the words "black dog" do not symbolically represent the animal, any more than it could be said that a rat's lever press represents a yellow signal light in a Skinner box. The problem with a word 'symbolizing' or 'representing' an object is that we then must explain what 'symbolizing' or 'representing' means in order to understand the verbal response. Instead, by saying that a tact is 'controlled' by a prior discriminative stimulus, the behavior can be explained by referring to the well-understood process of discrimination.

From a therapeutic viewpoint, the world can be divided into discriminative stimuli (Sds) located in the therapy session, in the client's daily life, or in both therapy and daily life. The primary focus of FAP is responses that are controlled by stimuli occurring in the therapy session. For example, this focus highlights the most important response among several emitted by a client whose presenting problems are depression and anxiety:

1. "I've been sleeping a lot lately and overeating junk food."
2. "I've been spending a lot of time playing videogames."
3. "I've been thinking about our session last week."
4. "I'm falling behind at work and feel stressed about it."

These responses would all be classified as tacts, but only response three is controlled by a within-session stimulus. It is therefore the most clinically significant response, assuming that all responses are equally related to this client's presenting problems.

Mands. Mands are speech involved in demands, commands, requests, and questions. They have the following characteristics: (1) they occur because they were followed by specific reinforcers in the past; (2) their strength varies with relevant deprivation or aversive stimuli; and (3) they appear under a broad range of discriminative stimuli. Thus, if one were to say, "I would like something to eat," this would be a mand because it would be reinforced by a specific reinforcer—namely someone giving you food or showing you where to get some. It would not be reinforced by a generalized secondary reinforcer such as, "Thanks for sharing that with me," or "I understand." The strength of this mand would vary with the intensity of one's hunger. Finally, one's mand for food can occur in almost any setting in which one is hungry and another person is present who can hear.

Detecting CRB1s in verbal behavior. In American culture, occasions in which clients say one thing but mean another tend to be CRB1s. Take for example the tact, "I'm feeling suicidal." The client may simply be reporting his or her feelings. This tact, however, may be a disguised mand, such as "Tell me that you care about me." Conversely, the mand "Do you care about me?" may be a request for reassurance, but it can also be a disguised tact for "I'm feeling suicidal." Figure 4.1 below indicates the way in which one statement (e.g.,

Fig. 4.1 Forms and functions of client statements

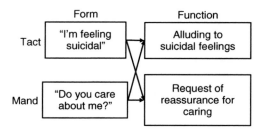

"I'm feeling suicidal") can have different meanings or functions (a description of feelings or a request for reassurance of caring), and different utterances ("I'm feeling suicidal" and "Do you care about me?") can be functionally similar (indicating a need for reassurance of caring).

In sum, clients' statements should not always be taken literally. A CRB1 may be occurring when a tact is in reality a mand, or a mand is really a tact. Of course, any verbal utterance may function as both a tact and a mand.

Furthermore, most verbal behavior is multiply determined. In addition to a primary controlling stimulus, additional supplementary controlling stimuli usually influence the response. Multiple causation may explain why a particular comment is being made at a particular moment, when many others are also possible. For example, a client who is supplementarily stimulated by irritation at his therapist may raise an incident in which he lost his temper at his partner. Or a client who is worried about her inability to pay for her mounting therapy bill may talk about her difficulty living within her budget.

Multiple causation and disguised mands and tacts are behavioral accounts of what have traditionally been referred to as 'hidden', 'latent', or 'unconscious' meanings, or simply cases in which clients can say one thing but mean another. These variables have their effects independent of client awareness, however an inner mechanism, such as the unconscious, does not need to be posited. Instead, in FAP such effects are considered to be the results of 'subtle' variables. In contrast, 'obvious' variables are those that correspond to the form of the response (e.g., a client stating he is angry at his partner, and being angry only at his partner and not at his therapist).

We define a 'metaphor' as a response controlled by subtle variables. For example, a negative experience with a massage therapist is the obvious variable that controls a client telling his or her therapist, "My massage therapist used too much pressure and bruised me." If this client is describing the experience because he/she has been pushed too hard emotionally by the therapist, then the subtle variable is the hurtful therapy experience. According to the above definition, the statement about her massage therapist is a metaphor because it is a multiply caused response under partial control of a subtle variable.

The key objective of this conceptualization is to provide therapists with a different perspective, acquired through an understanding of a behavioral approach to language, through which to interpret the meaning of client statements. Everything that is said, including the words on this page, should not be taken literally. Indeed, words, assertions, comments, explanations, reasons, and even theories such as behaviorism have meaning that best can be understood through knowledge of the context and history that led to their occurrence.

In this example of how a statement can be viewed as a metaphor, MT's client, an artist, begins the session by complaining how messy her studio is.

Client: I was just confronted with this mess, or this unclean, cluttered, burdened space in my studio. I set myself up, in a way for failure, by thinking I was going to have this wonderful day to clean my studio when it's probably going to take weeks actually. I should break it down into some smaller goals so I could feel a sense of accomplishment instead of confronting the entire chore, because it's still not workable. I didn't feel good by the end of the day. I started out optimistic in the morning and I ended up very grumpy, pessimistic, unhappy and cranky in the evening by the time my husband came home. I woke up in the middle of the night just like I had been awakened by a loud noise. I was startled awake and I was feeling so agitated about this studio mess...

Therapist: I'm wondering if what you just told me about your studio is a metaphor for your life and your therapy with me?

C: Hmm...

T: You said you didn't want to set yourself up for failure, that you thought you were headed that way by thinking you could do it all in one day, that it's important for you to break it up into smaller tasks so you can do it little by little, and that it was so important for you to have a sense of accomplishment. Do you think that applies to what we're doing here?

C: Possibly now that you put it that way, the idea of walking in the door and having to confront everything that's possible in the world. Where do we even start, and that's how I feel about that space. I have so many projects in there that I either don't care about anymore, I have to do something with. Yep, it's a very apt metaphor. Where do you start? I'm in this little yellow room here, I just don't even know where to start, I guess. I got my list of risks, and I've got my life history hanging out there, and I've got my outside life, how is that all going to get compressed in this 45 minutes of potentially very expensive time? I don't know the answer. So I could just leave at the end of 45 minutes and I won't think about it again 'til next week, like next Tuesday when I go back into my studio, and I have nothing scheduled for that day, amazingly.

T: So this just feels so wide open and you have so much to do, you need to break it down.

C: I guess. I mean, when you ask me to set an agenda, I don't even
            know what to say, what, where do I even start?

In this excerpt, the client's description of her messy studio was interpreted as a
metaphor for how she viewed therapy, leading to a fruitful discussion of ways in
which her therapy can be structured to be a more helpful and less overwhelming
experience for her.

The behavioral approach to interpreting language can be a powerful tool for
the detection of CRBs, and suggests that what a client says may in fact be a
metaphor that disguises a more important issue. Thus if a client is talking about
a relationship with a friend, consider elements in the therapy relationship in
common with the outside relationship that may be responsible for the client
bringing it up at this time. If the client describes feelings about someone else,
hypothesize that there is a similarity in his or her feelings about the therapeutic
relationship. If the client describes an event during the week, what in the
therapy relationship could be in common with that event? Are a client's dreams
relevant to what is happening in therapy? Using the FAP classification system
will help generate hypotheses about the subtle variables that may be influencing
a client's comments. Once the hypothesis is made, further information can be
collected to help confirm or reject it.

Although this approach is more typically associated with psychodynamic
treatment, it is an intervention based on well-established behavioral theory and
research. Similarly, slips of the tongue are viewed as caused by hidden factors
much in the same way that Freudian therapists interpret them. A crucial
difference, however, is that Skinnerian slips may or may not be clinically
relevant. In behaviorism, sometimes a cigar is, in fact, a cigar—not all in-session
behavior is clinically relevant. Overall, the FAP system for classifying client
verbal behavior enables therapists to explore alternative meanings to what has
been said, such that deeper and more significant interpersonal issues may be
identified.

Rule 2: Evoke CRBs (Be Courageous)

From a FAP standpoint, the ideal client-therapist relationship evokes CRB1s,
which in turn are the precursors for the development and nurturing of
CRB2s. CRBs are idiographic or pertain to the unique circumstances and
histories of individual clients, and thus the ideal therapeutic relationship will
depend on what a particular client's daily life problems happen to be. If a
client is anxious, depressed, or has difficulty committing to a course of action,
then almost any type of psychotherapy has the potential to evoke relevant
CRBs. FAP, however, also focuses on relationship and intimacy issues such
as the ability to deeply trust others, take interpersonal risks, be authentic,
and give and receive love. Thus FAP calls for therapists to be present and

to structure their therapy in a manner not typically found in other behavior therapies.

Implementing the steps necessary to create an evocative therapeutic relationship requires therapists to take risks and push their own intimacy boundaries. Such risks involve being courageous, and having the mental or moral strength to venture, to persevere, and to withstand fear of difficulty. When therapists are doing FAP well, they are most likely stretching their limits and venturing beyond their comfort zones.

The methods discussed under Rule 2 help therapists: (1) structure a therapeutic environment that evokes significant CRBs; (2) employ evocative therapeutic methods; and (3) use themselves as instruments of change. In behavior analytic terms these methods are best seen as establishing operations, in that they not only evoke CRBs (i.e., present discriminative stimuli for CRBs) but also establish the therapist as an effective reinforcer of client behavior. Without these operations FAP could not occur.

Structuring the Therapy to be Evocative

From the very first contact between therapist and client, whether that interaction is an initial phone call or an intake session, FAP therapists can begin structuring the therapeutic environment to prepare the client for an intense and evocative therapy that focuses on in-vivo interactions.

Describing the FAP rationale ('FAP rap'). In order for FAP to be most effective, it is important that clients understand its premise—that the therapist will be attempting to identify ways clients' outside life problems emerge within the therapy relationship, because such an in-vivo focus facilitates the most powerful change. This is an atypical idea, as most people believe they enter therapy to talk about problems and relationships outside of therapy. Thus, variations of the 'FAP rap' (FAP rationale) are presented in the initial phone contact, in the client informed consent form, and in the early sessions of treatment until the client understands it fully.

The following are two sample FAP rationale statements. The first is used by MT, but is considered a 'high therapist risk' version and we recognize that not all FAP therapists will use it. A second, moderate risk version used by RJK is subsequently provided. The rationale can of course be modified to reflect more accurately one's therapeutic stance. Remember that rationale statements are intended to be evocative, and thus all therapists' rationales should reflect some risk-taking and be a T2 (therapist target behavior).

What You May Expect in Our Therapy Work Together [MT's High Therapist Risk Version]
     Clients come into therapy with complex life stories of joy and anguish, dreams and hopes, passions and vulnerabilities, unique gifts and abilities. Your therapy with me will be conducted in an atmosphere of caring, respect and commitment in which new ways of approaching life are learned. Our work will be a joint effort; your input is

valued and will be used in the treatment plan and in weekly homework assignments. I will be investing a great deal of care and effort into our work together, and I expect you to do the same. I will be checking with you in an ongoing way about what is working well for you in our relationship, and what needs to be changed.

The type of therapy that I will be doing is called Functional Analytic Psychotherapy (FAP). It is a therapy developed at the University of Washington that is behaviorally based, but has the theoretical foundation to incorporate methods from other therapeutic modalities when appropriate. FAP emphasizes that the bond that will be formed between you and me will be a major vehicle in your healing and transformation.

The most fulfilled people are in touch with themselves and are able to be interpersonally effective. They are able to speak and act compassionately on their truths and gifts, and are able to fully give and receive love. FAP will focus on bringing forth your best self. In order to do that, you must first be in touch with yourself at a core level (e.g., needs, feelings, longings, fears, values, dreams, missions). You will have the opportunity to learn how to express yourself fully, to grieve losses, to develop mindfulness, and to create better relationships. All aspects of your experience will be addressed, including mind, body, feelings, and spirit. I will be challenging you to be more open, vulnerable, aware and present. There is an optimal level of risk-taking in any situation, however, and it's important that you and I monitor how much outside your comfort zone to be is best for you at any given time.

It will be important for us to focus on our interaction if you have issues (positive or negative) or difficulties that come up with me which also come up with other people in your life. When one feels the power in expressing one's thoughts, feelings, and desires in an authentic, caring and assertive way, one has a greater sense of mastery in life. Our therapeutic relationship will be an ideal place for you to practice being powerful.

I consider the space that you enter with me in therapy to be sacred—I am privileged to be embarking on a journey of exploration and growth with you, and I will hold all that you share with reverence and with care. I will be a genuine person in the room with you, and my main guiding principle is to do that which is in your best interest.

***

I accept the above statement, and have been given a copy for myself. I have had the opportunity to ask questions and to voice my reactions. I am committed to doing my best in this therapy. [client signature]

What You May Expect in Our Therapy Work Together [RJK's Moderate Therapist Risk Version]

Clients come into therapy with complex life stories of joy and anguish, dreams and hopes, passions and vulnerabilities, unique gifts and abilities. Your therapy with me will be conducted in an atmosphere of caring, respect and commitment in which new ways of approaching life are learned. Our work will be a joint effort; your input is valued and will be used in the treatment plan and in weekly homework assignments. I will be investing a great deal of care and effort into our work together, and I expect you to do the same. I will be checking with you in an ongoing way about what is working well for you in our relationship, and what needs to be changed.

The type of therapy that I will be doing is called Functional Analytic Psychotherapy (FAP). It is a therapy developed at the University of Washington that is behaviorally based but has the theoretical foundation to incorporate methods from other therapeutic modalities. For example, the therapy often includes the empirically supported Cognitive Behavior Therapy protocols for specific disorders. At the same time, FAP emphasizes that the therapist-client relationship is important for accomplishing significant life change. Thus in addition to a specific symptom focus as needed, FAP also provides the opportunity to bring forth your best self, to learn how to express yourself fully, to grieve losses as needed, to develop mindfulness, and to create better relationships.

It will be important for us to focus on our interaction if you have issues (positive or negative) or difficulties that come up with me which also come up with other people in your life. Our therapeutic relationship will be an ideal place for you to practice being more effective in your relationships with others.

I consider the space that you enter with me in therapy to be dedicated to the above, it will not be handled lightly. I consider it a privilege to participate in a process of exploration and growth with you, and I will hold all that you share with reverence and with care. I will be a genuine person in the room with you, and my main guiding principle is to do that which is in your best interest.

In addition to a written statement, the following are examples of 'FAP raps' that can be provided in-session.

(1) A primary principle in the type of therapy I do is that our relationship is a microcosm of your outside relationships. So I will be exploring how you interact with me in a way that is similar to how you interact with other people, what problems come up with me that also come up with other people, or what positive behaviors you have with me that you can translate into your relationships with others.

(2) Our connection provides an opportunity for you to explore how you are in a relationship, for you to experiment with different ways of relating, and then to take it to your other relationships.

(3) I understand that you are seeking treatment for depression. One reason why people get depressed is that they find it hard to express what they feel and to assert what they want from important people. Do you find that this is true for you? [The answer is usually "Yes."] Well, one focus of our therapy will be on how you can become a more powerful person, someone who can speak your truth compassionately and go after what you want. [The response is typically "That sounds good."] The most effective way for you to develop into a more expressive person is to start right here, right now, with me, to tell me what you are thinking, feeling, needing, even if it feels scary or risky. If you can bring forth your best self with me, then you can transfer these behaviors to other people in your life. How does that sound?

(4) Therapy has a greater impact when you talk about your experience in the present moment, like feelings of being depressed and anxious, or thoughts of being unsure of yourself—things that are happening in the session rather than just reporting about things felt during the week. When we look at something that is happening right now, we can experience and understand it more fully and therapeutic change is stronger and more immediate.

When and how to deliver the 'FAP rap' depends of course on the client. For some clients, a full FAP rationale in the first session may be too intense and confusing; for others it may be quite powerful and jumpstart a positive therapy process. The above examples are fairly generic, but it is always helpful when giving the FAP rationale for the therapist to use specific examples. Ideally such examples should relate events that have already occurred in-session to the client's out-of-session problems, so the client may experience the relevance of the therapeutic relationship rather than being convinced of it verbally. It is also vital for the therapist to gauge where the client is in terms of reaction to the rationale (Addis & Carpenter, 2000). Therapists should be flexible and open to client reactions to the rationale and also should recognize the possibility that FAP is not appropriate for all clients.

Creating a sacred space of trust and safety. The importance of fostering trust and safety can not be overstated in FAP. The therapist may choose to describe this process as 'creating a sacred space' for therapeutic work. According to the Oxford Dictionary, a 'sacred' space is dedicated, set apart, exclusively appropriated to some person or special purpose, and is protected by sanction from injury or incursion. Use of this term with clients may be quite powerful. Whether or not a FAP therapist chooses to use the term 'sacred space' with clients, the key issue is that, functionally, their relationship is indeed sacred as defined here, and creating trust and safety is essential. Refer to Chapter 7 (The Course of Therapy) for a detailed discussion of how to build trust and a sense of safety in FAP.

Using FAP process feedback forms and questionnaires. As an aid to enable therapists to become more sensitive to the different types of CRBs and also to evoke client CRBs, we have devised numerous forms and questionnaires to guide therapy, a selection of which are provided in the Appendix. We usually request that, after the first session, clients begin to provide weekly written feedback using the "Session Bridging Form" (Appendix D). This form includes questions about how connected they feel towards the therapist, what was helpful and unhelpful about the previous session, what they are reluctant to say, and what issues came up in-session that are similar to daily life problems. Questions that can be asked by the therapist to focus on the therapeutic relationship are listed in "Typical FAP Questions" (Appendix E). The "Beginning of Therapy Questionnaire" (Appendix F) is usually assigned by session three or four. The "Mid-Therapy Questionnaire" (Appendix G) evokes reactions regarding the middle phase of therapy. The "Grief Worksheet" (Appendix H), "Loss Inventory" (Appendix I), and "Crying Out in Your Poetry" (Appendix J) do not address the process between therapist and client directly, but rather facilitate the expression of grief, anger, and sadness at loss, emotions that many clients avoid. The willingness of clients to experience intense emotions in the presence of their therapist and to let themselves feel cared about as a result is typically a CRB2. The "End of Therapy Tools" form (Appendix K) has separate sections for clients and therapists, helping each to say goodbye in a meaningful way.

Using Evocative Therapeutic Methods

FAP is an integrative therapy (Kohlenberg & Tsai, 1994) and calls for varied therapeutic techniques that no single therapeutic orientation would predict. The adoption of particular techniques depends on the therapist's judgment of what will evoke client issues, and what will be naturally reinforcing of client target behaviors. This section discusses evocative techniques that spring from other therapies. Depending on one's training history, one may have been taught to avoid engaging in some of these techniques due to their non-behavioral origins. In FAP, however, what is important is not the theoretical origin of a specific technique but its function with the client. To the extent that a technique—any technique—functions to evoke CRBs, it is potentially useful to FAP. Several techniques are now presented that have been found to be useful in this regard. What these methods have in common is that they all create unusual contexts that may help clients contact and express to the therapist avoided thoughts and feelings.

Telling others about one's innermost thoughts and feelings is central to establishing intimacy and reducing emotional avoidance. In this context, it is useful to consider two general classes of avoided thoughts and feelings that may occur during the session. The first is about the therapist and the therapeutic relationship. These are the type of CRBs most often illustrated in this book. A second class, and the focus of our present discussion, is a more generic avoidance and involves the expression of thoughts and feelings that are emotionally laden but are not necessarily about the therapist. Nevertheless, the presence of the therapist evokes the avoidance. In our experience, the avoidance of such expression is a common outside life problem (O1). Being more emotionally expressive in the session is a CRB2 that can be naturally reinforced and thus generalize to an O2. These techniques are borrowed from other therapeutic approaches and are viewed functionally. That is, emotional expressions (e.g., grief or a remembered trauma) are not described as "a release of energy" or "getting out repressed feelings". Instead, a FAP therapist may ask whether the expression is a CRB2 related to being more open, that will act to build and strengthen closeness and intimacy. In this sense, FAP is a technically integrative therapy approach. These techniques do not define FAP and we encourage FAP therapists to use this section not as a blueprint for how to conduct FAP, but as a stimulus for exploring the possible clinical relevance of such techniques.

Free association. A mainstay of psychoanalytically-oriented therapies, free association involves the client saying out loud whatever comes to mind without censoring. This technique may be helpful for clients with self-identity issues, whose behavior is under the tight stimulus control of others' approval (see Chapter 5 on the Self and Mindfulness). Such clients are focused on gaining the approval of others and find it difficult to talk without immediate responses from the therapist. Once a strong therapeutic relationship has been established, if the client is willing to experience the anxiety of not receiving immediate feedback, free association can bring forth the CRB2 of authentic statements that are under private control.

Writing exercises. Exercises such as timed writing (Goldberg, 1986) can be used in-session or assigned as homework. In timed writing, the client is given a set amount of time (e.g., three minutes) to write whatever comes to mind without censoring. The written piece can be about a specific topic that is being addressed in therapy (e.g., feelings toward a parent, or fear of success or failure), or it can deal with whatever is on the client's mind. Other than a time limit and the task being written rather than oral, it is much like free association, as the aim is to express feelings and thoughts that are under private control (see Chapter 5) and that may be more difficult to contact and express under normal social conditions. Once strengthened in therapy, these expressions are more likely to occur in daily life.

Another exercise that may be introduced towards the beginning of therapy, sometimes even in the first session, is the non-dominant hand writing task. Writing with the non-dominant hand tends to elicit more potent, less ordinary responses. Because the cues are so different from normal writing (e.g., non-dominant hand, simple writing that looks like a child's handwriting, difficulty in writing more than a few words), there has been less historical opportunity to develop avoidance repertoires. Often, to the surprise of clients, more unusual and childlike responses tend to be expressed, which in turn can result in intense emotions, connections to old memories, and explorations of difficult and important material. These emotional expressions in the presence of the therapist are potential intimacy CRB2s (see Chapter 6). This exercise may be quite powerful and valuable in the service of evoking CRBs, depending on the client's problems. Instructions for the non-dominant writing exercise are as follows.

> This is a writing exercise for your non-dominant hand. I ask that you write with your non-dominant hand because it forces you to be more brief and to the point. Because it's not something you're used to doing, you can't be as verbose as usual. I will read you a stem sentence, and I'd like you to write whatever comes to mind without censoring it. You don't have to show your answers to me unless you want to, so be as honest with yourself as possible.

- I feel...
- I need...
- I long for...
- I'm scared...
- I'm struggling with...
- I dream of...
- I pretend that...
- It's hard for me to talk about/it's hard for me to tell you...
- If I had the money, I would...
- If I had the courage, I would...

Empty chair work. A fundamental technique in Gestalt Therapy (Perls, 1973) and Emotion Focused Psychotherapy (Greenberg, 2002), empty chair methods can be used to evoke avoided feelings and thoughts for willing and imaginative clients. The empty chair represents a person who typically evokes emotional avoidance. When effective, the empty chair shares enough stimulus properties in common with the 'real' person or Sd (discriminative stimulus) to evoke relevant feelings, but is different enough to reduce avoidance. From a behavioral standpoint, it does not matter that the stimulus does not exist 'in reality' because imagined stimuli may be very similar functionally to the real stimuli and thus can be useful in the therapy room. Furthermore, because the stimulus is imagined, any consequences that would follow from talking to the real stimulus will not occur, facilitating the expression of particularly difficult thoughts and feelings in the presence of the therapist. Thus empty chairs may evoke strong emotional responses because clients are contacting the aversive features of the source of their distress, rather than talking *about the source of their distress.*

For example, rather than talking about feelings of having been unloved by a parent, a client may talk directly to the imagined presence of that parent in an empty chair (e.g., "I feel like you abandoned me when I was two and you were really depressed"). Rather than talking about how a client feels conflicted about life goals, the different goals may be anthropomorphized by imaging them seated in different chairs, and encouraged to converse (e.g., "I want to climb the ladder of success" versus "I want to stay home and be a full-time mom"). Although such moves require a more extensive discussion involving relational frame theory (Hayes et al., 2001) to fully explain behaviorally, they may function to facilitate contact with genuine but hard to experience emotions. As stated previously, for many clients, such emotional expressions in the presence of their therapist are CRB2s.

Evoking emotion by focusing on bodily sensations. Clients can avoid their feelings using a variety of distraction techniques. They often readily will be able to tell a therapist the means they use to avoid emotion if asked, "Do you know what you are doing to keep yourself from feeling your feelings?" Responses we have heard include, "I count backwards from 1000 by 7s," "I shrink you down into a dot on the carpet and stare at it," "I stare at the space in between your front teeth," and "I dissociate—it's a sensation of floating above my body." While clients may be aware of their distraction strategies, they are often less aware of how they block the physical responses that are the source of their feelings. The excerpt below is from the 12th session of MT's therapy with a client named Victor, whose presenting problem was that he had difficulty contacting, labeling and expressing his emotions. MT was working with Victor to enable him to make contact with how he blocks feelings by calling attention to his avoidance behaviors, which included not making eye contact, smiling when he felt emotion and holding his breath.

Therapist:	You're looking at me like this (eyes looking up, tilted down), I'm wondering if you can look at me more directly? That would help me feel more connected.
Client:	All right.
T:	What are you feeling right now?
C:	I'm sad. When I start to think about the play I saw last night, there's sadness, crying, there are tears in me somewhere.
T:	You're smiling. What happens when you smile? Does it block your tears?
C:	Yeah I guess.
T:	See you're doing it, you're making your sadness go away. It's hard to be sad when you're smiling and kind of laughing. [MT is blocking avoidance repertoires.]
C:	It's true.

T: I'd like to hear more about your sadness.

C: All right. Anyway, the sadness is about loss, separation.

T: How do you experience it in your body right now? Get basic—
        lump in your throat, heaviness in your chest. What do you feel?
        You're blinking more right now.

C: Really? I didn't know that. I notice shallower breathing.

T: You're doing a good job of staying with yourself, and not smiling,
        not going into your head. I hear what you say about this play, it
        really moved you. What did it bring up for you about your life?
        [Reinforcing being in contact with his body.]

C: I thought about my father getting older, my parents getting older.
        At the very end of the play the main character ends up dying, and
        he and his friend finally tell each other they love each other, and he
        says, "If I had another son, I'd like him to be just like you." It's
        very loving. I'm going to stay with my emotion. I don't know how
        that connects to my folks. The love I got, I know they did the best
        they could. Is it ever enough? It was just a beautiful moment,
        and...

T: Let's go back to that statement, can you say it again? [MT noticed
        that the client seemed to block being emotional when he said 'If
        I had another son. . .', and it is evocative to suggest he say it again
        along with the implicit encouragement to feel.]

C: Um, if I had another son, I'd like him to be just like you.

T: What did you do to stop the emotion?

C: I don't know.

T: You're smiling. So the words "If I had another son I would want
        him to be just like you" really touched you. "If I had another son
        I'd want him to be just like you." [MT repeats this statement
        several times for its evocative power.] I'm not sure you had that
        feeling when you were growing up, that your parents wanted you
        to be just like you. I think it was probably the opposite, they were
        trying to medicate you, calm you down. You weren't okay the way
        you were. Are you holding your breath? [Evoking emotion, block-
        ing avoidance.]

C: Yeah, I'm holding my breath.

T: What would happen if you would just let yourself cry?

C: Nothing. I don't understand why I can't do it. I'd just get sad. I
        don't get it, I don't know why I can't do that.

T: You actually do that better than a lot of men. You let yourself get
        teary in the play, you've let yourself sob at times when you're
        alone. I think you'd feel much more liberated if you were in touch
        even more with your feelings and more expressive. The big thing
        for me about your emotional expression is the incongruence, the
        smiling. The first thing I want you to do is to cut that out. I don't

	know what it feels like for you, but it seems invalidating, a very effective way of cutting yourself off from your feelings. And I'm wondering how that came about. Did you have to smile for your parents, and let them know everything's okay?
C:	My breathing is shallow. I'm sweating in my chest and legs. I'm anxious.
T:	What's percolating that you're anxious about, what do you need to say that you're not saying? Just blurt it out.
C:	You said my smile cuts me off from my feeling. I was thinking I don't want to be cut off from my feelings. I don't want to put myself in my box. My parents contained me in a box.
T:	I feel sad when I hear you say your parents put you in this box.
C:	It is sad.
T:	Can you say '*I* feel sad'? [Evocative.] (Client smiles) You're smiling again.
C:	'I' statements, I feel sad.
T:	Say 'I feel sad when I think about my parents putting me in a box.' I feel sad too about your parents putting you in a box. Your voice is really low. Say it in your own voice like you mean it.
C:	I feel sad that my parents put me in a box.
T:	What do you notice in your body?
C:	I'm tight, I'm not breathing, I'm not really moving. Was that my own voice? No? What do you notice?
T:	I'm wondering what you are doing to cut yourself off from your feelings. You're not smiling which is really good, but you are constricted. It seems like you are in a box. What are all the ways they put you in a box?
C:	They gave me medicine, they didn't tolerate intense emotions, they were very protective, making sure the homework was done, plugged me into lots of activities.
T:	I'm really struck by how subdued you sound. I guess that's exactly what you are telling me about, being put in a box, being medicated. You seem to have so much grief under the surface. It seems like you are doing everything you can to keep it there.
C:	I'm clenching my teeth.
T:	You have an impressive array of techniques. You're not letting yourself smile so you are clenching your teeth instead.
C:	I think I'm mad too. There's anger in there.
T:	So have you ever told them you are mad at them for medicating you and so forth?
C:	No I don't think anything so direct. No. I was thinking if I ever told them I'm mad at them for not loving me for who I am. And I still get that message from my mother. My emotions are just gone. I'm dissociated, aren't I? This is fucking crazy.

T: I think you're a little hard on yourself, you're not fucking crazy.
          What do you expect? You grew up in this environment where
          they medicated you because you were a little too much for them.
          And what do you think you're going to do, emote like crazy?
          Not yet.
C: I am hard on myself. I keep thinking the last line, 'If I had a son I'd
          want him to be just like you.' So how do we do it?
T: Do what?
C: Just keep doing this? Looking at my defenses, try and get to the
          emotion... I want to emote.
T: I want you to.
C: (Cries briefly)

After a substantial time spent on evocative work focused on how he was
blocking his feelings, Victor was finally able to contact his emotions directly
in MT's presence, a behavior that facilitated a sense of closeness between them.
   Evoking a client's best self. One way to evoke CRB2s is to ask, "How do you
act and feel when you are at your best? How do you start doing that right here,
right now, with me?" It is sometimes helpful to lead the client in a visualization
or meditation in imagining this best self; often this visualization is taped so the
client can listen to it for homework. First, solicit some descriptions from the
client as to what sensations are experienced when in touch with his or her best
self. Sometimes clients prefer the term 'higher self' or 'wiser self'. Sometimes if
they are struggling with a particular issue outside of therapy, they can be told,
"At the end of the meditation, I'm going to ask you to write down a message
from your wiser self." In this next example, MT is working with a client named
Jessica who is devastated because a man she has fallen in love with, a recovered
alcoholic, has begun binge drinking again. Her friends are advising her to leave
him immediately, and she does not know what to do. In addition, other
stressors in her life are negatively affecting her sense of competence and con-
fidence as a social worker and as a mom. Here is a sample transcript of what this
process can look like:

Therapist: Close your eyes and focus on your breath. Allow yourself to feel
            whatever feelings you're having, and be with them gently. Let
            yourself be okay just as you are, being at peace with whatever
            you are feeling, resting gently in your heart. Just keep focusing on
            your breath, because that's very grounding and empowering for
            you. Allow yourself to feel more solid with each breath. With your
            feet planted firmly on the floor, let yourself feel grounding energy
            from the earth. Imagine yourself being rooted into the ground,
            roots reaching deep, deep into the earth and bringing up the
            solidness of the earth. Allow a sense of expansiveness to develop
            as you breathe, becoming more open and connected, not just with
            yourself, but with rhythms of nature, opening up to energy from

the sky. As you breathe, get more and more in touch with your wiser self and the voice that comes from your wiser self. I know that I've been in touch with your wiser self a lot. It's the part of you that keeps wanting to grow and move forward and is able to persevere despite lots of adversity. This is the part that got you through the tumultuousness and the anguish of your childhood. This part believes in you, knows that you have important gifts and contributions to make. And this part really helps pave the way for you to say yes to things that are scary, and to say no when it feels unsafe. This part really watches out for you, takes care of you, and has a perspective of what really matters in the long run. It helps you move forward, and is full of caring for you and for other people. It recognizes the ways you've been hurt and how you need to heal, and just as importantly, it recognizes the best of who you are.

See and feel yourself at your best. Feel how you carry your body, how you make eye contact with others, how you project your energy outward. Hear how clear your voice is. Feel how in touch you are with your core, how you feel compassionate toward yourself and others. You are in touch with your thoughts and feelings at a deep level, and you are willing to express these thoughts and feelings. Engage your senses right now in feeling bold and confident. How do you carry your body? How do you project your energy? How do you speak? What do you say? How do you make eye contact? Imagine how you interact with your clients and your children on a daily basis when you are in touch with your best self. And you can start being bold and confident with me, right here, right now. How can you be with me in therapy, so that you are speaking from your deepest voice, so that you are saying and doing the things that are hard for you? When you are in touch with this wise voice, it has important messages for you. See if you can let it talk to you right now. Let a message come through about what you need to know. When you have some clarity about what it is your wiser self wants you to know, you can go ahead and write it down.

Client: I wrote: 'Breathe, trust your gut, I know what I am doing. My way is the path of love, that is the core of who I am. Things will be okay. Things will work out.'

T: How does it feel coming from you, from your wiser self rather than from me?

C: Feels really grounding. It feels true in a sense that there's been a lot of experience behind it. My own personal experience where I've been through many different things, and this has held true, so this is the constant that holds true throughout my life. Whenever other people tell you that, there is no way for them to ever really know what it's like to be you. So it's reassuring when others say it, but it's reassuring in a much deeper sense when you say it to yourself, because you have all that history that's making that statement.

Using Oneself as an Instrument of Change

Once the setting, the therapeutic alliance, and the case conceptualization are established, to the extent that therapists can allow themselves to be who they really are, a more powerful and unforgettable relationship can be created. Giving some thought to the following questions may help you as a therapist to increase your potency as an agent of change.

- What are your unique qualities that make you distinctive as a person and as a therapist? How can you use your distinctiveness to your clients' advantage?
- Do any of your client's interests match yours? Do you have in common an interest in mountain climbing, quilting, playing a musical instrument, reading certain authors, spiritual pursuits, running, fine dining, international travel, poetry, sports? Consider disclosing this commonality. Similarly, do you have comparable life experiences, such as growing up Catholic, birth order, moving around a lot as a child, being a member of a minority group? As similar life experiences become more personal, a therapist may feel more vulnerable about disclosing experiences such as divorce, childhood abuse, or death of a family member. A major factor to take into account in making a decision to disclose is whether such disclosure will facilitate clients having greater contact with their issues, or whether it will take them away from their own focus. Other considerations include whether the disclosure will engender more closeness from the client, and whether the disclosure is a T1 (problem behavior) or T2 (target behavior) for the therapist.
- What is your experience of your client? What do you see as really special about this person, how does this person positively impact you, and how evocative would it be for you to mirror back to this client what is most special about him/her? Clients are often only in touch with their flaws and shortcomings; for you to consistently tell them how you experience their positive characteristics is an experience they may not have had before, creating a turning point in self-perception.
- What are the ways you care about your client? Anyone can say the words, "I care about you," but it is far more impactful to describe your behaviors that indicate caring. For example, you can talk about the ways they affect you outside of the therapy hour, such as, "I had a dream about you," "I was thinking the other day about what you said to me," or "I saw a movie and thought at the time, 'I've got to tell you about this movie because you would really like it,'" or "I went to a workshop on art therapy with you in mind because I thought the techniques would be really helpful in our work together." Statements such as these are likely to be both evocative (Rule 2) and naturally reinforcing (Rule 3).

- How can you take risks to deepen your therapeutic relationship in ways that serve the client's best interests? Are there topics you avoid addressing with your clients (e.g., his lateness, her behaviors that push you away, wanting him to say what he is feeling underneath his façade) because your discomfort would match your clients'? Are there ways you can ask your clients to be more present and open with you?

The above questions facilitate exploration of how one can become a more compassionate and transparent change agent through disclosing one's own thoughts, reactions and personal experiences. Such strategic disclosures can enhance the therapeutic relationship, normalize clients' experiences, model adaptive and intimacy building behavior (Goldfried, Burckell, & Eubanks-Carter, 2003), demonstrate genuineness and positive regard for clients (Robitschek & McCarthy, 1991), and equalize power in the therapeutic relationship (Mahalik, VanOrmer, & Simi, 2000). From a FAP perspective, the most important effect is that such behavior may evoke CRBs, block CRB1s and reinforce CRB2s. Thus disclosure should be undertaken strategically, with an awareness for how it may evoke, reinforce, or punish CRBs for a particular client. For example, clients whose problems include maintaining distance from others may become afraid of the intimacy of being allowed into the therapist's emotional world. In such cases, it would be helpful for them to explore their fears of closeness, and learn ways to stay connected despite these fears, a skill that can be generalized to daily life relationships. Alternately, a therapeutic disclosure with such a client may make it more likely the client would avoid the therapeutic relationship (i.e., drop out). Therefore such disclosures should be titrated to what the client can handle, and should almost always include a discussion of how the client is reacting to the disclosure and why the disclosure was offered. Strategic disclosure by the therapist can enhance the intimacy of the therapeutic relationship and establish it as more similar to outside relationships, thus facilitating generalization. The thoughtful use of oneself as a therapeutic instrument of change within the context of a client's case conceptualization can evoke CRBs and thus provide an exploration of emotions, themes, and relationship factors that can lead to client growth.

Obviously therapists have differing levels of comfort in terms of how much therapeutic intimacy they are willing to create; such individual differences are recognized here through the provision of examples of variations in procedures and forms. There is a clear expectation, however, that when therapists increase their risk taking in the service of evoking and reinforcing CRB2s, they in turn will be reinforced by their clients' growth.

Rule 3: Reinforce CRB2s Naturally (Be Therapeutically Loving)

An important distinction was made in Chapter 1 between natural reinforcement (which resembles and functions similarly to genuine and caring relationships in the client's community) and contrived reinforcement (the 'reward' most commonly associated with behaviorism, including purposely smiling, saying "that's good", and giving tokens or monetary reinforcers). Rule 3 is somewhat enigmatic in that FAP is based on the assertion that reinforcement is the primary mechanism of change, yet deliberate efforts to reinforce run the risk of producing contrived or arbitrary, rather than natural reinforcement. The following recommendations seek to resolve this conundrum by suggesting approaches therapists can use to be more naturally reinforcing and avoid using contrived reinforcement. Such naturally reinforcing behaviors are described as 'therapeutically loving.' Therapeutic love is ethical, is always in the client's best interests, and is genuine. Loving clients does not necessarily mean using the word 'love' with them, but it does mean fostering an exquisite sensitivity and benevolent concern for the needs and feelings of clients, and caring deeply. Factors that determine whether therapists' reactions are likely to be therapeutically loving and naturally reinforcing include: responding to CRB1s effectively; being governed by clients' best interests and reinforced by their improvements; having clients' goal repertoires; matching one's expectations with clients' current repertoires; and amplifying one's feelings to increase their salience. Because the blocking of CRB1s is so closely tied to the evoking and reinforcing of CRB2s, this discussion begins by describing the best ways for therapists to respond to CRB1s.

Responding to CRB1s Effectively

Addressing CRB1s often involves making therapeutic use of negative personal reactions representative of the client's community. One such example is provided in Kanter, Tsai, and Kohlenberg (in press), in which the FAP therapist let his client know that he was coming across rather ominously. It is important to underscore, however, that CRB1s are addressed in the context of therapist care and concern for the client, and a conceptualization of the client's problems in terms of historical and environmental factors rather than as something 'inside' or inherent in the client. It is also vital that the client concurs that certain behaviors are in-session problems connected with daily life problems, and that the therapist has a belief in the client's ability to produce more adaptive behavior in response to a CRB1 being pointed out.

It is best to address CRB1s after the client has experienced sufficient natural positive reinforcement and a solid therapeutic relationship has formed, and after a client has given permission for the therapist to do so (e.g., "We've talked about how it's a problem for people to track you when you go off on tangents. Is it okay for me to interrupt you when you do that with me?"). If possible, it is best to address or block a CRB1 after the client already has emitted a CRB2 counterpart. For example, a therapist can say, "You know how sometimes you are really able to let yourself feel your sadness with me? What's stopping you from doing that right now?" Tone of voice and other non-verbal cues (e.g., leaning forward, moving the chair closer) also act as reinforcers. In general, compassionately toned responses to CRB1 are appropriate unless that approach has not been effective in the past. Simply punishing CRB1s is almost never encouraged, except in the most extreme situations involving life-threatening behavior. In addition, punishment carries risks. In particular, it is well known that punishment in the absence of positive reinforcement for alternative behavior generally yields only temporary decreases in the targeted behavior. Further, the punisher, in this case the therapist, may elicit fear and frustration resulting in avoidance or termination of treatment. For more on how to work with client avoidance refer to Chapter 7, The Course of Therapy.

Being Governed by Clients' Best Interests and Reinforced by Their Improvements

Caring for clients means being governed by what is in their best interests and being reinforced by their improvements and successes. The characteristics of a naturally reinforcing therapist are reminiscent of what Carl Rogers called for in his client-centered therapy, namely genuineness, empathy, and caring. Known for his opposition to 'using reinforcement' to control others, Rogers would certainly not deliberately use it. Yet a careful analysis of his reactions to clients (Truax, 1966) indicates that Rogers reacted differentially to certain classes of client behavior. His caring and genuineness probably manifested as interest, concern, distress and involvement that naturally punished CRB1s and reinforced CRB2s. Thus we would suggest that Roger's call for genuineness and caring is an indirect method of enhancing the occurrence of naturally reinforcing contingencies.

The therapy relationship is one of unequal power, and thus it is important to focus on the question, "What is best for my client at the moment and in the long run?" Keeping this question at the forefront of treatment minimizes the likelihood of exploiting or harming clients through a host of situations that can be harmful to them, such as an unhealthy dependence on the therapist, sexual involvement, or interminable treatments where both parties are gratified by a relationship that is more like friendship than therapy.

Having Clients' Goal Repertoires

Therapists are more able to discriminate client CRB1s and foster CRB2s when they have client goal behaviors in their own repertoires. For example, if a client is feeling invalidated by something the therapist said and shuts down, a therapist who is avoidant of conflict and negative feedback is unlikely to discriminate that the client is upset and is engaging in a CRB1 of pulling away. This therapist also is unlikely to encourage a CRB2 involving an open discussion of what just occurred between them to help the client do the same in daily life relationships. Similarly, if a therapist is disdainful or afraid of client attachment and dependence (e.g., frequent emailing of the therapist, announcing feelings of dread at the therapist's upcoming vacation), he or she will find it difficult to use these as therapeutic opportunities. Helpful discourse may include exploring how a client's dependency behaviors play out in current relationships, and creating healthier ways of expressing attachment and dependency in both the therapeutic relationship and in daily life relationships.

Matching One's Expectations with Clients' Current Repertoires

Being aware of clients' current repertoires will help therapists to have reasonable expectations and to be tuned to nuances of improvement. Continuing with the example of the client who felt extremely dependent on her therapist, it is not helpful to expect her to cheerfully say, "Have a great vacation" given that she felt suicidal upon thinking about her therapist going away. Rather her behavior was shaped so that each step of the way, while difficult for her, the therapeutic task matched what she was capable of in terms of her current repertoire: (1) going into the hospital while her therapist was on vacation; (2) meeting with a back-up therapist while having telephone sessions with the primary therapist who was on vacation; (3) asking for a transition object (e.g., teddy bear) from the therapist and having sessions with a back-up therapist without having phone sessions with the primary therapist; (4) asking for a little object from where the therapist was going to let her know the therapist was keeping her in mind; (5) not needing contact while her therapist was away by arranging to have lots of get-togethers with friends. While challenging, these therapeutic tasks did not feel impossible to her because they took place over a period of ten years. The client has now reached a point in her therapy where she has a full social support network and sees her therapist once every two months.

Technically, the above strategy incorporates the principle of shaping successive approximations to a desired target behavior, and CRB1s and CRB2s should be defined with shaping in mind. For example, although the ultimate goal for the above client was non-dependency on the therapist, if strict non-dependency were seen as the CRB2, the client never would have emitted any behavior that could have been reinforced. The therapist's task is to identify graded improvements within the client's capability. What is an incremental improvement in terms of the client's current level of functioning? What would be a small, but real, stretch for this client?

The issue of shaping raises a certain complication for FAP. Specifically, although the therapist may be reinforcing CRB2s that are successive approximations to the target behavior, these CRB2s may not be reinforced by outside others. Thus behaviors that are occurring in the therapy relationship will not be maintained by others in daily life. For example, a very shy client's first attempt at assertiveness may be reinforced by the therapist, even though it was awkward and unlikely to meet with success in the outside world. Or a male client's first attempt at spending more time with his wife may be explained away by his wife as "You just want to get me off your back." This may be discussed directly with the client. The therapist may explain that the therapy relationship is an opportunity to practice and improve important interpersonal behaviors before 'going on the road' with them. The therapist may also explain that clinicians are probably more sensitive to subtle changes, and more reinforced by them, because their only purpose in the relationship is to help the client. Daily life relationships are more complicated, and relationship partners may require time and patience before they change as well. The therapist, by being sensitive to the client's progress and being naturally reinforced by small improvements over current functioning, may foster the client's appreciation for these small changes as well, such that they become self-reinforcing enough to allow the time needed for further growth even in the absence of positive responses from others.

Amplifying One's Feelings to Increase Their Salience

Sometimes it is helpful for therapists to add other verbal behavior to a basic reaction in order to increase therapeutic effectiveness. Amplification can help clients discern and be reinforced by subtle manifestations of therapists' private reactions that may not be noticeable otherwise. To illustrate, consider a male client who has difficulty in forming intimate relationships and who has taken a risk in revealing vulnerable feelings during the session. His disclosure results in mostly private and subtly observable spontaneous reactions of the therapist, including predispositions to act in caring ways and private respondent behaviors that correspond to 'feeling close.' If the client's CRB1, however, is a lack of sensitivity to the subtleties, such reactions will not be discriminated and will have weak reinforcing effects. In this case the therapist can describe private reactions by saying, for example, "I feel really moved by what you just said." Without this amplification, the therapist's reactions would have little or no reinforcing effects on the client's CRB2. With that statement the therapist may also be taking a risk, and may evoke additional intimacy-related CRBs in the client.

The next case material is from a session about six months into MT's work with her client SJ, a 41-year-old male who entered therapy seeking to work through the effects of childhood physical and emotional abuse and to develop intimate relationships in his daily life.

Therapist: So you are telling me that because of our interactions, your awareness of your impact on other people is really dramatically increasing. [MT has been reinforcing this awareness as CRB2.]

Client: Yes, Very much. I am more aware of how I interact with other
            people. But am I interacting in a healthy way? Is my neediness
            coming through, is my self confidence coming through?
T: What feels healthy to you about how you and I interact?
C: The only thing that's coming into my mind, I'm just going to
            throw the answers out, is that you see me for me. It's sort of like
            you're in an airplane. I'm sorry, but this is the mental image that's
            coming to mind. SJ is a lot like Safeco Field (Seattle's baseball
            stadium), okay, hang in with me, this is good. The roof is closed on
            Safeco field, but for Mavis I've opened up that rolling retracting
            roof and you are in an airplane flying around. You see SJ in the
            whole picture, you see the whole vision, the good, the awkward,
            the clumsy, everything. But you also see center field, you see the
            baseball diamond, the good stuff in baseball. And you have
            binoculars and you sort of look over here and you see all the
            good stuff but then again you see over in the stands, you see the
            rowdy face painted side, you see the reserved bleachers and the
            box seats. You see the entire picture of me. And you go 'Yeah, I
            want to hang out in my sunglasses with my little helicopter, I may
            even land and hang out with SJ.' It's a unique metaphor but it's
            true. You accept me for who and what I am–the good, the
            awkward, and the not so good. There's a comfort and a safety
            within you, within our dynamic, and that's how I feel. I feel safe
            when I'm here with you.
T: SJ, you're right. It's really a great metaphor, and I feel really
            moved by what you're saying. [Rule 3, Although MT felt she
            displayed subtle signs of being moved, she amplified expression
            of feelings with the intention of facilitating natural reinforcement
            and the evocation of CRBs. Rule 2.]
C: And I'm not going detract from what I just said, but I am going to
            ask you a question related to FAP. To the best of your ability you
            are supposed to represent in a general way the world outside so I
            can interact with you the same way that I interact out in the world.
            How do I get to that level of safety and that comfort in feeling
            okay with other people, other safe people who see SJ for who and
            what he is. [SJ is asking an important and relevant question, but is
            not acknowledging MT's response of feeling moved. This is a
            CRB1 and will be responded to later as shown below.]
T: Do you expect some kind of deep philosophical answer that's
            going to solve your problems?
C: Yes, immediately, right on the nose, within 30 seconds. Boom.
T: You already know the answer.
C: I have to take the personal risks. I've got to get out there and
            engage. [CRB3.]

T: SJ, having done it with me increases the possibility that you'll be able to do it with other people. I have every belief that you'll be able to do it with other people. You think this has been an easy ride for you? You've been really scared at times. You've really pushed yourself to take risks with me, and I know you can do the same with others. [Rule 3, natural reinforcement; Rule 5, facilitate generalization.]

C: Right.

T: Can we now sit with what transpired today... what stands out to you about today? Please give short answers. [MT is prompting the CRB2 of succinct responding.]

C: Quiet empowerment, that in fact I am doing what I need to do, that it may not be as big or bad or ugly as I think.. I feel encouraged by you.

T: What stands out to me is that I loved your metaphor, I was really moved by it, and I wonder if you sensed how moved I was. And you didn't create space for that. I told you I felt moved, I started getting teary, and you moved in with your talking. That's something I want you to watch, especially outside of here, especially when you're with your girlfriend, that there's a way you use your language to be in charge. Just be aware of that, to create more space for the other person, to be tuned into what's happening. How aware were you of what was going on? [Calling attention to the CRB1s of limited discrimination of MT's positive emotional responses, his lack of reinforcing intimacy building, and prompting O2s.]

C: Not very aware, but yet it triggers memories and things like that that have happened in the past.

T: What triggers things?

C: When you complimented me last week, and I didn't, I sort of rolled past it, like Paul at work..

T: Don't give me any examples right now, we're talking about you and me. [Blocking SJ's CRB1 of intimacy avoidance, but said with a gentle tone.]

C: You complimented me in the past and I had a hard time letting it in. Last week, it was like, okay, Mavis complimented me.

T: Before you couldn't take it in and you've started taking it in. You were talking about your awareness of other people and how it's skyrocketed. Keep working on that. That also increases your connection with me and others. [Rule 5, facilitate generalization.]

C: It does. Being with the silence. In other words, somebody says something that I've moved them or touched them, be with the stillness, be with the silence, accept what they've said. I can be that way with my girlfriend.

Rule 4: Observe the Potentially Reinforcing Effects of Therapist Behavior in Relation to Client CRBs (Be Aware of One's Impact)

Rule 4 highlights the importance of paying attention to client reactions and the therapist observing his or her effect on the client. By definition, the client has experienced therapeutic reinforcement only if his or her target behavior is strengthened. Therefore, it is essential that therapists assess the degree to which their behaviors that were intended to reinforce actually functioned as reinforcers. By continuing to pay close attention to the function of one's own behavior, the therapist can adjust his or her responding as necessary to maximize the potential for reinforcement. Here we discuss multiple strategies for enacting Rule 4, including explicit (therapist process questions) and implicit (paying attention) strategies.

Of course, the only way a therapist truly knows that a response that was intended to be reinforcing actually was reinforcing is by observing a change in the frequency or intensity of the target behavior. Explicit process questions, however, can serve to give clues about the reinforcing effects of the therapist's responses. These questions can be fairly straightforward, and often occur after a CRB2/Rule 3 interaction. For example, the therapist may simply ask, "How was that for you?" or, "When I responded to you in that way, how did you feel?" or, "Do you think my response made it more likely for you to do what you did again, or less likely?"

An important consideration when asking these questions is the timing. Although they should follow therapist attempts to reinforce CRB, they should not follow too closely. A CRB2/Rule 3 interaction in FAP may be quite intense, and immediate attempts to 'process' this interaction with Rule 4-type questions may truncate the natural interaction, and may represent a therapist's subtle avoidance of the intensity created. Thus a therapist should be sensitive to the natural end of a CRB2 interaction and only follow with Rule 4 behavior when the interaction has come to a natural conclusion. This may result in waiting until the next session to process the interaction.

Paying attention without explicit questioning is equally important. In this case example, SJ (the client described earlier), sent MT an email the afternoon prior to an 8:30 am appointment telling her of his diagnosis of severe periodontal disease and asking a question about his CRBs. MT opened the email at night, and had not responded because her appointment with him was in less than 12 hours. SJ began the session the following way.

Client: Did you get my email?
Therapist: I did. That's bad news about your periodontal disease.
C: Usually you just respond, saying I got it or something like that, so I was wondering if that was you not reinforcing bad behavior on my part. [Rule 1, because of his assertiveness difficulties, MT is thinking that SJ raising this issue of her not responding to him is a CRB2.]

T: No, I'm overwhelmed because I'm leaving the country day after tomorrow. I have a ton of emails and it was really late at night. You asked a question that I just didn't have time to even think about, so I apologize if you were waiting for me to say thanks for the email. [Rule 3, reinforcing CRB2.]

C: I wasn't sitting feverishly by the email.

T: I was thinking I'm going to see him in the morning and we can talk about it then.

C: Right, exactly, but...

T: But you're saying it would have been nice if I had said, 'I'll see you in the morning.' [Rule 3, again naturally reinforcing client's CRB2 by taking it very seriously.]

C: Yes, if you had acknowledged that you received it. That's kind of important to me, not a dissertation, but just an acknowledgement, 'copy received' or something like that. [Client is being more direct with his request, another CRB2.]

T: You're right, it would've only taken me two seconds to send something like that, and you wouldn't have been left wondering if I had gotten your email. [Rule 3, MT is again reinforcing his request.]
(...at the end of the session)

C: In your travels, if you could, I can't remember the name of the chocolate. [This is an unusual request from a client, suggesting that SJ was reinforced for his earlier request that MT acknowledge his email. Rule 4, noticing the effects of therapist reinforcement.]

T: You want me to bring you a chocolate bar? [MT was a little surprised, and could see how this request had both CRB2 and CRB1 properties. She gave a noncommittal response because she wanted some time to think about how she wanted to handle this request. Ultimately she decided she wanted to reinforce him for asking, that it was a tact disguised as a mand they could discuss at another time (he was probably anxious about not seeing her for two weeks), and that getting him this small item was an act of relationship building.]

T: I gotta run.

C: May I ask one more question on the way out, some of the studies that have been cited in the papers I'm reading on FAP are no longer accessible. Do you have copies of those on hard drive?

[T considered this request a CRB1 in which the client was not being aware of her needs—she had already indicated she was overwhelmed because of her overseas trip, and he had gone overtime in his session.]

T: I can't deal with that right now 'cause I'm way overwhelmed with all the tasks I need to do, so at some point, in the latter part of

August, make a note of whatever papers you're interested in and we'll see. [MT did not reinforce this request, but gave him the opportunity to bring it up again at another time.]

In the above sequence, following Rule 4, MT viewed SJ's requests as evolving from a CRB2 to a CRB2/1 to a CRB1. It seemed as if once his initial request was taken seriously, it was hard for him to 'put the brakes on' saying what he wanted. This highlights the fact that, due to the process of shaping, a CRB2 (making a request) can turn into a CRB1 (making a request at an inappropriate time). Thus a different CRB1 emerged, and the new target CRB2 involves SJ becoming more discriminating and sensitive as to when he makes his requests or what he asks for (Class B on the FIAT-Q). In the future, MT will be more aware of SJ's request-making behavior (Rule 1),and will raise the topic of how he deals with asking for what he wants and its impact on her (Rule 2). She will let him know when his requests constitute CRB1s, and will reinforce him for requests that are CRB2s (Rule 3). Adhering to Rule 4 would mean closely monitoring the trajectory of his request-making behavior so that ultimately SJ becomes more discriminating and sensitive as to when and how he makes his requests. MT will also help him generalize this behavior (Rule 5) in a way that facilitates a balance between focusing on his own versus others' needs, and receiving and giving in a way that optimizes closeness in his daily life relationships.

In terms of Rule 4, it also is important for therapists to focus on the role of T1s (therapist in-session problem behaviors) and T2s (therapist in-session target behaviors) because an increased awareness of oneself goes hand-in-hand with an increased awareness of one's impact on clients. We recommend that therapists set aside time to explore questions such as the following.

- What do you tend to avoid addressing with your clients?
- How does this avoidance impact the work that you do with these clients?
- What do you tend to avoid dealing with in your life? (e.g., tasks, people, memories, needs, feelings)
- How do your daily life avoidances impact the work that you do with your clients?
- What are the specific T2s you want to develop with each client based on the case conceptualization?

Rule 5: Provide Functional Analytically Informed Interpretations and Implement Generalization Strategies (Interpret and Generalize)

A great deal of talking occurs during therapy sessions and this rule identifies certain types of therapist talk of particular importance in FAP. A client might ask the therapist "Why did I do that?" or "Why am I so afraid of intimacy?" and the therapist is expected to give an answer. From a behavioral standpoint, the answer is just a bit of verbal behavior referred to as a 'reason.' FAP 'reasons' are designed to help clients find solutions to their problems and to help generalize progress in therapy to daily life. A functional analytically informed reason includes a history that accounts for how it was adaptive for clients to act in the ways they do. For example, being intimate and open not only is beneficial in forming and maintaining close relationships, but it also makes one vulnerable to punishment. For a particular client, his or her history might include a childhood and/or later period in which attempts at intimacy were punished. Clients who account for their lack of intimacy by referring to this history are better positioned to take risks in the future as a means to remedy the problem.

Parallels Between In-Session and Daily Life Behaviors

'Out-to-in parallels' take place when daily-life events correspond to in-session situations, and 'in-to-out parallels' occur when in-session events correspond to daily-life events. These parallels may facilitate the generalization of gains made in the client-therapist relationship to daily life as well as assist in identifying CRBs. Both are important, and a good FAP session may involve considerable weaving between daily-life and in-session content through multiple in-to-out and out-to-in parallels.

Facilitating generalization is essential in FAP, thus different case illustrations of this process will be provided. The first example is an interaction between MT and her client Alicia (described in Chapter 7) who participated in a 20 session treatment for depression and smoking cessation. In this session they are discussing an out-to-in parallel that Alicia is struggling with regarding her pulling away once she knows someone cares about her.

Therapist: You know how I've said to you a number of times in our work together that our relationship is very, very important, and that it's a microcosm of your outside life relationships. [Rule 2: Evoke CRB. MT hypothesized that Alicia cancelling her recent sessions due to back pain may be a CRB1 involving avoidance of the closeness that has been increasing in their therapeutic relationship. Rule 1: Be Aware of CRB.]

Client: Yeah I was thinking about that, and I kind of wrote about it on my session bridging sheet. When I think back to the relationships I've been in, all my boyfriends, I really relish the pursuit, but once they turn around and start liking me, I go 'Yuk.' Then I feel smothered. I realized I did that in this relationship too in a way.

T: With me?

C: Yeah it was like the excitement in the beginning, everything's new, then you really focused on me and turned your attention on me, and I froze. And I don't know why at a point when people reciprocate the energy I'm putting into it, then I freak out.

T: Close relationships involving intimacy can bring about a lot of hurt, which you've certainly experienced in your relationships with men. So it makes sense that you might want to be cautious and pull away. That gives you more of a sense of control over the relationship, but it can also bring about the very outcome that you are trying to avoid. [A Rule 5 interpretation.] It's so important that you can say this out loud, it's incredible, because I certainly felt you freaking out. [Rule 3, reinforcement of her being open.]

C: Yeah, I felt it really strong, when I met Jay, same thing, with Terry it was even worse. I really like you but I didn't want you to like me. Of course I have my terror of being rejected, so it solidifies the rejection.

T: So if you had just let me really like you and let yourself get closer to me, what would happen?

C: It's loss, the rejection thing, which ties in loss also. I would just be teetering on the brink worrying everyday of losing someone who likes me. Maybe I'm a lot slower in relationships than I think I am. I like to think I make friends really quick, but then I realize that my freak out feelings come up, what do I do, and then I think what if I wait it out, but I don't know how I am during that waiting out.

T: I think that the other person also has to wait it out, it's like I sort of knew what you were doing, we have a commitment to each other, I was hoping you'd talk to me about it, and you are. Were you able to say anything to these guys you were involved with?

C: No, because I was so terrified of losing them. When relationships get to the stage where they matter to me, I have some kind of psychic time gauge, I have to reject it before I get rejected. If I sit it out and I'm convinced I won't be rejected right off the bat, I'm able to recommit myself.

T: Does it feel like we kind of went through that, you and I?

C: Oh yeah.

T: What does it feel like on your end?

C: It feels comfortable now, but it was so weird, I went through exactly that. For the first four and a half months I was so psyched you cared so much about me, then I did it, I went through this freak out thing.

T: I think I really precipitated you going into this when I was calling you every morning to help you in the process of quitting smoking. So we're talking about the idea of you being honest about it while it was happening. For me it felt important that I stayed pretty steady.

C: That's true, and then I was convinced that you weren't going to dump me or turn your back on me.

T: It seems that when you talk about it, the pressure's off. So for you to say, I'm get scared and overwhelmed, and...

C: I haven't done that, except for here.

T: I felt so much better when you told me. [Amplifying feelings.]

C: I'll have to make a mental note of this.

T: This is really important. I can't wait for you to get into a relation-ship, have this issue come up, and talk about it. I can't emphasize enough how connecting it is to have someone tell you what's going on, to have you tell me, this whole conversation we are having is just awesome. [Rule 3, more natural reinforcement, Rule 5, encouraging an in-to-out parallel.]

This second case example is Michael, a brilliant researcher, who suffered from severe depression as he increasingly found it more difficult to obtain grants to fund his research projects. He had been in therapy with MT on and off for about five years. For the last two years he had been generally avoidant of intimate interpersonal stimuli and noted a particular disappointment that this resulted in an absence of sexual desire. The transcript segment below illustrates how MT reinforced his CRB2 of contacting sexual stimuli. She then directed attention to the O2 of sexual intimacy that is possible between Michael and his wife (an in-to-out parallel).

Therapist: You're not making very much eye contact with me today. Is there something you're avoiding?

Client: Okay, maybe, I'm certain because of your mother's death (T has come back to work after attending her mother's funeral), I'm maybe holding back, not deliberately, but maybe I'm holding back because I feel you need a gentle time.

T: What are you holding back? What would you be like if you weren't worried about giving me a gentle time?

C: I would tell you I can see you've had a haircut, that I really like what you said when I first came in about how I gave you an important gift. (Client had promised in last session not to commit suicide.)

T: Tell me more about that.

C: It's... uh... part of me gets aroused, part of me starts feeling sad, it's a strange combination.

T: Sexually aroused? [Addressing Michael's sexual arousal in-session is evocative. MT wants to evoke the CRB2 of contacting and expressing intimacy related feelings, including sexual ones. Asking this question was anxiety provoking, took courage, and was an example of a T2 on MT's part.]

C: (Nods)

T: That's interesting. How often do you experience that combination of being aroused and sad?

C: I'd say very rarely.

T: Tell me more. So you really liked what I said, that your promising not to commit suicide is one of the best gifts that anyone has ever given me.

C: See, it doesn't make any sense. I understand why I feel sad. I always feel sad when someone says nice things about me. But why I get aroused I have no idea.

T: So are you aroused right now?

C: Mm-hmm.

T: What's that feel like for you?

C: Slightly embarrassing. But I can't be that embarrassed or else I wouldn't tell you, would I? It's not a topic of conversation I normally tell people when these things happen.

T: We're so far beyond what's polite social conversation. I just really value that about you, that you can tell me anything.

C: I think my body's beginning to tell me it wants sex.

T: It's been a long time since you have felt that.

C: Mm-hmm.

T: So what's it like for your body to tell you that it wants sex?

C: It can be distressing.

T: Before interpreting it, just tell me what the sensations are like. What's your body saying to you? How do you know it wants sex?

C: I spend a lot of time in shops looking at young ladies, admiring them, even older ones...

T: That's wonderful! Michael. Are you eying J (his wife) differently? I hope she's still open to being physically intimate with you—'cause you've rejected her a lot.

C: Yep.

T: You think she's still open to it?

C: I'm going to say yes.

T: What makes you think so?

C: Oh every now and then I give her a hug and hold her breasts from behind.

T: And what does she do when you hold her breasts?

C: She doesn't reject me.
        [Overall, MT was careful to not risk punishing the CRB2s involved with having and expressing sexual feelings by doing the typical 'it's okay to have feelings in here but there is a strict rule of no touching.']

Assigning Homework

FAP ultimately is a behavioral therapy and success is achieved when the client has changed his or her behavior in daily life. Thus provision of homework assignments is also important to Rule 5. The best homework assignments in FAP are when the client has engaged in a CRB2 during the session, and the assignment is for the client to now take the improved behavior 'on the road' and test it with significant others in his or her life. For example, the therapist might say, "Allowing me to help you without pushing me away went well, why don't you try it with your partner this week if an opportunity arises?" Homework assignments in FAP are likely to involve another person in the client's life, and the therapist cannot guarantee how this person will respond. This is particularly an issue when the in-session CRB2 is an approximation of the desired behavior—such behaviors are CRB2s in-session but are not yet ready for daily life, and this can be discussed with the client.

This next case is an example of how a client of MT's was able to focus on feeling present and grounded in-session, and then was asked to practice the specific behaviors associated with those feelings in his outside relationships.

Therapist:	Can you feel the difference when you are feeling your 'mojo' (client's term for when he is feeling 'on')?
Client:	Yeah, okay, good. I practiced what we talked about with Jennifer. I can kind of feel that physically. So I really paid attention to my body. And I paid attention to how I was on the date. I tried not to speak too quickly, get kind of tumbling up here in my head. Staying centered here in my solar plexus, and yeah I could feel it. I know that centered feeling.
T:	You're really different. You exude your energy differently when you are centered.
C:	Mm hmm. You can feel that confidence coming from me.
T:	Yes, I can feel that confident energy coming from you.
C:	Yeah, it's interesting, I've really come to that place where I can tell the differences in those two states of being.
T:	And I think all these women are responding.
C:	I think that's part of it. I'm getting positive responses from several women who have responded to me as a person, not just my email. I can feel it now. I was feeling that centeredness, and it helped me keep there, rather than getting too caught up in the anxious machinations of my brain.
T:	You're such a quick study. We focus on something, and you just get it right way. It's very exciting.
C:	Well, you and I have really achieved something here that I've been looking for in therapy for a long time. The last couple times in therapy I've been looking for somebody to help me find out what I might be bringing to the table. This is a testament to our work together, it's a testament to you as a therapist, it's a testament to FAP. 'Cause what we did is you helped me pay attention to my behavior in the room, I paid attention to what was going on with me. That was a key piece of this is that I could talk a good game about what's going on in my relationships, but we're talking about it rather than focusing on something I could take out of the room. In this case, it was a feeling, a centered, locked in feeling I got in touch with that I was then able to take out of here, so thank you.
T:	Well it's thrilling to me.

Ethical Issues and Precautions

FAP seeks to create a deep and profound therapeutic experience; the degree of thoughtfulness, care and caution that FAP therapists bring to their work must be equally deep and profound. Ethical codes developed to guide therapists in general, such as the APA Ethical Guidelines (American Psychological Association, 2002) are relevant and applicable to FAP. Specific characteristics of FAP ensure some of these guidelines are particularly salient.

The following sections delineate several precautions in terms of areas of potential ethical concern and the ways they relate to FAP. Additional issues are also discussed that are specific to the competent practice of FAP.

Avoid Sexual Exploitation

The intensity and emotional intimacy that are often present in FAP relationships may increase the chances that sexual attraction will develop. FAP therapists must therefore have the best possible boundaries in this area. As described in the feminist code of ethics (feminist-therapy-institute.org/ethics.htm), therapists must not exploit clients sexually in an overt manner, but also should be aware of more subtle forms of sexual exploitation. For example, if a client has a CRB1 of seeking approval from others through sexualized behavior in a way that is detrimental to his or her sense of self, the FAP therapist must be able to identify this behavior and avoid reinforcing it.

Be Aware of Cultural Biases

All of us have been shaped by the cultural contexts in which we have lived. Given that, FAP therapists must guard against defining client behaviors as CRB1s or CRB2s based solely on cultural expectations. When we are unaware of our biases, we may inadvertently reinforce a client for a behavior that is actually a CRB1. For example, if the therapist expects men to be stoic, he/she may subtly punish emotional expression in a male client, even if such expression is a CRB2 for that person.

Do Not Continue a Non-Beneficial Treatment

FAP-informed treatment does not help all clients. Research also clearly supports the importance of therapist-client match. Having therapy not work well is often emotionally evocative for therapists, and can result in problematic behavior such as blaming of the client, directly or indirectly distancing from or being rejecting toward the client, becoming overly apologetic, self-critical or tenaciously continuing therapy without acknowledgement of the lack of progress. At times, having a client decide not to continue treatment may represent an important CRB2, and FAP therapists must be able to reinforce this behavior.

Competence in Conducting FAP

In the above discussion of FAP rules, the factors that are important in conducting FAP were noted. Here we reiterate the most significant variables for FAP therapists to develop in themselves.

Importance of thorough understanding of the client. FAP therapists take risks, evoke CRBs, and create intense therapeutic relationships. All of these experiences have the potential to be beneficial but also may be stressful and challenging, or even harmful for the client. The therapist therefore must proceed with caution, and make careful use of principles of shaping. This requires knowing the client well, and knowing what behaviors exhibited by the therapist will encourage growth and change at a level that the client is ready for, versus what behaviors will be overwhelming or off-putting in a way that leads to disengagement, undue distress or even termination of therapy. FAP therapists are encouraged to carefully inform the client of the nature of the treatment (refer to the previous section 'Giving the FAP rationale') but also to titrate the move into in-session focus in a way that the client can tolerate.

Importance of being controlled by reinforcers that are beneficial to the client. From a FAP perspective, a primary source of ethical violations is the situation of the therapist being controlled by reinforcers that are not beneficial to the client. For example, the therapist may be reinforced by frequent expressions of gratitude and praise from a client for whom such behavior is a CRB1. If the therapist is unaware of this process, he/she may respond in a manner that reinforces and helps maintain the client's problem. Thus it is exceedingly important that therapists recognize areas where they may be vulnerable to reinforcers that are not helpful to the client.

Importance of therapist self-awareness. FAP encourages therapists to take risks; such risks must be taken in a context of clarity and self-awareness. Effective FAP therapists must have a high level of self-awareness, openness to examining their own motives and reinforcers, and an ability to recognize and respond to their own T1s non-defensively. Although this kind of self-awareness is important for all therapists, we believe it is particularly important in FAP because the therapist is being encouraged to take risks and evoke CRBs. For example, a therapist who is lonely or lacking intimacy in personal relationships may overly rely on therapeutic relationships for a primary source of closeness, and be attracted to FAP as a means of increasing or justifying that intimacy. Such a therapist may place subtle or not so subtle demands on the client for greater closeness, under the guise of following FAP rules. It is crucial that FAP therapists examine their own responses and TIs in an on-going way. Consultation and supervision are often a crucial part of such exploration.

Importance of having the client target behavior in one's own repertoire. Traditional psychodynamic theories have emphasized the importance of the development of autonomy as a sign of psychological health, and the importance of minimizing dependence in the therapeutic relationship. Ethical guidelines have similarly focused on establishment and maintenance of boundaries. Humanists, feminist therapists and others have emphasized the relational nature of human development, the importance of psychotherapists being able to engage in genuine, deeply caring relationships with their clients, and not assuming that highly relational people are necessarily overly dependent. FAP therapists must be able to balance flexibly these perspectives, depending on the issues and needs of the client.

Many clients have difficulty accepting care and help, and have trouble being vulnerable, open, close or intimate with others. With such clients, the FAP therapist needs to create a context in which there are opportunities to engage with the therapist in new, more connected ways. A therapist who is uncomfortable with closeness, and is not addressing that limitation, is not likely to engage in behaviors that evoke connection or intimacy with his or her client at a level that feels risky or threatening. The client may not be given the opportunity to work on essential issues around closeness in relationships, or be reinforced for CRB2s in this area. Similarly, a therapist who is uncomfortable with intimacy, closeness or vulnerability may be inclined to interpret a client's request for more connection, personal questions about the therapist or expressions of reliance on the therapist as CRB1s in a broader class of dependence or neediness in relationships. For some clients, this may be the case, but it is clearly problematic if the therapist's own TIs are leading him/her to mistakenly assume the client's behavior reflects a CRB1 if it does not.

Alternatively, clients who have difficulty tolerating separation, solitude or acting independently may need the therapist to help evoke and reinforce those behaviors. Again, a therapist who has difficulty with distance, autonomy or separation in relationships may inadvertently reinforce the client's CRB1s. He/she may not recognize these behaviors as CRB1s or create opportunities for CRB2s to occur.

These relationship capabilities involving both closeness and independence are examples of a wide range of behaviors that the FAP therapist ideally would strengthen in order to help clients develop similar behaviors. Just as a therapist who is phobic of heights is hindered in conducting an in-vivo treatment for height-phobic clients, FAP therapists are more likely to be effective if they can engage in the behaviors they are helping their clients develop. FAP therapists must carefully evaluate the types of client problems they can effectively help by taking into consideration their own histories, behavioral repertoires and current life limitations. They are strongly encouraged to address areas of limitation in their own psychotherapy and/or in supervision and consultation.

Conclusion

In concluding, we would like to underscore that, in the service of client growth, we not only shape our clients' behavior, but allow ourselves in turn to be shaped by our clients. As Martin Buber (n.d.) stated, "All journeys have secret destinations of which the traveler is unaware." Allow yourself to experience each therapeutic relationship as such a journey.

We would also like to emphasize that the behaviorally defined rules described in this chapter are not rigid and formulaic as typically implied in common usage of the term 'rule.' No procedures from other therapies are ruled out, but rather at any moment the FAP rule-governed approach can lead to the awareness and utilization of a therapeutic opportunity. We fully endorse Greben's (1981) viewpoint, expressed below.

> Psychotherapy is not a set of elaborate rules about what one may not do: rules about when to speak or not to speak, how to handle vacations, how to deal with missed hours, and so on. It is something much more simple than that. It is the meeting and working together of two people; it is hard honest work. You might say, it is a labor of love. (p. 455)

References

Addis, M. E., & Carpenter, K. M. (2000). The treatment rationale in cognitive behavioral therapy: Psychological mechanisms and clinical guidelines. *Cognitive and Behavioral Practice, 7* (2), 147–156.

American Psychological Association. (2002). Ethical principles of psychologists and code of conduct. *American Psychologist, 57*, 1060–1073.

Barnes-Holmes, D., Barnes-Holmes, Y., & Cullinan, V. (2000). Relational Frame Theory and Skinner's Verbal Behavior: A possible synthesis. *The Behavior Analyst, 23*, 69–84.

Buber, M. (n.d.). *Martin Buber quotes.* Retrieved February 14, 2008, from thinkexist.com/quotes/martin_buber/

Callaghan, G. M. (2006). The Functional Idiographic Assessment Template (FIAT) System: For use with interpersonally-based interventions including Functional Analytic Psychotherapy (FAP) and FAP-enhanced treatments. *The Behavior Analyst Today, 7*, 357–398.

Goldberg, N. (1986). *Writing down the bones: Freeing the writer within.* Boston, MA: Shambhala Publications.

Goldfried, M. R., Burckell, L. A., & Eubanks-Carter, C. (2003). Therapist self disclosure in Cognitive-Behavior Therapy. *Journal of Clinical Psychology, 59* (5), 555-568.

Greben, S. E. (1981). The essence of psychotherapy. *British Journal of Psychiatry, 138*, 449–455.

Greenberg, L. (2002). *Emotion-focused therapy: Coaching clients to work through their feelings.* Washington, DC: American Psychological Association.

Hayes, S. C., Barnes-Holmes, D., & Roche, B. (Eds.). (2001). *Relational frame theory: A post-Skinnerian account of human language and cognition.* New York: Kluwer Academic/Plenum Publishers.

Kanter, J. W., Tsai, M., & Kohlenberg, R. J. (Eds.). (in press). *The practice of FAP.* New York: Springer.

Kohlenberg, R. J., & Tsai, M. (1991). *Functional analytic psychotherapy: Creating intense and curative therapeutic relationships.* New York: Plenum Press.

Kohlenberg, R. J., & Tsai, M. (1994). Functional analytic psychotherapy: A radical behavioral approach to treatment and integration. *Journal of Psychotherapy Integration, 4*(3), 175–201.

Mahalik, J. R., Van Ormer, E. A., & Simi, N. L. (2000). Ethical issues in using self-disclosure in feminist therapy. In M. Brabeck (Ed.), *Practicing Feminist Ethics in Psychology* (pp. 189–201). Washington, DC: American Psychological Association.

Peck, M. S. (1978). *The road less traveled.* New York: Simon & Schuster.

Perls, F. (1973). *The gestalt approach and eye witness to therapy.* Palo Alto, CA: Science and Behavior Books Inc.

Robitschek, C. G., & McCarthy, P. R. (1991). Prevalence of counselor self-reference in the therapeutic dyad. *Journal of Counseling & Development, 69*(3), 218–221.

Skinner, B. F. (1957). *Verbal behavior.* New York: Appleton-Centery-Crofts.

Truax, C. B. (1966). Reinforcement and nonreinforcement in Rogerian Psychotherapy. *Journal of Abnormal Psychology, 21*(1), 1–9.

Zettle, R. D., & Hayes, S. C. (1982). Rule governed behavior: A potential theoretical framework for cognitive-behavioral therapy. In P. C. Kendall (Ed.), *Advances in cognitive behavioral research and therapy* (Vol. 1, pp. 73–118). New York: Academic Press.

Chapter 5
Self and Mindfulness[1,2]

Robert J. Kohlenberg, Mavis Tsai, Jonathan W. Kanter, and Chauncey R. Parker

I think therefore I am.

Rene Descartes

Descartes' statement has given birth to countless philosophical theses, books and scholarly papers. In the present context our interest is in the psychological level of analysis, more specifically, functional analysis. From this functional perspective several speculations can be made about Descartes based on his statement. First, it seems he knew who he was and that his experience of 'I' the thinker, was stable. Thus we would not expect Descartes to request therapy to discover 'who he is' or complain that he feels like a chameleon who changes his persona depending on the circumstances in which he finds himself. Descartes' statement also implies that he was self-observant or aware of the private experience of thinking as an activity or process independent of the content of his thoughts. It suggests that he could step back and objectively observe the raw data of his experience. The act of being non-judgmentally aware of the process of thinking enters into the definition of *mindfulness*, an increasingly popular strategy in treatments for psychological problems (e.g., Linehan, 1993; Hayes, Follette, & Linehan, 2004), and one that plays an important role in many FAP cases.

The goals of this chapter are to provide a behavioral account of self and mindfulness, explain how a lack of sense of self may interfere with mindfulness, and provide suggestions to shape treatment interventions that target the self and mindfulness in FAP.

R.J. Kohlenberg (✉)
Department of Psychology, University of Washington, Seattle, WA 98195-1525, USA
e-mail: fap@u.washington.edu

[1] The authors are indebted to Madelon Y. Bolling, Ph.D. for her contributions—they greatly improved this chapter while we take full responsibility for its shortcomings.
[2] Portions of this chapter are based on Parker, Bolling and Kohlenberg (1998).

M. Tsai et al., *A Guide to Functional Analytic Psychotherapy*,
DOI 10.1007/978-0-387-09787-9_5, © Springer Science+Business Media, LLC 2009

A Behavioral View of Self

Let us begin with a simple two-step exercise. Do step 1 right now—look at your hand for approximately five seconds. Now do step 2—look at your hand again for a few seconds, but while doing so, try to become aware that *you* are looking at it. If this exercise worked effectively, the steps should have involved two forms of awareness. During step 1 you were simply looking at your hand—noticing the hand itself. You may have noticed certain features and wondered what we wanted you to see. Such awareness involves simple discriminations that all creatures make, verbal or otherwise. It is pure awareness, automatic and unconscious. The second step, however, incorporated an additional type of awareness. Not only were you seeing your hand, but you were *seeing that* you were seeing your hand. That is, you were aware of a 'you' a 'something' or 'someone' that was looking, noticing or wondering. You might have even tried to metaphorically step back in order to observe you looking at your hand. The experience of a 'you' that is observing is what the general public and most social scientists refer to as 'the self.' Deikman (1999) defines this self as an 'I' with an abiding, resting awareness, featureless and unchanging, a central something that is witness to all events, both exterior and interior.

The Experience of Self

In this chapter the terms 'consciousness,' 'self-awareness' and 'self observation' are used interchangeably to refer to the second type of awareness described in the exercise above. Skinner posited that, "...a person becomes conscious in a different sense when a verbal community arranges contingencies under which he not only sees an object but 'sees' that he is seeing it. In this special sense, consciousness is a social product" (Skinner, 1974, p. 220). Skinner thus emphasized the way in which a particular social history is required for one to learn to see *that* one sees. To the extent that this history is normative in our culture, commonalities can be expected in descriptions of a 'normal' or 'ideal' self. Not everyone, however, develops the purported ideal self. That is, despite some similarities, a sense of self is learned and thus is dependent on the vagaries of this learning history; consequently the experience of self should vary a great deal. We conceptualize a continuum of experience; on one end an ideal experience of continuity and selfsameness, a 'central something' corresponding to the descriptions and experiences of Descartes and Deikman; on the other an empty or unstable sense of self, corresponding to the experiences of clients who state, "I don't know who I am," or who report multiple selves.

Our behavioral view is that the experience of self consists of a 'central something' that is experienced, and the process of being aware of or perceiving that 'central something.' The functional analysis of the experience of self thus focuses on the discriminative stimulus (Sd) that one becomes aware of and identifies as this 'central something.' This focus on self as an object is congruent with its use by clients and conventional self psychologists. Our task is thus to identify the experienced thing that is self. This analysis is guided by Skinner's discussion of the self (1953, 1957) and functional analysis of the verbal behavior of labeling stimuli (e.g., ball, car) known as tacting (Skinner, 1957; Barnes-Holmes, Barnes-Holmes, & Cullinan, 2000). This approach is complementary with the contemporary behavior-analytic innovator Steve Hayes and his colleagues' analysis (Hayes & Gregg, 2000; Hayes & Wilson, 1993). Although we focus on the self as an experienced or perceived object, we do not give it agency properties (e.g., the psychoanalytic concepts of id, ego and superego) and then use it to explain self problems. Rather, we attempt to understand the self functionally, by elaborating the nature of the interpersonal environments that influence how the self develops and the conditions under which 'normal' and problematic experiences of self occur.

In non-technical language, suppose we are trying to understand a person's *experience* of being hot. We could put a man in a temperature-controlled room, vary the temperature, record body temperature, and find out what temperature is required for this person to report that he is hot. This report would be a tact, a response controlled by the specific discriminative stimulus of the experience of heat. Our understanding would be even greater, however, if we knew more about this person's previous experience (history) with hot and cold surroundings. If he grew up in the desert, a considerable increase in room temperature might be required for him to say he is hot, more than would be needed for someone born and raised in Alaska. The more known about the historical and contextual variables that result in the individual reporting that he is hot, the more we can say we 'understand' his experience. This approach to understanding a person's experience is connected intimately to understanding the stimulus (the thing) that led to the verbal report, and the assumption is that the same factors that affect one's inner private experience also affect the verbal report of that experience.

Our approach to understanding the experience of self parallels that of heat described above. Just as we would explain the experience of heat by identifying the stimulus and history for the response "hot," we explain the experience of self by describing the stimuli and history that account for the words used to identify the self. These words include 'I,' 'me,' 'baby,' or the child's proper names such as 'Davie' or 'Dottie' (when used to refer to one's self), and 'you' (as commonly misused by very young children to refer to themselves). We would contend that such terms are all members of the same equivalence class. For illustrative purposes the following discussion will use the generic 'I' to represent this class. Thus the analysis of 'I' can be viewed as a prototype for the analysis of other verbal responses associated with the self. Indeed, an understanding of 'I' in particular does appear to account for a wide range of experiences of self. Specification of the stimuli for 'I' thus illuminates the 'phenomenon' or the illusory 'central something' that is experienced as the self.

Development of the Sense of Self

When learning to talk, children actually are learning to tact, or to say the sounds or words evoked by specific discriminative stimuli (Sds). The process begins with the learning of the meaning of individual utterances (in FAP, 'functional units'). As an example, consider how a child learns the tact 'apple.' A parent may show his or her child an apple and then encourage the utterance 'apple.' It is obvious to the parent (as an observer) what object the child should be attending to that is referenced by the term 'apple.' To the pre-verbal child, however, it is at first a confusing situation. Consider the myriad of potential discriminative stimuli that are present that could mistakenly be linked to the word 'apple.' For the infant, the situation is a stimulus soup consisting of irrelevant publicly observable stimuli that happen to be present in concert with the prompt to say 'apple.' To confuse the issue, there is also a myriad of private stimuli (e.g., bodily sensations associated with neural and hormonal activity) that are available only to the child. Nevertheless, remarkably, the child learns to identify the publicly observable apple from the stimulus soup as the Sd that evokes 'apple.' Of course for this to occur the parents (the 'verbal community') need to be consistent and use contingent reinforcement to ensure that 'apple' is only applied when an apple is present, and is not an appropriate response to other stimuli (e.g., mommy, daddy, particular bodily responses, or any of the other objects in the environment). The child learns to say 'apple' because it was the one stimulus that was consistently present on each occasion saying 'apple' was reinforced. Verbal behavior researchers suggest that what is learned at this stage is the behavior of bidirectional verbal relating (e.g., the word 'apple' shares equivalence with the object apple, and vice versa) (Lipkens, Hayes, & Hayes, 1993).

Linguists and developmental psychologists call the period of life from about six months to two years the 'single-word speech period.' (Cooley, 1908; Dore, 1985; Fraiberg, 1977; Peters, 1983). At this early stage, even multiple word phrases such as 'Mommy come' and 'juice all gone' serve as single functional units and are not understood as individual words. To illustrate, consider the case of a parent trying to teach the phrase 'I see apple,' once the child has learned to tact 'apple.' The parent intends for the child to report his or her private experience of 'seeing an apple.' If the parent is successful, 'I see apple' can be used to report both physical and imagined apples, such that the child can describe and be aware of his or her private activity of seeing the apple even if there is no public apple stimulus present. In order to have the child's 'I see apple' reflect this subtlety, the parent has the difficult task of teaching the child to come under the control of the private activity of seeing an apple when saying, 'I see apple.' This task is difficult because the parent cannot tell with certainty if the child is really having the intended private seeing experience. Instead the parent relies on public stimuli for this purpose, including the overt orienting of the child toward the apple by head-turning, pointing, widening of the eyes and intense staring in the direction of the apple. The public stimuli would vary slightly depending on the location of the apple, child, ambient lighting and so on. If the parent is successful, however, the private stimulus associated with the private seeing will gain control over 'I am seeing apple,' as it is the one stimulus consistently present each time saying 'I see apple' was reinforced.

Although we have taken poetic liberty in the above description by implying that the parent is purposely attempting to teach the child the difference between the public stimulus 'apple' and the private stimulus of seeing an apple, it is likely there is no such pre-conceptualization involved when parents interact with their children. The fact, however, that most of us can report when we are seeing an imaginary apple or having a private visual experience is evidence of this prior learning. Although others may well disagree with our view on this matter, we do not believe we are born with the ability to see or report private images; instead we would argue that we have our parents or caretakers to thank for teaching us how to do this. This same complexity is present whenever we or our children are taught to tact or to identify any private event such as feelings of hunger, sadness, happiness or anger.

Kohlenberg and Tsai (1991) provide a detailed behavioral account of the three stages of language development leading to the tact 'I' emerging as a separate functional unit (pp. 125–168). The three stages are shown in Fig. 5.1.

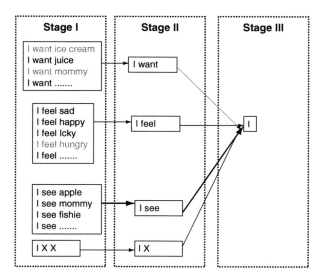

Fig. 5.1 The three stages of verbal behavior development that result in "I" emerging as a small functional unit show how variations in learning experience might ultimately influence one's experience of self (the "I"). For example, the bold letters and lines stand for "I x"s that are privately controlled, and then combine with publicly controlled responses (shaded letters and lines), leading to a somewhat weakened sense of self

As illustrated in Fig. 5.1, during Stage I the child learns larger independent units that are the basis of the more abstract intermediate-size units of Stage II. Then the 'I' of Stage III emerges from the medium-size units of Stage II. As an example that illustrates the variability in emergence of 'I,' the terms in bold represent the strength or degree of private control that may be in place for a given individual. Thus the phrase 'I want juice' occurs when the child truly 'wants juice' and is experiencing the private aspects of 'wanting juice.' In contrast, the phrase 'I want ice cream' is prompted by the mother (who actually wants ice cream at the time). The net result is that in Stage II, the 'I want' is only partially under the control of private stimulation and partially under the control of the child's perception of what the mother wants.

The experience of 'I' that emerges in Stage III can be thought of as the experience of a 'perspective' or 'locus' as defined by Hayes (1984). This perspective is the one stimulus that remains constant across all 'I want x' and 'I see x' statements, as the activity (wanting or seeing) and the object (the 'x' that is wanted or seen) varies. Hayes, Barnes-Holmes, and Roche (2001) argue that additional verbal behavior is necessary for the complete experience of self as a perspective to develop. In particular, the growing child learns to distinguish 'I' from 'you,' 'here' from 'there,' and 'now' from 'then.' The self as perspective emerges from this more complex relational verbal behavior. For example, sometimes the child may be five feet from the parent and at other times 50 feet, but the child is always 'here' and never 'there.' The private stimulus that is always 'I, here, now,' and which includes some sensations within the body, seems likely to gain control. Thus, the response 'I' as a unit over time comes under the stimulus control of the perspective (the locus) from which other behavior emanates.

It is crucial to recognize that this locus from which behavior emanates is not the body, although it observes things that happen inside the body. 'I hurt my finger,' 'I have a tummy ache,' and the like teach us this discrimination, as the 'I' observes the body but can not be the body. Because the perspective from which these observations occur appears to be located behind the eyes, however, the 'I' is experienced as within the body. Activities under private control—activities attributed to the 'I'—are experienced as coming from within. The experience of self as continuous over time (e.g., you at your 10th birthday party is the same you as now, even though your body is completely different) adds to a learning history that distinguishes the sense of self as something other than the body, but that emanates from within the body (Hayes, Strosahl, & Wilson, 1999). Ideally, the self comes to be experienced as relatively unchanging, centrally located, and continuous, and a sense of interiority develops.

Our theory that the self develops as a result of language acquisition (and the meaning of 'I' emerges from the meaning of larger phrases in which 'I' is embedded) is not new. In 1908, Cooley collected data on the acquisition of 'I' as a child was learning to talk. Although not stated in behavioral terms, his theory is remarkably similar to ours. Cooley concluded that at age 26 months, 'I' phrases such as 'I don't know,' 'I want. . .' and 'Come see me' seem to have been learned as 'wholes' (p. 355)—in our terminology, large functional units. Cooley states, "From these she probably gets the 'I' idea by elimination, (that is) the rest of the sentence varies but the pronoun remains constantly associated with the expression of the will, the self attitude" (p. 355). In our terminology, 'I' emerges as a small functional unit.

Although ideal development leads to a large degree of control of the 'I' response by private (within the skin) stimuli, more problematic development involves the opposite—the development of a small degree of control of 'I' by private stimuli. In such situations a number of 'I x' Stage II responses have come under public control (as illustrated in Fig. 5.1). This usually will have come about through some parents or other early caretakers inadvertently teaching children to receive their cues for 'I' statements from public stimuli (people or situations outside themselves), rather than from the private events and responses that only the child can access.

Take as an example a young girl, Tammy, in a grocery store with her mother. Tammy says, "I wanna candy bar." Her mother, in a hurry to finish shopping, says, "No you don't." This statement prevents Tammy's private experience of 'wanting' from gaining control over her 'I want' response. If this occurs regularly in a wide variety of circumstances, 'I want' will increasingly come to be under public control. For example, Tammy's 'I want' behavior may eventually be influenced heavily by the presence of any important person who looks anxious or hurried. Public discriminative stimuli will come to control whether she really wants something or not, and the experience of wanting, which ideally would come to control Tammy's report of wanting, will go wanting (if we may), and finally have no control over Tammy's behavior. This process operates outside of Tammy's awareness.

If similar invalidations of Tammy's other 'I x' statements occur, her problems with her experience of self may become more severe. For example, imagine the statement "I feel sick today," receiving the response, "Nonsense, you're perfectly fine." Or the statement, "I am hungry," is returned by, "No you aren't, it's not lunch time yet!" Such exchanges may pervade the history of people who eventually say their actions do not come from within, or that they are not doing what they appear to be doing. This may still sound a little far-fetched, but how many times have you heard interactions such as "Do you want to go out tonight?" "I don't know, do you?" Or "Do you want dessert?" "Well, I'm not sure, do you?"

Although the above statements are relatively non-pathological, they illustrate self-referent behaviors that are being spoken of (tacted) as being under public control. There is a continuum of severity of problems with self, depending on the degree of private control of the functional unit 'I.' Keep in mind that this situation does not involve someone suppressing a verbal report of feelings or needs. Rather, this section involves pinpointing the developmental antecedents of being aware of one's feelings (private stimuli) and needs (reinforcers), and how one comes to notice them in the first place. In addition, note that this discussion does not simply refer to unassertive individuals—such people may know what they would prefer but are reluctant to speak their wishes. In contrast, people whose 'I's are under public control actually do not know what they want, what they can do, what they feel etc., unless they discover what significant others want or will allow. Under ideal conditions, the 'I' emanates from within, and thus in cases such as those described above, a strong sense of emptiness, a void where the self should be, may well be reported if most of what a person refers to as 'I' is actually under the control and subject to the modifications of others.

Kanter, Parker, and Kohlenberg (2001) report on the development of a measure of public versus private control over the experience of self (the Experience of Self Scale, or EOSS). The EOSS was administered to a sample of undergraduate students and participants diagnosed with borderline personality disorder (BPD). BPD participants reported significantly more public control over the experience of self, and EOSS scores also correlated strongly with measures of self-esteem and dissociation, such that more public control predicted lower self-esteem and more dissociation. These findings provide preliminary empirical support for the above theory.

A vast body of literature also supports the basic premises of the behavioral theory of the self, dating back to Asch's (1951) classic studies investigating social influences on basic perceptual processes. These early studies demonstrated that the public can exert strong influences on how individuals report perceptual experiences. In addition, early research on locus of control (Rotter, 1966) identified that individuals differ to the degree they experience their behavior to be controlled internally (by themselves) or externally (by others). These social psychological theories, however, do not offer an account of how these individual differences develop. For instance, why do some people respond to public influence in the Asch experiments while others do not? What developmental issues account for these differences between people? Our current theory provides an account of how this pattern of behavior might develop. Real life processes, of course, are much more complex and not as linear as suggested by the framework provided above. We acknowledge the above theory is a mere sketch of a rich continuum of phenomena (for a more detailed description of this process, refer to Kohlenberg and Tsai, 1991, 1995).

The sense of self, in summary, develops in partnership with language. Under ideal conditions, the sense of self is an internal, stable perspective under the control of private stimuli. If one's tendency to behave a certain way is consistently checked by a punishing or invalidating environment, however, one may perceive that one's own behavior does not come from within. Indeed, in a sense it does not if it is always (or nearly always) determined by what is going on outside—if the tendency to behave is under public control. This history of invalidation leading to public control of the sense of self is a major factor in the development of disorders of the self in our culture.

Mindfulness

As an introduction to what is meant by mindfulness in a therapeutic setting, consider the clinical example in the following quote from Germer (2005) in Germer, Siegel and Fulton's (2005) book *Mindfulness in Psychotherapy* (p. 3–4).

> People are clear about one thing when they enter therapy: they want to feel better, they often have a number of ideas about how to accomplish this goal, although therapy does not necessarily proceed as expected. For example, a young woman with panic disorder, let's call her Lynn, might call a therapist hoping to escape the emotional turmoil of her condition. Lynn may be seeking freedom from her anxiety, but as therapy progresses, Lynn actually discovers freedom in her anxiety. How does this occur? A strong therapeutic alliance may provide Lynn with the courage and safety to begin to explore her panic more closely. Through self-monitoring, Lynn becomes aware of the sensations of anxiety in her body and the thoughts associated with them. She learns how to cope with panic by talking herself through it. When Lynn feels ready, she directly experiences the sensations of anxiety that trigger a panic attack and tests herself in a mall or on an airplane. This whole process requires that Lynn first turn toward the anxiety. A compassionate bait and switch has occurred.

What may be surprising to some readers is that Germer does not mention therapeutic interventions such as sitting still and focusing on a thought, mantra or breath. Such techniques often are referred to as meditation and are considered prototypical mindfulness interventions. In fact, it appears that Lynn received something along the lines of a traditional CBT (Cognitive Behavioral Therapy) treatment for panic. Here we extract several generalizations from Lynn's case that are relevant to the discussion of mindfulness: (1) patients may enter therapy wanting to 'get rid of' negative feelings and thoughts; (2) nevertheless, the treatment process involves facilitating the patient coming into contact and being present with avoided negative thoughts and feelings; (3) the therapeutic relationship provides a safe environment and fosters the courage needed for the client to come into contact with situations that evoke these avoided thoughts and feelings; and (4) 'remaining present' in evocative situations may occur under the guise of doing the opposite—the therapy is presented to the client as a means of getting rid of negative thoughts and feelings. Therapists themselves may or may not be aware of this contradiction, and hence unknowingly participate in the so-called 'bait and switch.' We contend that a variety of techniques lead to greater mindfulness, remaining present and improved outcomes. Consistent with this sentiment, we suggest that mindfulness-promoting interventions often occur naturally during all types of psychotherapy, whether intended or not.

A Behavioral View of Mindfulness

Our behavioral view of mindfulness is intended to help therapists decide how and when these interventions might help. Techniques to increase client mindfulness are suggested, many of which are easily integrated into current CBT as well as other treatment modalities. A case example below illustrates how to tweak CBT interventions to enhance the naturally occurring mindfulness that occurs in most therapies. Although we avoid defining mindfulness as a specific intervention, a particular meditation procedure based on Herbert Benson's relaxation response (Benson, 1975) is presented, and we discuss how it can be used in a manner consistent with FAP.

Not surprisingly, mindfulness is considered a behavior in the context of FAP. That is, being mindful is considered a type of self-awareness that also plays a role in the development of self. Consistent with the functional analytic approach, we eschew topographical descriptions of mindfulness and instead examine its effects or consequences. The focus is on those effects that have therapeutic implications. We fully recognize that defining mindfulness in terms of therapeutic effects excludes many commonly accepted notions and topographic descriptions, particularly in contexts such as spiritual practice or self-development. To avoid confusion, we will refer to the phenomena of interest as 'therapeutic mindfulness.' Keeping this limitation in view, we begin by considering how others define mindfulness and then attempt to extract the implied functions or effects of its practice.

Alan Marlatt, among the first cognitive behaviorists to recognize the therapeutic potential of mindfulness (Marlatt & Marques, 1977), has researched and written about its clinical application. Recently, Witkiewitz and Marlatt (2005) defined mindfulness as a metacognitive state of nonjudgmental awareness, with a focus on moment-to-moment direct experience of ongoing thoughts, feelings and physical sensations. In this conceptualization, attention is focused on the breath as a touchstone of awareness, and if one becomes distracted, one returns attention to the breath as soon as one realizes that awareness has shifted to other cognitive events.

Janet Surrey's (2005) description of mindfulness emphasizes the interpersonal aspects of mindfulness while doing relational psychotherapy.

> Connection, whether to her own experience or to others, is never static. It is a process of successive moments of turning toward, turning away, and returning. Mindfulness cultivates awareness of this movement, informed by the intention to return to connection again and again. In mindfulness, the object of our investigation is our connection to whatever arises in awareness. (p. 94)

She then describes the process from the therapist's perspective and notes its therapeutic effects.

> ...the therapist remains attentive to moment to moment changes in his or her own sensations, feelings, thoughts, and memories... Through the relationship, the therapist offers the patient the possibility of staying emotionally present with the therapist, perhaps staying with difficult feelings for 'one more moment,' thus enhancing the patient's capacity for mindful awareness of self-in-connection. The therapist's empathic attunement helps to draw out the truth of the present moment without flooding or shaming the patient—with acceptance. (p. 94–95)

Both Marlatt and Surrey describe mindfulness as a type of awareness or consciousness that has two characteristics: (1) it is non-judgmental; and (2) it has a focus on the here and now. These elements are found in nearly all definitions of mindfulness (Germer, 2005). First, we discuss the non-judgmental element of mindfulness.

Non-judgmentalness. In keeping with the clinical relevance of this analysis, the 'judging' of interest is defined as an evaluative tact that is under the control of an aversive stimulus. For example, the tact 'bad' indicates that an aversive S^d (such as being criticized) was contacted. This aversive Sd could be a thought, feeling, an action by others, or other real world occurrences. The associated response repertoire evoked by aversive Sds includes avoidance, escape, attack and related actions to control or eliminate the aversive Sd. Such tacts and responses often are functional; think of avoiding the aversive Sd of a car racing down the street towards the spot where you are standing. Here we restrict our analysis, however, to those instances when negatively charged judgments and associated response repertoires are problematic for the client. The implication is that being mindfully and therapeutically non-judgmental involves an absence of avoidance or other attempts to control the aversive Sd, also known as acceptance.

This view is consistent with Hayes et al. (1999) discussion of acceptance in Acceptance and Commitment Therapy (ACT), although these authors emphasize experiential avoidance (avoidance of aversive Sds that are thoughts, feelings and other private experiences). From their perspective, acceptance involves making contact with the automatic or direct stimulus functions of experiences without acting to reduce or manipulate those functions and without acting on the basis of their derived or verbal functions (Hayes, 1994). Hayes and colleagues' behavioral analysis of language (Hayes et al. 2001) provides an elegant, empirically supported and comprehensive account for how a verbal tact (e.g., 'bad') can become functionally aversive in and of itself—through stimulus equivalence and related processes—and evoke avoidance. Their analysis also provides a model describing how such tacts can serve other stimulus functions that contribute to clinical problems. FAP therapists are encouraged to learn ACT theory and interventions.

Focus on the here and now. A focus on the here and now is the second element in mindfulness definitions. Some data suggest that a here and now focus (also referred to as 'being present in the moment') has similar functions to those of acceptance (Brown & Ryan, 2003). The widely read author, Tolle (2004), expressed this sentiment by pointing out that giving "fullest attention to whatever the moment presents... implies that you also completely accept what is, because you cannot give your full attention to something and at the same time resist it" (p. 56). Thus, although being non-judgmental and focusing on the here and now may imply different topographies in the various definitions of mindfulness, their primary therapeutic function is defined here as reducing problematic avoidance repertoires.

Therapeutic Mindfulness

We define therapeutic mindfulness functionally as a type of self-awareness that
helps the client to remain in the presence of aversive Sds (such as negative
thoughts, feelings and events) that typically evoke avoidance repertoires. In
turn, this provides an opportunity for new, more adaptive behavior to emerge
and be reinforced. Using a functional definition can help reduce the considerable confusion in the mindfulness literature resulting from the failure to distinguish specific techniques from a psychological process (Hayes and Wilson
(2003).

One possible approach intended to help the client remain present can be
ruled out summarily, namely interventions aimed at blocking escape or otherwise forcibly blocking the avoidance. Over and above ethical and therapeutic
alliance issues, such interventions would be nearly impossible to implement as
avoidance still can occur in the private realm and is not subject to external
control. Instead, we focus here on techniques to change the stimulus functions
of those aversive Sds that typically evoke avoidance. For example, consider a
client, Millie, who fears contamination and avoids touching doorknobs. The
doorknob serves as an aversive Sd that evokes negative evaluative tacts and
avoidance repertoires, thus depriving her of the opportunity for extinction of
anxiety and the emergence of new productive behavior. Assume that Millie is
asked to give up 'trying to get rid of thoughts' and instead is encouraged to
observe (e.g., 'step back and see') her own thinking as a process rather than as
content.

The observation of thinking as process is a function of the emergence of 'I
think' as a functional unit (Stage II), the client tacting the private activity of
thinking as an independent unit regardless of thought content. The same applies
to other 'I x' Stage II behavior, such as 'I feel' and 'I sense.' Thus Millie might be
asked to notice (be aware of) other events when in the presence of the doorknob.
She might momentarily shift her attention and become aware of the flow of her
breath, the ticking of a clock, the taste of garlic on her tongue, and other bodily
sensations. Being mindful transforms the original doorknob aversive Sd (in
Relational Frame Theory (RFT) terms, there has been a transfer of discriminative functions (Hayes et al., 2001)), reducing its aversive properties and
evoked avoidance and thus providing an opportunity for productive behavior.

Clinical Implications for Problems of the Self

In broad terms, clients with extensive problems of the self begin treatment
displaying in-session behaviors such as being wary, overly attentive and concerned about the therapist's opinion of them. They do not confidently describe
feelings, beliefs, wants, likes and dislikes. All these behaviors are likely to be
CRB1s, and indicate a lack of control over the experience of self by private

stimuli. If treatment is successful, clients' within-session behaviors should become more confident and trusting, and include the CRB2s of freely describing thoughts, feelings, wants and beliefs.

The description of client behaviors in the foregoing paragraph could pass for the generic psychotherapeutic endeavor. A primary source of such clients' difficulties is a lack of private control, and thus treatment by a therapist who is accepting, responsive, and who encourages expression of feelings naturally can provide the contingencies to strengthen private control. Such a generic therapeutic environment is the antidote to the invalidating early environment that failed to reinforce control by private stimuli. In addition, the FAP behavioral model leads to some specific suggestions for treatment.

Reinforce Talking in the Absence of Specific External Cues

For clients with self problems, much behavior is under the tight stimulus control of others. They appear vigilant and are focused intently on the therapist, watching for nuances in facial expression and voice inflection. Although often not obvious at first, almost everything these clients say about themselves and what they think and feel may be heavily influenced by the therapist as Sd. The therapy procedure described below is aimed at loosening this control by encouraging and reinforcing talking in the absence of specific external cues. In other words, treatment consists of strengthening the CRB2s of privately controlled 'I x' statements, which will also aid in the eventual emergence of private control over 'I.'

One means of helping clients establish private control is for the therapist to sit mindfully in silence—simply be present, listening without judgment— rather than structuring each moment of the session with questions. A variant of the psychoanalytic free-association task may be given to the client to enhance the chance of evoking CRB2s in the form of 'I x' responses under private control. It is problematic to use this strategy during the early stages of treatment, as it can evoke a strong CRB1 of avoidance in the client. Numerous clients have complained about previous treatment failures because of their former therapists' passivity.

Additionally, rigidly adhering to a rule of therapist silence is likely to preclude reinforcement of CRB2s should they occur. For example, a client might say, "I can't stand this." This is an 'I x' response that the therapist should take seriously, thus reinforcing private control of an 'I x' statement. FAP therapists often use strategies from other therapies, provided they address the functions of problematic behavior in the client's life. It is essential, however, that the therapist be clear that the topography of the strategy (e.g., therapist silence) is less important than its function, in this case that of evoking private 'I x' statements.

In the early stages of treatment therapists will benefit from a mindful, present-moment focus so that they can respond flexibly and appropriately when clients emit CRB2s. Later in therapy, after clients have made progress in gaining a privately controlled repertoire of 'I x' responses, more passivity on the therapist's part can be useful. The following case involving a client named Terry is illustrative.

During the initial months of therapy with RJK, Terry focused primarily on his medical treatment and the medications he was using to control a psychosomatic symptom. When RJK posed more general questions about mood or an emotional state, Terry became stymied and anxious. Early in treatment RJK would suggest an answer based on specific public stimuli. For example, when a severe medical symptom appeared that was similar to one that resulted in a relative's death, it was suggested that Terry was feeling fear (thus RJK provided the public stimulus by saying "fear"). This is similar to what parents do when they impart to their children the tacts for emotions. Gradually over the next few months, however, the specificity was reduced. Rather than continue to name a feeling, RJK would provide Terry with a list of emotions to choose from (e.g., pain, fear, anger, disappointment, irritation or frustration). In other words, RJK was still prompting a response based on public stimuli, but the specificity of the stimuli was broadened. Terry was assured that he would not be punished for answering as he was given an 'approved' answer in the first case, and a list of approved answers in the second. The general idea is that structure was gradually reduced to allow more private stimuli to gain control.

Match Therapeutic Tasks to the Level of Private Control in Client's Repertoire

Unstructured free association. Just as the general strategy of a therapist can vary from passive to highly structured, this free association task (adapted from traditional psychoanalysis) can be presented with more or less structure. In its most unstructured form, the free association instructions are as follows.

> Tell me everything that enters your mind—all thoughts, feelings, and images. It's important not to censor anything. Report whatever comes up, even if you think it's unimportant, nonsensical, trivial, embarrassing, or whatever.

The client is asked to continue without feedback and may even be asked to sit so the therapist is out of sight. Interestingly, this is similar to some mindfulness exercises, except that instead of allowing thoughts, feelings and images to arise and pass uncensored solely in the private realm, the client is asked to tact them aloud. Indeed this 'tell me everything' technique may be a prerequisite for later mindfulness practice for persons who lack private control over the experience of self.

This task requires talking to the therapist with a minimum of external cues, making it possible for clients to say 'I feel x' or 'I see this image' under conditions that favor control by private stimuli. Clients with extensive self problems likely will become anxious and be unable to perform this task because of the lack of public stimuli. They may experience a 'loss of self' in the absence of therapist cues. A similar phenomenon occurs when therapists use relaxation or meditation techniques and find that their clients become highly anxious when the task is too unstructured. FAP therapists using free association can vary the classic unstructured format depending on the client's level of private control.

Structured free association. More structured tasks that call for a gradually increasing degree of private control can be used, such as sentence completion and word association. Another more structured variant of free association is the 'movie theater in your mind' task, where clients are asked to close their eyes and imagine they are sitting in a movie theater. First they are instructed to see a blank screen in their mind's eye. When the movie begins, the first scene is stipulated to be of the client and the therapist sitting in the office at that moment. Next, the movie is described running backward, with the client walking backwards out of the office and back into his or her car. The movie is then said to run faster and faster, turning into a blur. The client is asked to view the blur, and then have it suddenly stop and to describe the scene at that point. It is still vital to reinforce any 'I x' responses that occur because they are likely to be under at least a modicum of private control. A wide variety of such imagery tasks used in gestalt therapy, psycho-synthesis and hypnotherapy can be adapted for FAP.

Another more structured adaptation of free association involves the use of a computer and word processor. The client is asked to type everything that crosses her or his mind and not to censor anything. An advantage of this method is that it lends itself to shaping the process. At first, the client is given the option of erasing any or all of the material before the therapist reviews it. In order to reinforce talking (typing) in the absence of public stimuli, the therapist uncritically reviews the word processing file during the session. Over time, the client is encouraged to erase as little as possible.

In summary, four adjustments can be made to imagery or free association tasks borrowed from other therapies. First, they should be presented to the client as a task whose value is derived from the process (e.g., imagining and describing in the presence of the therapist). Ideally, clients should be told in everyday terms that what is important about the task is that it is likely to evoke CRB2s under private control. Second, the task should be selected or modified to vary the degree of private control required to match the level of the client's repertoire. For example, the 'movie theater' task could begin with no image present on the screen or could be time-limited. Third, the client should be reinforced for making 'I x' statements. Fourth, the therapist should keep in mind that CRBs other than those related to self problems could be evoked and thus provide therapeutic opportunities. A case study illustrating the clinical application of imagery and free association tasks can be found in Kohlenberg and Tsai (1991, pp. 161–164).

Reinforce as Many Client 'I x' Statements as Possible

When clients have self problems, it is particularly important for therapists to treat with respect differing ideas and beliefs. In this context 'respect' is defined such that the client's behavior should be strengthened or reinforced by a therapist's reaction even though he or she may indicate different beliefs. Special significance is given to those client 'I x' statements that differ from the therapist's own feelings and impressions, because it is precisely these behaviors that are most likely to be under private control. Ideally the therapist should reinforce as many 'I x' statements as possible.

As noted previously, if a client's self problem is related to a lack of private control over 'I want,' it is critical to reinforce if at all possible such a response if it occurs. One important clue that a client's 'I want' is under private control (as opposed to public control) is the therapist's inclination to reject the request. For example, a client whose self problem was that she did not know what she wanted asked RJK to try hypnosis to find out what she wanted. RJK's first reaction was to turn her down and give the reasons why he did not use hypnosis. This inclination to reject her request signaled the possibility that her 'want' was under her private control and that her request was a CRB2. Realizing that this was something that she truly wanted, RJK agreed to hypnotize her.

A delicate juncture is broached when a client whose self problems include a paucity of 'I feel' responses says, "I feel you don't care about me." Such a comment is not unusual and should be treated as a CRB2 (assuming it is not a disguised request for reassurance). The most reinforcing response would be to validate the client's response by reviewing interactions in the therapy that may have led to his or her feeling that way. For example, the therapist may have been distracted or preoccupied during the session or even may have been irritated by the client. Needless to say, this validation of the client's tact does not preclude the importance of the therapist emphasizing his or her caring about the client in general. Even more difficult situations are encountered when a client makes 'I x' statements that are counterproductive, self-maligning, suicidal, or homicidal. The following suggestions for dealing with these types of statements are more relevant for clients with self problems who are just beginning to develop private control over 'I x' statements, rather than clients who chronically engage in destructive behaviors.

1. Counterproductive statements. Client behaviors that lead to avoidance often appear counter-productive to the therapist. For example, MT supervised a case in which the client said, with tears in her eyes, "I don't want to talk about my mother's death. It's just rehashing old stuff and it doesn't get me anywhere." Appropriate therapist responses would include emphasizing that she does not have to talk about the issue (non-judgmental acceptance on the therapist's part) and exploring the situation further (in the service of being present). Here are three variants of such responses.

- You look like you are about to cry, like you're really hurting inside... What are you feeling? Are you afraid that if you keep talking you'll start crying? How did your Mom and Dad deal with you when you cried as a child?
- What do you mean by 'rehashing old stuff'? What's happened before when you talked about your Mom's death?

- I'm feeling conflicted because I really want to respect your feelings about not talking about your Mom's death, and yet I don't want to collude in your avoiding grief feelings because I think that avoiding them is related to your avoiding close relationships in general. What do you think would be more growth-enhancing for you right now—to push yourself to talk and to feel your feelings about your Mom, or to respect your feelings of not wanting to talk about her even though you know that's what I want? How can we honor both your desire of not wanting to talk right now, which is important in developing your sense of self, and also your desire to make progress in therapy in general by feeling your feelings?

2. Self-maligning statements. "I am a whore and a slut. I feel like the scum of the earth. I'm scared I'm going to become schizophrenic because my Mom was." These were all statements made by a client to MT. MT's initial reaction was to reassure the client that these statements were not true, but she felt angry and invalidated by MT's response. She acknowledged that while reassurance was important, it cut her off from describing feelings with which she was getting in touch. Gradually the client trained MT to combine her reassurance with allowing her the opportunity to explore her feelings. For instance, "You're definitely not a slut, but tell me all your feelings and thoughts about being a slut before I tell you why I don't think you are... The research on schizophrenia indicates that if you haven't developed it by now, it's highly unlikely that you will. But it must be scary for you to have that fear. Tell me about it."

3. Suicidal or homicidal statements. Although suicidal and homicidal fantasies are too aversive for most therapists to listen to in any detail, it is not uncommon for clients with self problems to get in touch with these feelings because their histories are so replete with unmet needs. It is important to reinforce these expressions by helping the client tell his or her story until the therapist thoroughly understands why it makes sense for the client to feel this way. Furthermore, it is important that the therapist forbid these harmful actions not just by mandate, but by helping the client separate feelings from actions (i.e., the connection between thinking about suicide, feeling suicidal, and engaging in suicidal behavior is that of a behavior-behavior relationship and one need not lead to the other), and by exploring in depth the consequences of suicidal or homicidal actions. If these suicidal or homicidal statements are threats made because more attention is wanted from the therapist, then the client should be confronted and taught how to ask directly for what is wanted without threatening hurtful behavior.

Clinical Implications and Techniques for Promoting Mindfulness

Self-Observation or 'Being Aware That You Are Seeing'

We will now turn our behavioral lens to understanding and using mindfulness. Earlier in this chapter a distinction was drawn between two types of consciousness, illustrated through use of the exercise 'seeing your hand' and 'being aware that you are seeing your hand.' We refer to the 'being aware that you are seeing' as consciousness or self-observation. Self-observation of an event is under the control of a different Sd (discriminative stimulus) than the Sd for the event itself. Thus, if a client is anxious, the aversive Sd that evokes that anxiety (a bodily state) is different from the Sd that controls the self-observation of that anxiety. Typically, anxiety motivates problematic avoidance and escape whereas self-observation of that anxiety as 'noticing bodily sensations as sensory phenomena' reduces its control over avoidance and thus allows for more productive responses. It is a shift in stimulus control that provides the opportunity (referred to as 'giving space' in the mindfulness literature) for new behavior to emerge and for openness to experience to occur. Similarly, the thought, "I am stupid," an automatic response to an aversive Sd that may in turn evoke problematic avoidance, is different from the stimulus control (Sd) resulting from self-observation of the thinking (i.e., "I am having the thought I am stupid"). In the latter case presence to experience is enhanced, avoidance is reduced, and there is an opportunity for more effective behavior to occur. Consistent with our earlier analysis of the sense of self, there is considerable individual variation in the ability to self-observe. Accordingly there is overlap between being mindful (being aware that you are seeing, feeling, etc.) and having a stable sense of self. Both involve strengthening private control over the repertoires, 'I see, I feel, I x.'

We contend that strengthening of self-awareness naturally is reinforced by therapists during most therapeutic encounters. For example, the ubiquitous therapeutic move of asking clients to report what they are feeling is an opportunity for self-observation and for improving the private control of their 'I x's.' Not surprisingly, at the beginning of treatment clients may have difficulty answering the question, "What are you feeling right now?" With a therapist's compassionate prompting, attunement and sensitivity, clients are reinforced for both contacting private feelings and being aware that they are doing so (self observation or self-awareness). Similarly, the thought record routinely used in cognitive therapy asks clients to label and rate thoughts, feelings, and even how much they 'believe' a thought. All of this requires self-observation—awareness that one is having thoughts. As therapists help clients become more skilled at using the thought record, they are also prompting and reinforcing them to become more skilled at self-observing, first in the presence of the therapist. This skill of self-observing is then more likely to generalize to corresponding daily life situations.

Noticing (being aware of) bodily sensations when in the presence of an aversive Sd also changes the Sd somewhat and thus aids in being present. Transfer to daily life of this noticing will be enhanced when reinforced in an interpersonally evocative therapist-client environment (e.g., being asked to take risks and develop trust). Progressive muscle relaxation training or body scanning strengthens this observational skill and makes it more likely to occur when the client is confronted with aversive Sds. Similarly, asking clients to notice and describe the qualities of external visual and tactile stimuli produces a shift in the controlling Sd (the stimulus they are attending to). This attention shift can then aid in being present to the experience of the aversive Sd that evokes avoidance.

Awareness/Relaxation/Acceptance Exercise (ARA)

In concert with opportunities for remaining present that occur during the course of therapy, specific exercises can be introduced to help clients be mindful. The following exercise is based on three sources—Herbert Benson's relaxation response (Benson, 1975), an ACT (Acceptance and Commitment Therapy) awareness exercise in Woods, Wetterneck and Flessner's (2006) treatment manual, and a respondent conditioning model for producing a self-induced, rapid anti-anxiety response. In keeping with the interpersonal emphasis in FAP, the ARA is taught in-session where encouragement and reinforcement of self-observation enhances the possibility of transfer to daily life. In addition, the exercise emphasizes the utility of awareness, relaxation and acceptance skills in the presence of others, particularly during difficult interpersonal situations. During in-session trainings therapists should watch carefully for negative reactions and frequently ask clients how they are reacting. The therapist also should remain alert for CRBs that this exercise might evoke, and alter the technique depending on client response.

The following is a rationale for the ARA exercise. Therapists may choose to paraphrase this rationale and emphasize those issues most relevant to their clients.

(1) It increases your ability to stay with your awareness of moment-to-moment experience, even when in the presence of another person or evocative situation. (2) It increases your skills in noticing having thoughts as a process, and accepting thoughts and feelings without having to avoid them or change them. (3) It increases your ability to observe sensations in your body and stimuli around you. (4) It provides a cue to break a chain of automatic unproductive responding and sets the scene for more productive behavior even when in difficult situations involving other people. (5) It provides a cue that can be used for momentary coping with stress or strong negative feelings so that you can remain in the situation and not show avoidance. (6) According to Benson (1975), it reduces your accumulated daily arousal/stress.

An example of a paraphrased rationale is as follows.

Often the buzz of mental activity and daily life routine dominate, and we get thoroughly caught in it. We forget to pay attention in the moment, to pause and reflect on what we are doing and what our choices are. The following meditation practice and the conditioning of a cue word [explain classical conditioning if it is appropriate] allows us to practice observing the buzz of mental activity and gives us a tool to help us become aware of choices—even when being with, noticing, and interacting with other people. (Based on Woods, Wetterneck, & Flessner, 2006 and modified for use in FAP.)

The instructions for the ARA exercise are as follows.

STEP ONE: Pair Breath (Exhale) with Cue Word or Phrase

Always start each practice session with this step. You can be in any position—standing, sitting, or even in an uncomfortable position. You can be alone or with others like you are now. Select a cue word or phrase that you will be using. It can be a fairly neutral word or one that has meaning for you. Examples are 'blue sky,' 'moonlight,' 'canoe,' 'let it be,' or the first few words of a familiar prayer. You will be using this same word or phrase throughout your daily practice sessions.

    With your eyes open, focus your attention on your breath. Breathe naturally. After noticing one to three breaths, say the cue word or phrase (e.g., 'moonlight') to yourself as you exhale.

STEP TWO: Brief Muscle/Body Scan (approximately a minute or two for this step)

Sit in a comfortable position. Close your eyes if you would like—it's not critical that you follow these instructions exactly. Do a brief inventory or mental scan of muscle tension in your body. Spend only about ten seconds on each of areas listed below. See if you notice any muscle tension. If you have tension, try to release it. If you can't release it, that's okay, move on to the next area.

> Feet, legs, and thighs.
> Buttocks and pelvic area.
> Abdomen, stomach, and lower back.
> Chest and upper back.
> Shoulders, arms, hands.
> Neck, back and top of head.
> Jaw (it's okay if your mouth is open).
> Eyes and eyebrows, forehead.

STEP THREE: Mindfulness/Acceptance

Breathe naturally, focus your attention on your breath. Follow a breath as it comes in through your nose, travels through your lungs, moves through your belly in and out, and leaves back through your nose. Ride the waves of your breathing without attempting to alter it; just notice it as it happens. Each time you exhale, say the cue word or phrase to yourself (the practice). Assume a non-judgmental, passive or 'let it happen' attitude. Do not evaluate how you are doing. There is no need to 'make it happen,' 'do it right' or to be critical of yourself (either for not following these instructions or for anything else that comes to mind). If you notice that you have stopped doing the practice, just notice the distraction, and gently return to your breath or cue word. When distracting thoughts go through your mind, notice whatever thoughts you are having and say, "Oh well, those are just my thoughts," and gently return to the practice. Your distracting thoughts may be judgmental, self-critical and/or other-critical and it is likely you will go back and forth between various distractions and doing the practice.

    Allow yourself to completely experience the present moment. Be deeply present with yourself. Even if you are having thoughts or feelings you don't like, do not push them away. Adopt an attitude of acceptance and curiosity towards all parts of your experience: treat every experience, thought and feeling gently, even if it is undesirable or distressing. Gently be present with yourself. Continue this process for ten to twenty minutes. It's okay to peek at a clock or watch. Do this mindfulness/acceptance procedure twice a day, preferably in the morning and the evening.

Although Benson suggests doing this exercise for twenty minutes, twice a day, in reality any practice is better than none. The ARA, when practiced in-session, is an interpersonal situation that has the potential to evoke CRBs. For example, considerable interpersonal vulnerability and risk can be evoked by asking clients to close their eyes, shift attention to bodily sensations and relax while in the presence of a therapist. Thus if taking interpersonal risks and trusting others are daily life problems, the ARA has the potential to provide therapeutic opportunities to evoke and shape CRB2s. Correspondingly, inadequate mindfulness repertoires (e.g., weak or absent 'I see' responding) might appear as CRB1s during ARA.

Similarly, the ARA has a component that resembles free association, in that the patient is instructed to let thoughts occur, to notice them, and to let them pass in and out of awareness. This may be particularly beneficial for individuals whose interpersonal vulnerability is based on inadequate private control over 'I x' repertoires. As discussed earlier, this task could evoke CRBs related to being in touch with one's own private experiences, as opposed to relying on cues from the therapist. In this case, the therapist might observe that the ARA evokes anxiety and avoidance, and could be restructured along the lines suggested for altering traditional free association instructions. Another potential benefit of the ARA is that the client learns a way to cope with situations that evoke very strong anxiety (bodily) responses. When this happens during the session, the client is prompted to momentarily shift attention to his or her breath and then return to being in contact with the therapist and the evocative content. Momentary focus on the breath provides an alternative to complete avoidance and can facilitate the expression of more productive behaviors. Similarly, if naturally occurring thoughts during ARA practice in the presence of the therapist are related to aversive stimuli that evoke anxiety and avoidance, the process resembles desensitization. That is, the thoughts can be considered items on the hierarchy that are paired with relaxation.

In contrast to the emphasis on the role of the client-therapist relationship presented above, the highly interpersonal nature of mindfulness-based therapeutic interventions are rarely discussed (although for an exception refer to Surrey, 2005). Interestingly, Fischer (1999) points out that traditional meditation-based forms of Buddhist practice are built on the student-teacher relationship and "cannot be learned from books and is impossible to do alone." He goes on to say, "For me, the magic of the teacher-student relationship lies in trust" (p. 2).

Case Example: Exposure and Response Prevention, FAP and Mindfulness for Obsessive Compulsive Disorder

The empirically supported treatment for Obsessive Compulsive Disorder (OCD) is Exposure and Response Prevention (ERP). Although OCD is usually not viewed as an interpersonal problem, Kohlenberg and Vandenberghe (2007) underscored interpersonal issues present for clients with OCD and reported using the therapist-client relationship to shape CRBs relevant to OCD treatment. Even the straightforward implementation of ERP requires a strong therapeutic alliance and a client who is able to trust the therapist enough to engage in previously feared activities. In essence, an ERP therapist is saying to the client, "Trust me—if you follow my suggestions, you can deal with the negative emotions and thoughts evoked by remaining present."

Self-awareness, self-observation or mindfulness as discussed in this chapter plays an important role in remaining present—the essence of ERP. Thus, one way to look at OCD is that the client lacks necessary self-observation repertoires. Given our behavioral conception of self-observation is that it occurs to the degree it has been encouraged and shaped by others, therapists can reinforce tacts that underlie a stable self and evoke and nurture self-awareness.

In the present case example, the client Jane, age 25, was fired from her job as a medical laboratory technician due to excessive checking and contamination anxiety. Although Jane had an extensive history of being assured by others that her fears were irrational, she did not trust the assurances enough nor did she have a readily available self-observation repertoire to help her stay present in evocative situations. Instead, when confronted with the possibility of making an error (and being discovered by others) or becoming contaminated with germs and inadvertently making others ill, she displayed checking behaviors and avoided contact with contaminated objects.

Her treatment involved nurturing self-observation (the core of mindfulness) and enabling the development of 'trusting' others (at first her therapist RJK) that underlie exposure and response prevention. Jane agreed that it would be helpful for her to work toward the goal of being able to observe herself having thoughts and feelings and telling RJK about them. Specific treatment elements included: (1) being prompted and encouraged in-session to step back, notice and describe bodily sensations, negative feelings and thoughts as an aid to remaining present with evocative stimuli; (2) using the ARA to develop a coping response that could be used during interpersonal situations (e.g., at work) as a means of reducing high levels of anxiety and facilitating ERP; (3) using FAP to establish a safe therapeutic environment that facilitated the trust and courage required for exposure work; and (4) generalizing trust of the therapist that enabled in-session ERP to others in her daily life.

It was explained to Jane (Rule 5) that her avoidance and other OCD behaviors were reinforced by an immediate reduction in anxiety. Contributing to the problem was the support she received from her husband and others that reinforced avoidance behavior. The goal was to trust RJK's and others' reassurances that she could deal with her fears, remain present in evocative situations, and thereby be positioned to be emit more productive behavior (e.g., working in her chosen profession).

Trust issues that immediately surfaced and were dealt with included her belief that RJK was holding her in low regard because she was not able to do 'normal' life activities. During ARA training, she was anxious when asked to notice bodily sensations and relax with her eyes closed, as she would be deprived of the public stimuli needed for sense of self and also was concerned that RJK would be looking at her with pity or degradation.

The context for the session described below was occasioned by Jane's discovery of a sanitary pad in a hallway in her condominium. Although the pad appeared to have been washed, it evoked contamination anxiety and avoidance of that hallway. She asked her husband to dispose of the pad. Based on the strength of her therapeutic relationship with RJK, Jane subsequently asked her husband to retrieve the pad from the trash container and risked bringing it to session (enclosed in a ziplock baggie and an additional plastic bag) with the understanding it would: (1) be used for exposure; and (2) provide an opportunity to practice and learn to be mindful in the service of remaining present. In the session prior to the one excerpted below, at the urging of RJK, Jane opened the plastic bag, stared at the ziplock baggie and pad, touched the outside of the baggie, but did not open it.

Transcript Excerpt 1 from Session 6

Therapist: Okay, are you willing to do some work on the pad? [Implied: Are you willing to trust me enough to go along with my urging you to remain present, to practice self-observation, and be willing to have negative feelings and thoughts?]

Client: Sure.

T: How about taking the ziplock baggie out of the plastic bag and tell me how far you are to willing to go. Then try to follow through while stepping back and watching yourself having thoughts and feelings. [Jane is asked to help structure the exposure and provide an opportunity to self-observe while remaining present and committing to an action.]

C: Sure. (She gingerly takes out the baggie and looks at the pad inside)

T: You're looking at it. [An attempt to emphasize the observer role—of her seeing herself looking.]

C: Yes. I am looking. There is a spot of some kind there.

T: You are *seeing* a spot, is that right? [Emphasizing the activity of 'seeing,' as opposed to whether a spot is there or not.]

C: Yes, I see there is a hair. I feel the anxiety. [An improvement—reporting "I feel the..." rather than "I am anxious."]

T: Alright, that's good—you notice yourself feeling the anxiety. [Emphasizing the observation rather than the feeling.]

Excerpt 2

T: As you are touching the bag, do you notice if you are feeling something on your hands? ['Noticing' a feeling is self-observation.]

C: Yeah, I do, my hands get sweaty right away. I think it contributes to feeling dirty. It's sticky.

T: So you are noticing the sweatiness. What other sensations do notice you are feeling right now? [Encouraging self observation—a shift in focus to other stimuli while remaining present.]

C: My breathing feels kind of tense, my chest is kind of tight.

T: Where do you feel the tightness? [Objectifying the sensation, adding the stimulus control of location, thus encouraging a shift in stimulus control aimed at enabling her to remain in contact with the baggie.]

C: (Places hand on her chest.)

T: Okay, that is the place you feel it. Anything else you notice?

C: Um, my eyes feel kind of damp, not like I'm going to cry, but just a little extra damp.

T: Okay, let's just take a moment, continue touching the baggie, and at the same time take a few breaths, saying "on the beach" [client's cue word used during ARA practice] to yourself each time you breathe out. [Historically for her this particular eye symptom occurs with high anxiety and interferes with the perception needed to do her laboratory work, thus RJK is cautiously using the ARA response as a coping strategy; the downside is that it momentarily strengthens the avoidance of feeling.]

C: With my eyes open?

T: Yes, this is something you can do on the spot. It isn't going to get rid of the anxiety or the tears, but it does give you a diversion for a moment. [An attempt to validate the ultimate importance of remaining present with the feeling even though the purpose of the relaxation response is to attenuate the intensity. This also an example of using attending to an immediate experience of breath as a means of aiding the "process of successive moments of turning toward, turning away" (Surrey, 2005).]

C: Okay (takes two breaths).

T: Now let's stay with what you are doing with the baggie. [Emphasizing using the momentary shift in attention in the service of remaining present and continuing with the task at hand—the exposure.]

C: Okay. I think I should touch it and take it out of the ziplock bag at the least.

T: You are being courageous and are doing great.

C: I think this is how far we got last week. I feel like I don't want to touch the inside of the bag. I feel like it has been dirty up here (indicating the upper inside portion of the baggie).

T: And are you aware of the sensation of something being on your fingers? Anywhere else?

C: I don't know, I think I am aware it is on my sleeve. I don't want to do this—can you help me. [CRB2, asking for help in remaining present rather than support for avoidance.]

T: I think it's important to stay with what you are doing. I am sensing how intense your feelings are and how difficult this is for you. I can't stop the feelings but I will be here with you [Emphasizing the

T: trust and caring established in the client-therapist relationship.],
        and you will get through this. [Reinforcing her asking for help
        without directly supporting avoidance.]

C: (Pulls pad out of baggy.) Aaag! Okay, so there it is.

T: Did you notice your strong negative response—even though you
        had it you still went ahead with taking out the pad? Okay, so why
        don't you just hold it (the pad) for a while and look at it. What do
        you see?

C: It's not quite white, and there is a little spot. Or maybe it's a little
        flower embroidered in the cotton. Yeah, now it looks like it might
        be crunchy, and of course I don't want to touch it there.

T: So, you are having the thought that it's crunchy. Can you step
        back from yourself and watch yourself having the 'crunchy'
        thought. [Practicing seeing herself see.]

C: Okay, I'm getting better at doing that.

T: If you touched it there, what would happen?

C: It would get on my fingers, and then my finger would be tainted,
        dirty (laughs).

T: You are able to be amused by your negative thought. So you were
        aware that it was just something you were thinking.

C: (Client holds up her hands and pad for RJK to see and smiles.) See
        what I am doing? I was careful to keep my sleeves away from it, but
        now I'm touching them to it. [Acknowledges the interpersonal
        support for remaining present and self observing.]

T: So, what you have done here is go beyond what most people would
        do when they are confronted with touching a used sanitary pad—
        even though it has been washed. And here you are, an OCD client
        who is aware of all these thoughts and feelings, and you are willing
        to trust me enough to still touch and handle it.

C: Wow, yeah. But now I am starting to get anxious and I would like
        to run out of here.

T: You notice that feeling of wanting to run out of here, but you are
        not running out of here, you are staying here with me and your
        feelings (and the pad).

C: Yes.

T: I think you are doing great, because you are not trying to avoid
        these feelings, but just learning to notice them, to stand back,
        watch them and tell me about them. And you seem to be doing
        okay.

C: Right, yeah. I think I'd rather be doing something else, but I'm
        doing okay.

T: Are you willing to try some of this [being aware of her thoughts,
        feelings, sensations, and remaining present] and accept Bill's (hus-
        band's) support?

In Jane's evaluation of the above session (from her session bridging form, see Appendix D), she stated, "I touched the pad to my clothes all over, I never thought I would be able to do that." She reported that high points for the week were accepting Bill's support and trusting his reassurance that she would not get contaminated, being able to remain present while touching the pad, and not asking Bill to help her avoid evocative situations.

Conclusion

Being mindful involves being aware of the private activity involved in such behaviors as seeing, feeling, thinking and hearing. Therapeutic mindfulness occurs when being aware alters the stimulus control of those events that evoke dysfunctional behavior and creates opportunities for the development of more productive responses. In FAP, client mindfulness is nurtured and shaped in the context of the therapist-client relationship. Therapist mindfulness is also an important T2 (therapist target behavior). Indeed, the most important guideline for practicing FAP is awareness—Rule 1. As stated by Kohlenberg (2004), "My job as a FAP therapist is to remain present in the moment so I can be sensitive to the needs of the client and be aware of my own reactions such that I can nurture CBR2s and not strengthen CRB1s."

Being aware of these private activities (self-awareness) occurs if the private activities themselves have acquired discriminative properties, and thus function to evoke tacts about them. It follows that clients with inadequate private control of 'I' will have difficulty acquiring mindfulness repertoires. Treatment in such cases should be staged with an initial emphasis on developing private control ('I x').

This behaviorally based interpersonal view of self and mindfulness was designed to be consistent with the emphasis in FAP on the development and use of the therapist-client relationship. When one's sense of self is stable, one is more able to be in the present moment, increasing connection not only with oneself, but with others.

References

Asch, S. E. (1951). Effects of group pressure upon the modification and distortion of judgment. In H. Guetzkow (Ed.), *Groups, leadership, and men* (pp. 177–190). Pittsburgh: Carnegie.

Benson, H. (1975). *The relaxation response.* New York: Morrow.

Barnes-Holmes, D., Barnes-Holmes, Y., & Cullinan, V. (2000). Relational Frame Theory and Skinner's Verbal Behavior: A possible synthesis. *The Behavior Analyst, 23,* 69–84.

Brown, K. W., & Ryan, R. M. (2003). The benefits of being present: Mindfulness and its role in psychological well-being. *Journal of Personality and Social Psychology, 84*(4), 822–848.

Cooley, C. H. (1908). A study of the early use of self-words by a child. *Psychological Review, 15*(6), 339–357.

Deikman, A. (1999). "I" = awareness. *Journal of Consciousness Studies, 3*, 350–356.

Dore, J. (1985). Holophrases revisited: Their "logical" development from dialog. In M. Barrett (Ed.), *Children's single word speech* (pp. 59–83). New York: Wiley.

Fraiberg, S. (1977). *Insights from the blind. Comparative studies of blind and sighted infants.* New York: Basic Books.

Fischer, N. (1999). *The teacher in the west.* Retrieved April 15, 2007, from http://www.shambhalasun.com/index.php?option = com_content&task = view&id = 1857&Itemid = 244.

Germer, C. K. (2005). Mindfulness: What is it? What does it matter? In Germer, C. K., Siegel, R. D. Fulton, P. R. (Eds.), *Mindfulness and psychotherapy* (pp. 3–27). New York: Guilford Press.

Germer, C. K., Siegel, R. D., & Fulton, P. R. (2005). *Mindfulness and psychotherapy.* New York: Guilford Press.

Hayes, S. C. (1984). Making sense of spirituality. *Behaviorism, 12*(2), 99–110.

Hayes, S. C. (1994). Content, context, and the types of psychological acceptance. In S. C. Hayes, N. S. Jacobson, V. Follette, & M. J. Dougher (Eds.), *Acceptance and change: Content and context in psychotherapy* (pp. 13–32). Reno, NV: Context Press.

Hayes, S. C., Barnes-Holmes, D., & Roche, B. (Eds.). (2001). *Relational frame theory: A post-Skinnerian account of human language and cognition.* New York: Kluwer Academic/Plenum Publishers.

Hayes, S. C., Follette, V. M., & Linehan, M. (2004). *The new behavior therapies: Expanding the cognitive behavioral tradition.* New York: Guilford Press.

Hayes, S. C., & Gregg, J. (2000). Functional contextualism and the self. In C. Muran (Ed.), *Self-relations in the psychotherapy process* (pp. 291–307). Washington, DC: American Psychological Association.

Hayes, S. C., Strosahl, K. D., & Wilson, K. G. (1999). *Acceptance and commitment therapy: An experiential approach to behavior change.* New York: Guilford Press.

Hayes, S. C., & Wilson, K. G. (1993). Some applied implications of a contemporary behavior-analytic account of verbal events. *Behavior Analyst, 16*, 283–301.

Hayes, S. C., & Wilson, K. G. (2003). Mindfulness: Method and process. *Clinical Psychology: Science and Practice, 10*(2), 161–165.

Kanter, J. W., Parker, C. R., & Kohlenberg, R. J. (2001). Finding the self: A behavioral measure and its clinical implications. *Psychotherapy: Theory, Research, Practice, Training, 38*(2), 198–211.

Kohlenberg, R. J. (2004). Using functional analytic psychotherapy when treating a client with anxiety and depression. In *World Grand Rounds, Annual Convention of the Association for Advancement of Behavior Therapy*, New Orleans, November 2004.

Kohlenberg, R. J., & Tsai, M. (1991). *Functional Analytic Psychotherapy: Creating intense and curative therapeutic relationships.* New York: Plenum Press.

Kohlenberg, R. J., & Tsai, M. (1995). I speak, therefore I am. *The Behavior Therapist, 18*(6), 113–116.

Kohlenberg, R. J., & Vandenberghe, L. (2007). Treatment-resistant OCD, inflated responsibility, and the therapeutic relationship: Two case examples. *Psychology and Psychotherapy: Theory, Research and Practice, 80*, 455–465.

Linehan, M. M. (1993). *Cognitive-behavioral treatment of borderline personality disorder.* New York: Guilford Press.

Lipkens, R., Hayes, S. C., & Hayes, L. J. (1993). Longitudinal study of the development of derived relations in an infant. *Journal of Experimental Child Psychology, 56*(2), 201–239.

Marlatt, G. A., & Marques, J. (1977). Meditation, self-control, and alcohol use. In R. B. Stuart (Ed.), *Behavioral self-management* (pp. 117–153). New York: Bruner/Mazel.

Parker, C. R., Bolling, M. Y., & Kohlenberg, R. J. (1998). Operant theory of personality. Chapter 7. In D. Barone, M. Hersen, & V. B. Van Hasselt (Eds.), *Advanced personality* (pp. 155–171). New York: Plenum Press.

Peters, A. N. (1983). *The units of language acquisition.* London: Cambridge University Press.

Rotter, J. B. (1966). Generalized expectancies for internal versus external control of reinforcement. *Psychological Monographs: General & Applied, 80*(1), 1–28.

Skinner, B. F. (1953). *Science and human behavior.* New York: Macmillan.

Skinner, B. F. (1957). *Verbal behavior.* New York: Appleton-Century-Crofts.

Skinner, B. F. (1974). *About behaviorism.* New York: Knopf.

Surrey, J. L. (2005). Relational psychotherapy, relational mindfulness. In C. K. Germer, R. D. Siegel, P. R. Fulton, & E. Tolle (Eds.), Mindfulness and psychotherapy (pp. 91–112). New York: Guilford.

Tolle, E. (2004). *The power of now: A guide to spiritual enlightenment.* Vancouver, BC: Namaste Publishers.

Witkiewitz, K., & Marlatt, G. A. (2005). Mindfulness-based relapse prevention for alcohol use disorders. *Journal of Cognitive Psychotherapy, 19*, 221–228.

Woods, D. W., Wetterneck, C. T., & Flessner, C. A. (2006). A controlled evaluation of acceptance and commitment therapy plus habit reversal for trichotillomania. *Behaviour Research and Therapy, 44*(5), 639–656.

Chapter 6
Intimacy

Robert J. Kohlenberg, Barbara Kohlenberg, and Mavis Tsai

Intimacy is the state of being [inter]personally intimate, defined as the "inmost thoughts or feelings; proceeding from, concerning, or affecting one's inmost self: closely personal" (Oxford English Dictionary, 1989). Our behavioral restatement of this definition is that intimacy is an interpersonal repertoire that involves the disclosure of one's innermost thoughts or feelings, and results in a sense of connection, attachment and close relationship with another. This definition will be elaborated during this chapter by referring to themes or features derived from our clinical experience and the relevant literature.

Along with interpersonal sharing, the notion of 'interpersonal connection' is incorporated in Laurenceau, Rivera, Schaffer and Pietromonaco's (2004) definition, namely that "intimacy is best conceptualized as a personal, subjective (and often momentary) sense of connectedness that is the outcome of an interpersonal, transactional process consisting of self-disclosure and partner responsiveness" (p. 62). A similar theme is voiced by Popovic (2005), who notes that "the noun 'intimacy' derives from the Latin term 'intimus' which means 'innermost' and refers to sharing what is innermost with others. Its 'core sense' concerns close familiarity or friendship" (p. 31). Kovacs (1965) also conveys the inherent personal risk and therapeutic relevance associated with intimacy by asserting, "Much that we do as therapists can be conceived of as attempts to participate in and to influence our patients' struggles and conflicts about intimacy" and "intimacy is something which seems to terrify us" (p. 99). In addition, Kovacs writes that "parties to an intimate relationship are interested in and derive pleasure (tinged with some anxiety to be sure) from a progressive exposure of themselves to each other."

We parse the above into three themes. First, intimacy issues are clinically important. That is, they are meaningful to many people who seek psychotherapy, and are carefully attended to by psychotherapists. Second, intimacy involves a mutual exposing or revealing of the self (expressing thoughts and feelings), that can feel difficult and even terrifying. Third, intimacy involves

R.J. Kohlenberg (✉)
Department of Psychology, University of Washington, Seattle, WA 98195-1525, USA
e-mail: fap@u.washington.edu

M. Tsai et al., *A Guide to Functional Analytic Psychotherapy*,
DOI 10.1007/978-0-387-09787-9_6, © Springer Science+Business Media, LLC 2009

attaching or connecting emotionally to others. Each of these ideas will be explored in more detail. Before doing so, however, the concise behavior analytic consideration of intimacy proposed by Cordova and Scott (2001) is described, as their work provides important groundwork for our behavioral approach to the understanding of intimacy.

Cordova and Scott define intimacy as a process involving two steps. First, an individual emits a behavior vulnerable to interpersonal punishment. Second, the other person responds in such a way that the interpersonally vulnerable behavior is reinforced. The authors point out that expressions of sadness, love and hurt share a commonality with making love, caring for a loved infant, and being totally open and honest with your romantic partner or a close friend. Each intimate expression is characterized by risk, that is, the possibility of censure or punishment by another person. Of course each of us has different histories with these types of intimate behaviors. The extremes are represented by those of us who have extensive histories involving abuse and rejection and those fortunate enough to have been exposed to unconditional acceptance and love. Interpersonal vulnerability occurs when a person acts in ways that in the past was punished, and yet emits the previously punished behavior regardless. Thus, when interpersonal vulnerability is reinforced, these reciprocal events are the core processes that establish intimacy. We now turn to the three themes of intimacy identified earlier.

Intimacy is Clinically Important

Ongoing interaction with close others (or the lack thereof) influences the development of (all) interpersonal relationship processes (Gable & Reis, 2006). These processes, in turn, are implicated in the onset, maintenance and/or relapse of most clinical disorders (Pielage, Luteijn, & Arrindell, 2005; Van Orden, Wingate, Gordon, & Joiner, 2005), and attachment and interpersonal intimacy problems are also related to substance abuse (Thorberg & Lyvers, 2006). Engaging in a satisfying, intimate relationship is reported to be the most important source of happiness and well-being (Russell & Wells, 1994); conversely, being in a distressed relationship constitutes a major risk factor for psychopathology (Burman & Margolin, 1992). It is well known that early childhood trauma, particularly physical or sexual abuse from a trusted caregiver, can lead to significant interpersonal difficulties (Kohlenberg, Tsai, & Kohlenberg, 2006). In his seminal paper, McAdams (1982) describes intimacy as a fundamental social motive. He notes that the benefits and virtues of warmth and closeness long have been recognized, as has the fact that individuals differ markedly in their ability to achieve such relationships. He elaborates further that intimacy can enhance psychological growth for all individuals and provide an experience that is profoundly therapeutic in times of distress. In the arena of physical health, Prager (1995) reports that a lack of intimate relationships is associated with increased mortality rates, mental and physical illnesses, stress-related symptoms and accidents.

Social support is a key interpersonal process related to the prevention and recovery of nearly all forms of psychopathology—it is also integral to intimate interactions. Two types of client responses can 'spoil' the positive effects of social support. One such response blocks the client from accepting the interpersonal support offered. Coyne (1976) argues that depressed individuals, for example, interact in ways that negate the offering of support. In particular, they doubt the sincerity of caring and feedback offered by others. A second response is that they discourage others from giving such support and, when it is provided, tend to react in a frustrating or irritating manner. When the offering of social support is an interpersonally vulnerable behavior and is punished by the recipient, intimacy is thwarted.

From a FAP perspective, the above process occurs during the therapeutic interaction when clients do not accept the caring, concern or therapeutic love offered by the therapist. Quite commonly, clients may even express their doubt directly as to the sincerity or genuineness of these expressions by suggesting that the therapist is paid to make caring comments. It is this dynamic (thwarted intimacy, as we define it) that forms the core of Coyne's (1976) interpersonal theory of depression. The therapist's expression of caring might even be a T2 (therapist target behavior), particularly if the therapist is emitting behaviors that feel interpersonally vulnerable for him or her.

Intimacy Involves Expressing Thoughts and Feelings That Can Feel Difficult and Risky

According to Cordova and Scott's (2001) formulation, sharing thoughts and feelings becomes an intimate event when these very behaviors have been punished in the past. In other words, in a situation in which an invitation to self-disclose is offered, there is a risk that the self-disclosure could be punished if that has been the case in previous interactions. Thus an invitation to self-disclose might in fact be an aversive stimulus that evokes tendencies to escape, avoid and attack. Given such a history, the behavior of self-disclosing would be difficult, even frightening. In the right relationship, of course, interpersonally vulnerable behavior is prompted, nurtured and reinforced, and intimacy occurs. One such relationship is provided in FAP where the therapist actively creates an environment in which intimacy building behavior can be shaped and reinforced.

It is important to note that the therapy relationship of course is imperfect. That is, there are boundaries which clients might have clinically relevant reactions to, such as session time limits, overall session limits, not seeing the therapist outside of therapy, and so on. There is indeed a power imbalance in psychotherapy, with the client revealing far more information than the therapist. Furthermore, the therapist inadvertently can punish intimate self-disclosures on the part of the client. For example, the therapist might forget something important to the client, which could make a self disclosure feel invalidated and punished. Or the therapist could simply not attend closely to an emerging self-disclosure, thus losing the opportunity to behave in a reinforcing manner.

We would contend that these imperfections actually add to the effectiveness of the psychotherapy session by providing opportunities (evoking CRB) for our clients to learn intimacy skills. That is, it is illusory to believe that any human interaction can be 'perfect' and provide a totally safe place in which intimate interactions always will be encouraged and nurtured. For this reason intimate behaviors should occur when a reasonable assessment of risk has been made. We believe that an effective therapeutic relationship has a very high ratio of reinforcing therapist responses to punishing therapist responses. Yet there is always some risk. Intimate behavior involves proceeding with self disclosure, even when the possibility of punishment exists.

Intimacy Involves Being Attached or Connected to Others

The experience of being attached or connected to others is an important part of human experience, and there are those (like Kari, discussed below) who have difficulty in identifying with this experience. There appears to be little discussion of the experience of attachment in the behavioral literature. Although not emerging from a behavioral tradition, there is an extensive literature on attachment theory (Bowlby, 1969) that is consistent with a behavioral conceptualization. Bowlby's fundamental hypothesis is that the contingencies of survival (natural selection) have pressed mothers and infants into each other's arms. In other words, there were powerful reinforcers for attachment behaviors (e.g, clinging, turning toward the primary caregiver in times of distress). According to Konner (2004), both Freud and Skinner essentially shared this view.

Early studies of attachment tended to examine the attachment process during childhood. More recently, the focus has extended to adult expressions of attachment, particularly in romantic and close relationships. Based on an individual's history of experienced contingencies of intimate behavior, there would be a wide range of attachment behavioral repertoires that can influence their propensity to engage in effective intimate relating. For example, the fear of rejection and how this impacts the development of close relationships would be a clear result of an individual's history of reinforcement and punishment with regard to intimate behavior. Attachment theorists have classified these behavioral repertoires in terms of "secure, anxious-ambivalent and anxious-avoidant attachment styles, which describe whether patients (and therapists) tend to be comfortable and confident in relationships, fearful of abandonment, or defensively separate" (Meyer & Pilkonis, 2001, p. 466). In Meyer and Pilkonis's brief review of the literature, they suggest that there are similarities between: (1) the way children attached to caregivers; (2) how adults attach to romantic partners; and (3) how clients can be said to attach to their therapists. They also conclude that a client's attachment style influences therapeutic alliance and outcome. Pielage et al. (2005), using a large community sample, found that security of attachment was negatively related to loneliness and depression, but positively related to satisfaction with life. Although problematic attachment repertoires appear to engender an enduring vulnerability for psychopathology (Van Orden et al., 2005), Meyer and Pilkonis suggest that FAP has potential to modify clients' attachment styles.

Therapeutic Implications

Intimacy in psychotherapy includes inviting clients to be open and to reveal deeply held secrets of the heart. This basic element of therapy sets the scene for evoking interpersonally vulnerable behavior. The therapist is implicitly requesting that clients take risks and to trust that they will not be punished for taking such risks. Given its broad clinical implications, we believe that many, if not most, clients can benefit from improving intimate relating repertoires. Further, it is not unusual to discover that intimacy problems extend back into a client's early history. Thus from a FAP standpoint, the therapeutic relationship ideally would evoke (Rule 2) client behavior that prevents intimacy from developing (CRB1s) and prompt and reinforce improvements (Rule 3) in intimacy behaviors (CRB2s). It is for this reason that a warm, active therapist who emits interpersonally vulnerable behavior is usually better positioned to evoke the client's problems and set the stage for improvement. A client who wishes to develop close relationships, and yet is frightened by warmth, can clearly benefit from a therapist who expresses warmth. Of course a caring but aloof therapist may also evoke CRB1s, and clients learning to discriminate more aloof but no less caring behaviors on the part of the therapist may also find that their interpersonal risk-taking repertoire is reinforced.

Reinforce Interpersonally Vulnerable Behavior

In the service of improving clients' emotionally intimate expressions, it is essential that therapists naturally reinforce their interpersonally vulnerable behavior (CRB2s). In clients' daily lives, intimate expressions generally are reinforced by the other person's increased interest, focused attention and reciprocal self disclosures. Contrived or arbitrary responses such as "Thanks for sharing," probably would not be a natural reinforcer. Thus a client who discloses and expresses grief about the loss of a child might best be served by a therapist who responds by revealing his or her deepest feelings of sadness about how to endure such a loss, along with willingness to hear the depths of such overwhelming grief.

In addition to taking the risk of self-disclosing, the client must learn to reinforce the intimate interpersonal behavior of others in order to create and maintain close relationships. Thus the therapist's interpersonally vulnerable expressions must also be reinforced. Take the example of a therapist expressing caring and concern about a client by disclosing that he or she thought about the client a great deal during the week. The client response, "That is what I pay you for," would punish such disclosures on the part of the therapist. This would be an opportunity for the therapist to point out a CRB1, that the client has blocked an opportunity to deepen the relationship. A CRB2 might be the client saying, "I am so moved, even a little frightened by the intensity of your caring for me. It is so new for me to have anyone care in this way, it even feels hard to trust it."

It is also the case that therapists never will be able to perfectly reinforce client interpersonal risks, and may inadvertently punish a client's vulnerable expression. If these events are recognized in the context of Rule 2 (evoke CRBs), they provide opportunities for clients to learn the recovering and repairing skills required to deal with the inevitable disappointments associated with intimate relating. While the notion of relationship rupture and then repair is clearly part of all close relationships, the concept of therapeutic alliance problems leading to rupture and repair is a general principle that is meaningful across many types of therapy (Kohlenberg, Yeater, & Kohlenberg, 1998; Safran, Crocker, McMain, & Murray, 1990; Safran & Muran, 1998, 2005).

Specific Techniques

Given our emphasis on functional analysis, we are reluctant to suggest specific exercises or techniques independent of the context of a particular client-therapist relationship. We strongly believe that the therapy relationship, as it stands, is highly evocative of intimate behavior and its avoidance. We recognize, however, that it may be useful at times to implement specific exercises in the service of evoking and intensifying interpersonal risk-taking (see Chapter 4). In this vein, examples of experiential exercises that can help explore the theme of intimacy in therapy are now discussed.

The open heart meditation, adapted from Deida (2001), is one such exercise. In this meditation the client is asked to:

> Focus on your breathing, soften your belly and relax your jaw as you breathe. Feel your heart beating in your chest, and feel its rhythm radiating outward, pulsing in your hands and feet and neck. Right now, and in every moment, you are either closing or opening your heart. See if you can feel your heartbeat, and allow yourself to relax and open your heart as if offering your heartbeat to the world. With your heart open, you can offer without holding back, you can receive without pushing away. Let yourself feel our connection, let yourself feel my caring for you.

The idea of opening your heart is a metaphor for the act of being vulnerable that corresponds to the behavior involved in developing an intimate or close relationship. The heart historically is seen as the most essential organ required to maintain life. Thus opening your heart to others risks the greatest vulnerability of all, namely the loss of life itself. The following popular song lyrics illustrate this metaphor:

> "You won't find a thing
> Until you soften your heart." Keith Green ("Soften Your Heart")

> "Ah, ah, ah, ah
> Open your heart, I'll make you love me.
> It's not that hard, if you just turn the key." Madonna ("Open Your Heart")

> "Baby, open your heart.
> Won't you give me a second chance
> and I'll be here forever." Westlife ("Open Your Heart")

There is even a reference to the heart metaphor in the Bible:

> God hardened Pharaoh's heart (Exodus 9:12), and the hearts of the Egyptians.
> (Exodus14:17)

Additional connection exercises are described by Surrey (2005, p. 108-110), in which one can 'breathe with' a client, 'co-meditate in the flow of connection and disconnection' and 'learn to see each other.' When these exercises are combined, the basic instructions involve: (1) sitting face to face at a comfortable distance; (2) attuning to one's own breath; (3) opening one's field of attention to include the presence of the other with a soft respectful focus on his or her breathing; (4) noticing thoughts and feelings that arise, but staying with being and breathing together; (5) expanding attention to the flow of connection and disconnection, including uneasiness, self-consciousness or emotional reactions; (6) looking into each other's eyes and feeling these words in your heart, "May you be happy. May you be free from suffering. May you touch the deepest joys of life. May you dwell in peace." (p. 109); (7) noticing what it feels like to connect, to send and to receive; (8) processing what it was like to share this exercise with each other.

Asking your clients to open their hearts also can take place spontaneously during a therapeutic interaction, as in this example of MT and her client Cindy, who is working on letting in others' caring, a cornerstone of building social support.

Therapist: Let's focus right on this moment. Basically in any moment you can choose to open into a feeling of worthiness and caring that others feel about you, or you can shut down and dislike yourself. Are you open to my caring for you right now?

Client: I want to be.

T: Be tuned into the energy I'm sending you. What are you picking up from me?

C: There's like a fight going on in my head. There's a warmth coming from you, but there's an underlying fear of accepting it. If I open up to your love, I have to feel all of this pain over here with it, the loss of when I didn't receive. If I open up, I'll feel this huge tidal wave of pain.

T: So you have this feeling that if you let in my love, you're going to get a tidal wave of pain. Can you sit with that contradiction, can you just be loving with yourself around it? 'Cause what I'm feeling isn't that you have to accept my love. What I'm feeling is simply love, it's like love for the contradiction that you are feeling for this intense dilemma you're in, and being with you. Can you be with yourself around it, that it's quite a dilemma. Really, really anguishing.

C: And admitting not only my pain, but also my sisters and brothers are in their 30s and 40s, and seeing the pain on my brothers' and sisters' faces and seeing the pain in their lives.

T: There's way, way too much. All I'm asking is for you to breathe and be with me in this moment.

C: There's one thing that's helped the last couple of days.

T: Cindy, Cindy. [Blocking her CRB1 of avoidance.]

C: Okay.

T: You don't want to do this, do you? You want to talk, and you want to be with the last few days and be with your brothers and sisters. You don't want to breathe and be with me in this moment? (Said in a gentle tone of voice.)

C: Yeah, it's tough to be in this moment.

T: Just feel your breath.

C: (Cries.)

T: It's okay, you can make sounds, you don't have to be quiet.

C: (Cries for a couple of minutes.) There's so much pain I'm scared of opening the door too far.

T: Is it okay to open it a little just by feeling your breath? What was it like to open the door a tiny bit?

C: It was okay.

T: So there's the pain, then there's also the exhilaration and the freedom to let yourself feel whatever is there. I feel really blessed that you allow yourself to be in your fullness, in your vulnerability, and in your trust of me. [Reinforcing her CRB2s.]

C: Well, this has been one of the few really safe places in my life.

Discuss and Assess Attachment and Connection

Given the amorphous nature of the topography of attaching and connecting, it can be useful to assess these concepts with your client. This discussion can be facilitated by asking the client to fill out the "FAP Experiences of Closeness in the Therapist-Client Relationship" questionnaire after each session (FAP-ECR, Appendix L). The FAP-ECR is a modified version of the widely used Experiences in Close Relationships Questionnaire (ECR; Fraley, Waller, & Brennan, 2000) that assesses adult attachment. Whereas the ECR gauges pist Session Report (PTSR) on Relationships" (Appendix M), both created at the University of Washington, can alert therapists to potential CRBs.

Case Example

Kari, a 25-year-old graduate student, sought treatment from RJK for depression and smoking cessation. She reported that she had been depressed since early childhood and in fact did not remember ever not being depressed. She had a few friendships and had engaged in brief romances that were emotionally distant, but had established no intimate relationships. Her ratings of the FAP-ECT item "I prefer not to be too close to my therapist" went from 5.5 (agree) to 2.2 (disagree) on a 7 point scale after the session discussed below. In the previous two sessions RJK and Kari briefly discussed her lack of 'connection' or attachment to RJK, even though she was aware that he felt connected to her and cared about her.

Segment 1

(Kari has been lamenting how poorly she is doing in school and does not have friends.)

Therapist: Well let me offer some solutions or ideas.
Clients: I need to lower my goals, I know this sounds dramatic and ridiculous, and I don't mean it seriously, but I need to find a good new life that's happy and meaningless and quiet. I obviously don't want to be in a trailer park with eight kids, but I need to give up my hopes and dreams and getting a Ph.D. that will serve no purpose whatsoever.
T: Okay, so let me throw this out to you. You pretty much steadfastly refuse to feel much of a connection to me [brings up the topic of attachment]... even though I feel connected to you. [T2, emitting interpersonally vulnerable behavior.]
C: I don't mean to refuse.
T: Well, I would say you refuse, that is, somehow you stop yourself. It's not just with me, you do this in general, but I do feel there is a real block that you put between the two of us. You tell me I am a professional who is being nice to you because it's my business to like you—that is really a way to protect yourself from connecting, so I just think that's the piece that's missing.

C: I do feel a huge obligation and even though I could not stop smoking, it's getting so I can feel better and get more done, but I'm not really on the path. I think you're doing everything possible to help me, giving your time and attention.

T: I am giving you my time and my attention and the thing that is missing is somehow you haven't connected with me. I know if that's there, it would help, it would provide the glue so that we could really start working together.

C: I don't know how to do what you're asking. I think I can do it, but I don't know how, or how I can not do it. Even with friendship it's similar. My roommate yelled at me yesterday, and that whole relationship I built, and I trusted her, and I cut her off. It's ridiculous, she didn't even yell at me; she just thought I did something I didn't do.

T: And you cut her off?

C: She was so mad at me. That was so upsetting, I just can't be her friend anymore. I won't be her friend (tearfully). I won't do it.

Segment 2 (later in the session)

T: That is why you won't connect with me. This lack of commitment that you have is deeply ingrained. Your roommate got angry at you and you got so upset you couldn't deal with it. That shows you why you need to protect yourself against connecting to people. You actually do like people, but then you are at risk for getting hurt in that way. I wish you would say you were willing to risk being hurt in this relationship with me. I'd like you to look at this relationship as a place to experiment getting close, even though I'm not going to be seeing you every week for the rest of your life.

C: Yes clearly.

T: But I will never forget you, and I will continue to see you, and do whatever it takes to try and help you make that connection with me. I think I can really be a resource. [Interpersonally vulnerable T2.]

C: I just need one step. I'm just not sure how to do that, I really don't know. [CRB2, taking a risk, being open, reinforcing the therapist for being therapeutically intimate.]

T: Well one thing is trying to take in that I believe you have great potential, the real talent to do good in the world. I know you well enough and I care too much about you to not try to help you get there.

C: I wish I could figure out a way because I don't mean to be cold and distant all the time.

T: I think you are very engaging in terms of you and me just right now. But you ignored me telling you how much I care. [Brings up a CRB1, client not responding to his expression of caring.]

C: I am. I don't think I could ever really care about someone.

T: So you don't think you could really feel this connection with me.

C: I don't know, because you see I don't know what the barrier is.

T: So how about this, will you let me in, that is, emotionally be close to you.

C: I just don't know how. It must be clear to you that I have this problem.

T: I think this is a central key—something that's related to all parts of your life that you're unhappy about right now.

C: I never have really been with anybody who hasn't hurt me.

T: I feel close to you. I don't know exactly what you feel, but I feel very connected to you. I look at you like a daughter, somebody that I really care about, so that's here. You might get hurt in this relationship but I can promise you this, it will get repaired.

C: It will be easier in here, wouldn't it. I will think about it. I'm not sure what's going on, I don't feel connected to you, but I do feel comfortable with you, and I do respect you a lot.

T: But no connection?

C: I guess that I don't even know what that means. I think there is a connection, I feel like I know a little bit about you—you drive a hybrid.

T: Is there anything else you want to know about me?

C: No, I don't have to know details.

T: I would answer almost anything that you asked about.

C: I don't know what my problem is, and I guess there is a connection. I feel like I know who you are.

T: Well that's a pretty good start. Now my caring for you, makes you uncomfortable.

C: But I appreciate it.

T: But it's real?

C: It's real, but it's not about me, it's you wanting to help people.

T: So this is really depersonalized.

C: I think you really do want to help. I don't think you realize that I really appreciate it, that you think about me, and try to help me. I really do appreciate these things, I'm just not sure what part I'm missing.

T: It's the emotional attachment part that's not there.

C: Yeah, like I'm thinking back to boyfriends, if they would break up with me I would be really upset for two days, and then just forget it. I didn't think about them, I didn't think about it, I was called the Ice Queen in high school for that very reason. I feel like I am a caring person, but if something happens and I don't see that person anymore, then a day or two, and it's done, you know.

T: That's what you gain by not connecting, however it is that you do that.

C: There are very few people who stay with me that I care about.

T: I have stayed with you in this therapy, and this is where I would like us to try and have you experience more of a connection. I'm really interested in how you are able to keep the distance since I can't help feeling the closeness.

In the subsequent session Kari said that she realized for the first time that RJK was on her 'team.' She said this changed the way she was seeing RJK, and that she no longer felt that she needed to oppose him. At the end of that session Kari's ratings of closeness dramatically improved for the first time in four months and remained that way. Four weeks after the above session she began a new relationship and mindfully was using intimacy building skills. She pleaded with RJK not to let her 'cut it off,' as she was inclined to do so even though this was the best relationship she has ever been in. RJK promised that he would do his best by helping her develop her attachment to RJK, to her partner, and to others she cares about.

Conclusion

Emotional intimacy can be a source of our greatest joys and deepest pain. Intimacy is the act of sharing one's deepest, most protected secrets with another person and reinforcing others for doing the same. It is the act of self revelation in the context of a compassionate, yet imperfect relationship. It is the act of risking hurt, and even being hurt, yet also experiencing efforts to repair these hurts. There are times when those experienced hurts cannot be repaired, such as when an intimate other dies or for other reasons the relationship ends before the intimate feelings have ended.

In psychotherapy, emotional intimacy on the part of the client is invited and nurtured across many therapeutic modalities. Emotional intimacy is a focus of FAP, and is evoked and naturally reinforced when such an endeavor is called for by the case conceptualization. In FAP, as in all psychotherapies, boundaries such as session time limits, treatment termination, therapist departure, client yearning for an extended relationship with the therapist (e.g., physical intimacy or friendship beyond what occurs in therapy), are all opportunities for the client to learn to risk vulnerability even in the face of painful longing and other known risks.

FAP helps to create a compassionate, evocative and reinforcing environment in which clients learn to improve their intimacy skills. It is also a context in which many of the conflicting and incongruous features that interfere with the development of daily life intimacy are present. There is a functional equivalence between imperfections and boundaries in daily life and some features of the therapeutic relationship, such as expecting payment for sessions, ending the session on time even if the client is not ready, and therapist imperfections. Despite such challenges, FAP therapists are committed to creating an environment that is a 'sacred space' (see Chapter 4) in which clients can take interpersonal risks in being vulnerable, and in which they can care and be cared for, so that they can reclaim the daily life intimacy that is their birthright.

References

Bowlby, J. (1969). *Attachment and loss*. New York: Basic Books.

Burman, B., & Margolin, G. (1992). Analysis of the association between marital relationships and health problems: An interactional perspective. *Psychological Bulletin, 112*(1), 39–63.

Cordova, J. V., & Scott, R. L. (2001). Intimacy: A behavioral interpretation. *Behavior Analyst, 24*(1), 75–86.

Coyne, J. C. (1976). Depression and the response of others. *Journal of Abnormal and Social Psychology, 85*, 186–193.

Deida, D. (2001). *Naked Buddhism: 39 ways to free your heart and awaken to now*. Austin: Plexus.

Fraley, R. C., Waller, N. G., & Brennan, K. A. (2000). An item response theory analysis of self-report measures of adult attachment. *Journal of Personality and Social Psychology, 78* (2), 350–365.

Gable, S. L., & Reis, H. T. (2006). Intimacy and the self: An iterative model of the self and close relationships. In P. Noller & J. A. Feeney, (Eds.), *Close relationships: Functions, forms and processes* (pp. 211–225). Hove, UK: Psychology Press/Taylor & Francis.

Kohlenberg, B. S., Tsai, M., & Kohlenberg, R. J. (2006). Healing interpersonal trauma with the intimacy of the therapeutic relationship. In V. Follette & J. Ruzek (Eds.), *Cognitive-behavioral therapies for trauma* (2nd ed., pp. 173–197). New York: Guilford.

Kohlenberg, B. S., Yeater, E. A., & Kohlenberg, R. J. (1998). Functional analytic psychotherapy, the therapeutic alliance, and brief psychotherapy. In J. D. Safran (Ed.), *The therapeutic alliance in brief psychotherapy* (pp. 63–93). Washington, DC: American Psychological Association.

Konner, M. (2004). The ties that bind – Attachment: The nature of the bonds between humans are becoming accessible to scientific investigation. *Nature, 429* (6993), 705–705.

Kovacs, A. L. (1965). The intimate relationship: A therapeutic paradox *Psychotherapy: Theory, Research & Practice, 2* (3), 97–103.

Laurenceau, J.-P., Rivera, L. M., Schaffer, A. R., & Pietromonaco, P. R. (2004). Intimacy as an interpersonal process: Current status and future directions. In D. J. Mashek & A. P. Aron (Eds.), *Handbook of closeness and intimacy* (pp. 61–78). New Jersey, US: Lawrence Erlbaum Associates Publishers.

McAdams, D. P. (1982). Intimacy motivation. In A. J. Stewart (Ed.), *Motivation and society: Essays in honor of David C McClelland* (pp. 133–171). San Francisco CA: Jossey-Bass.

Meyer, B., & Pilkonis, P. A. (2001). Attachment style. *Psychotherapy, 38* (4), 466–472.

The Oxford English Dictionary. (1989). (2nd ed.) OED Online. Oxford University Press. http://dictionary.oed.com/cgi/entry/50119926 (accessed December, 2007)

Pielage, S. B., Luteijn, F., & Arrindell, W. A. (2005). Adult attachment, intimacy and psychological distress in a clinical and community sample. *Clinical Psychology & Psychotherapy, 12* (6), 455–464.

Popovic, M. (2005). Intimacy and its relevance in human functioning. *Sexual and Relationship Therapy, 20* (1), 31–49.

Prager, K. J. (1995). The psycholgy of intimacy. New York: Guilford Press.

Russell, R., & Wells, P. A. (1994). Predictors of happiness in married couples. *Personality and Individual Differences, 17* (3), 313–321.

Safran, J. D., Crocker, P., McMain, S., & Murray, P. (1990). Therapeutic alliance rupture as a therapy event for empirical investigation. *Psychotherapy, 27* (3), 154–165.

Safran, J. D., & Muran, J. C. (1998). The therapeutic alliance in brief psychotherapy: General Principles. In J. D. Safran & J. C. Muran (Eds.), *The therapeutic alliance in brief psychotherapy* (pp. 217–229). New York: APA Press.

Safran, J. D., & Muran, J. C. (2005). Brief relational therapy and the resolution of ruptures in the therapeutic alliance, *Psychotherapy Bulletin, 40*, 13–17.

Surrey, J. L. (2005). Relational psychotherapy, relational mindfulness. In C. K. Germer, R. D. Siegel, & P. R. Fulton (Eds.), *Mindfulness and psychotherapy* (pp. 91–112). New York: Guilford.

Thorberg, F. A., & Lyvers, M. (2006). Attachment, fear of intimacy and differentiation of self among clients in substance disorder treatment facilities. *Addictive Behaviors, 31* (4), 732–737.

Van Orden, K., Wingate, L. R., Gordon, K. H., & Joiner, T. E. (2005). Interpersonal factors as vulnerability to psychopathology over the life course. In B. L. Hankin & J. R. Z. Abela (Eds.), *Development of psychopathology: A vulnerability-stress perspective* (pp. 136–160). Thousand Oaks, CA: Sage Publications Inc.

Chapter 7
The Course of Therapy: Beginning, Middle and End Phases of FAP

Mavis Tsai, Jonathan W. Kanter, Sara J. Landes, Reo W. Newring, and Robert J. Kohlenberg

Each phase of FAP, the beginning, middle, and end, has distinctive focal points and evokes different types of CRBs. For example, at the beginning of therapy, therapists can explore how clients typically begin a new relationship or activity (e.g., ignoring reservations and jumping in quickly, moving cautiously, starting out with high hopes and getting disappointed), how this relates to the way they are beginning therapy, and what they can do to increase the likelihood of having a good therapeutic experience. The substantive work takes place in the middle phase of therapy, where clients confront the emergence of core life and relationship issues in the therapy environment, and where 'ideal FAP interactions' that generalize to daily life are the focus. The end phase of therapy, a time to consolidate gains, may bring up feelings and memories of previous transitions and losses. Clients often learn to say goodbye meaningfully in a way they never have done before.

The duration of FAP may vary from a relatively brief treatment to several years depending on the severity of the client's presenting problems and the availability of the therapist in the setting in which it is conducted (e.g., a university clinic versus private practice). As discussed in Kanter, Tsai and Kohlenberg (in press), FAP techniques may also be used to enhance other treatments, including Cognitive Therapy (Kohlenberg, Kanter, Bolling, Parker, & Tsai, 2002), Behavioral Activation (Kanter, Manos, Busch, & Rusch, in press) and Acceptance and Commitment Therapy (Callaghan, Gregg, Marx, Kohlenberg, & Gifford, 2004). In research studies (e.g., Kohlenberg et al., 2002; Holman, Sanders, Kohlenberg, Bolling, & Tsai, 2006), effective FAP or FAP enhanced therapy has been conducted in 16–20 sessions. In this chapter the therapeutic interactions described involve relatively short-term FAP of approximately 20 sessions.

There is no one absolute way to conduct FAP. This chapter presents one approach, based primarily on the successful therapy experiences of the authors. It is important to note, however, that above all else FAP is a functional

M. Tsai (✉)
3245 Fairview Avenue East, Suite 301, Seattle, WA 98102, USA
e-mail: mavis@u.washington.edu

M. Tsai et al., *A Guide to Functional Analytic Psychotherapy*,
DOI 10.1007/978-0-387-09787-9_7, © Springer Science+Business Media, LLC 2009

treatment. Thus the specific techniques and tools suggested in this chapter should be implemented, or not implemented, in the context of a sound functional rationale linked to FAP's five rules (see Chapter 4 on Therapeutic Technique). In other words, how will technique A affect client X? Will it help in the observation of CRBs (Rule 1)? Will it function to evoke (Rule 2) or reinforce (Rule 3) CRBs? Will it assist in determining if CRBs have been reinforced by the therapist (Rule 4)? Or will it aid in the generalization of gains (Rule 5)? If the therapist is not clear how a certain technique could generate one of those functions, the method can certainly be applied, but it is arguably not a FAP technique in that inst-ance, functionally speaking. In a complementary fashion, many procedures not described in this chapter may be applied functionally in the service of the five rules.

Prior to Therapy

If possible, a telephone conversation with potential clients prior to the first session may set the stage for a very intense FAP process that begins immediately during the first session. As is typical of many therapy beginnings, this phone conversation may include a discussion of what the client is seeking from therapy and whether FAP is a good match for him or her. In addition, the therapist may probe for and assess initial CRBs by asking clients how they feel about schedul-ing their first appointment, and their initial reactions to the phone conversation.

The intensity of a full FAP experience dictates that clients provide informed consent and enter the relationship knowingly. Thus, if a therapist is planning to conduct FAP in a very explicit, evocative and emotional manner, it may be useful also to mail to clients prior to the start of therapy a statement describing the FAP rationale (the 'FAP rap'; for a sample statement and examples of FAP raps, refer to Chapter 4).

Beginning Phase of Therapy

In the initial sessions, in addition to assessment and case conceptualization (see Chapter 3), the goal is for the therapist to establish oneself as a positive reinforcer, to launch an authentic and memorable relationship, and to set the stage for a meaningful and transformative therapy. Every interaction the therapist has with a client, whether via telephone, email, or in person, has the potential to build the relationship and to evoke or reinforce CRBs.

A number of tasks are important to initiate in the first session, including creating trust and safety and instilling hope. These tasks may be considered important in any type of therapy, but they are particularly important in FAP in terms of building a foundation for the therapeutic relationship.

Creating Trust and Safety

Trust, behaviorally speaking, may be seen as a predisposition to approach another person in a situation in which one could potentially get hurt. Thus, trust essentially describes a situation in which one person is predisposed to take risks in the presence of, and toward, another person. Instilling trust and safety are crucial in FAP because clients are shaped and reinforced to take risks, to be vulnerable, to push beyond their boundaries of comfort, and to take more steps to trust the therapist. That said, the behavior of trusting may very well be a goal of therapy and it is the rare client indeed who will trust fully from the first session. Indeed, such blind trust may be as problematic as an inability to trust.

How to foster a sense of trust and safety, as everything else in FAP, is an idiographic process. Thus, for many clients, a host of what have been referred to as 'nonspecific' behaviors, such as accurate empathy, warmth, reflective listening, and validation, may be very important early therapist behaviors toward this end. Although many theorists, particularly Carl Rogers (1957), argue that the important quality of such nonspecific therapist responses is that they are unconditional (not contingent on particular client responses), the FAP therapist takes a different stance. As described more fully by Follette, Naugle, and Callaghan (1996), these responses are seen as potentially reinforcing broad classes of behaviors (e.g., trusting and other therapy-facilitating and relationship-building behaviors). The therapist behaviors are seen as generalized contingent reinforcement for the class of behaviors necessary for therapy to occur and a relationship to develop. This class includes behaviors like showing up on time, disclosing important personal information, paying attention and responding appropriately to questions, demonstrating caring and concern for the therapist's feelings, and being engaged in-session.

For the typical FAP client, however, fostering trust and safety may move beyond these basic therapy skills and into areas that are much more personal and genuine. Therapists can foster a sense of trust and safety with these clients by being more forthcoming with their thoughts, reactions, and observations (not hiding behind a therapist persona), and by encouraging clients: (1) to ask questions (e.g., What are your questions about me, my training, my background? or What qualities do you most seek in a therapist?); (2) to voice their reactions to the therapist (e.g., What reactions do you have to my gender, age, ethnicity?); and (3) to voice their feelings related to the appointment (e.g., What are your thoughts and feelings evoked by having this appointment today? or What would make this a really good first session for you?). The FAP therapist, however, remains open to the possibility that these therapist behaviors may be aversive to clients depending on their histories, so assessment of the therapist's stimulus functions (Rule 4) is important from the very beginning of therapy.

Numerous behaviors can help to engender another's trust. These trust-building behaviors are not specific to the therapy situation, because in FAP we do not believe the therapist becomes a different person when stepping into a therapy room. Rather, behaviors that are well practiced and integrated outside therapy are more likely to occur in the therapy room. These trust-enhancing behaviors may include: (1) providing accurate empathic reflections; (2) being honest and genuine; (3) keeping one's word; (4) being consistent and predictable, or explaining why one is being inconsistent and unpredictable so that the behavior makes sense; (5) recognizing another's expectations, and correcting them if not accurate, or explaining why one is not meeting them; (6) admitting when one does not know the answer; (7) seeing what's in someone's best interest and not taking advantage of or hurting him or her; (8) remembering the important things someone has revealed—people, events, memories; (9) being willing to match the other person's vulnerability; (10) being able to admit and take responsibility for mistakes, to repair ruptures; and (11) treating client truths and disclosures with care and reverence.

The importance of fostering trust and safety cannot be overstated in FAP. The therapist may choose to describe this process as 'creating a sacred space' for the client in which the therapy work may occur (refer to Chapter 4). A sacred space is dedicated exclusively to facilitating the client's growth. Whether or not a FAP therapist chooses to use the term 'sacred space' with clients, the FAP therapy relationship is indeed sacred, as defined here, and creating trust and safety is essential.

Instilling Hope

Therapists are generally taught to avoid raising client expectations excessively and not to make promises about the efficacy of treatment in case clients are disappointed. It is important, however, to focus on what is possible, to consistently see the best in one's clients, to validate their strengths and the difficulties they have overcome, to believe in what is possible for them, and to believe in one's own strengths and efficacy. Positive statements (e.g., "I'm excited about working with you because you seem so motivated" or "I really respect how tenacious you've been working to overcome your childhood abuse") can be experienced by clients as evocative (Rule 2) and/or reinforcing (Rule 3). It is helpful to ask about the impact of these statements. Note that whatever affirmative statements you make to your clients, however, need to be true for you, because a typical CRB1 is "You're just saying nice things because I'm paying you." It is thus important that therapists mean what they say, so that if a client doubts the statement, it can judged as truly a CRB1 rather than the result of a T1 (therapist problematic behavior).

Taking the Time to Form a Meaningful Relationship

It takes time to create a meaningful relationship, although the length of time required will vary from client to client. Often FAP therapists will experience the therapeutic relationship as a real relationship before their clients do. Most clients enter therapy not expecting to form the kind of real and genuine relationship with the therapist that occurs in FAP, while the FAP therapist does expect this. For example, SJL treated Allie, a warm, likable young woman with depression and borderline personality features, for approximately 20 sessions. Quite early in therapy SJL began to care about Allie and was genuinely concerned about her well-being and progress in treatment. Allie would remark, however, that the therapist could not really know her and therefore could not care for her. Despite Allie's skepticism, SJL continued to respond to her in a genuine manner and to express her caring. It was not until session 12, when discussing a recent sexual encounter with her ex-boyfriend, that Allie appeared concerned about the therapist's reaction to her behavior and asked, "Are you mad at me?" This was the first instance of Allie demonstrating that she viewed the therapeutic relationship as real.

As demonstrated in the above example, a client initially may be unwilling to accept that the therapist cares for him/her. The therapist may have to distinguish between a 'normal' period, during which the client does not care about the therapist, from not caring about the therapist as a CRB1 of blocking or avoiding relationship growth. There is no set rule for determining the normal or average time to build a relationship, thus it may be difficult to distinguish between these repertoires. The therapist may simply choose to ask the client if this is a problem behavior for him or her (e.g., "Are you having trouble trusting me?"). Therapists also can use the "Beginning of Therapy Questionnaire" (see Appendix F) to assess if the therapy relationship bears similarity to the beginning stages of the client's other relationships.

Some clients entering therapy with histories of abuse, neglect or other forms of punishment will avoid attempts at relationship building. These more emotionally wounded clients will require that great care be taken when building trust and in aspiring to the behaviors listed above. We are all flawed individuals, and thus if we fail these clients, what is most important is our ability to repair any harm we have done.

Therapy Forms

As an aid to help therapists become more sensitive to the different types of CRBs and to evoke client CRBs, numerous forms and questionnaires (discussed in Chapter 4 and included in the Appendix) can help to guide therapy. In this first phase of therapy, clients begin providing weekly written feedback using the "Session Bridging Form" (Appendix D). This form includes questions asking how connected clients feel toward the therapist, what was helpful and not helpful about the previous session, what they are reluctant to say, and what issues came up in-session that are similar to daily life problems. A more in-depth assessment of attachment and closeness can be obtained after each session through use of the "FAP Experiences of Closeness in the Therapeutic Relationship" questionnaire (FAP-ECR, Appendix L) and the "PTSR (Patient-Therapist Session Report) on Relationships" (Appendix M). By session 3 or 4, the "Beginning of Therapy Questionnaire" (Appendix F) should be assigned. At the end of the beginning phase of therapy (between sessions 5–8), the case conceptualization (Appendix A) is presented to the client for feedback (see Chapter 3). All of these forms facilitate a focus on clinically relevant behaviors.

Beginning Therapy with 'Alicia'

To impart a sense of what one may expect in each phase of therapy, below we provide transcript excerpts from the beginning, middle, and ending phases of MT's 20 session treatment with 'Alicia.' Alicia was a 34-year-old Caucasian female who entered treatment for depression and smoking cessation. This transcript of the first session illustrates the concept of creating a sacred space of safety and trust. This took place through MT's encouragement of Alicia's questions and reactions, by MT being forthcoming with her own thoughts and reactions, by instilling hope, and by beginning to focus on the therapeutic relationship. Possible CRBs are also indicated.

Therapist: What's it been like for you leading up to our first appointment? Looking forward to it? Too long to wait?
Client: I was looking forward to it.
T: Any thoughts, feelings leading up to coming here; what were you thinking today?
C: Not very much at all, it was a crazy day. It kind of stuck in the back of my mind. [Possible CRB1 of avoidance.]
T: You've had a ton of stuff to fill out; what's been your experience doing all that?
C: Kind of feeling like opening a door, someone opening my head, all the questions are repeated and rephrased. It's interesting...
T: You're definitely doing a lot of work... we're going to make this as effective as possible for you.
C: I'm a really good actress. I've had to be since I got depressed, to get through life. [Possible CRB1, being an actress in the session.]
T: What feels important to you today for us to get to that you want to talk about? Did you have certain ideas about what would make this a really good session?
C: No. [Possible CRB1, not being proactive.]
T: So you're going to leave it up to me?
C: I can help you figure it out [possible CRB2], the first session is always hard, 'cause there's so much of me that you don't know about...

T: The first session is hard, you don't quite know what to expect. I have a long list of things of things to get to today, but one of the things is what's important to you, because it's very important to me that this treatment be tailored to you. So you read about the therapy, right?

C: Yeah, I really like what you wrote.

T: I want to go over that and answer any questions you have... You can let me know what you like and don't like, we can go over... your smoking quit date, although that may be too overwhelming to do right now.

C: Yeah, that would be overwhelming. [Possible CRB2, assertion.]

T: Okay, we'll wait on that. [Reinforces CRB2.] And I want to answer any questions you have about me. You don't know that much about me.

C: I see that you are also affiliated with the University of Washington in addition to being in private practice. What do you do there?

T: I'm a clinical instructor, I supervise graduate students, I teach a class there on FAP, and I'm also involved in treatment research.

C: Oh great.

T: Any questions about my training, my background?

C: Yeah.

T: I got my doctorate here in 1982, did my undergraduate training at UCLA. In 1976 I came here for graduate school and thought I'd go back to southern California and never did.

C: That's interesting.

T: Do you have reactions to my being a woman, being Asian American?

C: I'm thankful you are a woman, since I saw a male psychiatrist, and his whole schtick about his being a guy, very strange man... accent. Since then I probably sought out female therapists.

T: How do you like your therapists to be, it seems you like your psychiatrist a lot. Do you want me to be directive, nondirective?

C: I really like people to be directive with me, but at the same time I'm ultra sensitive... (Client goes on to give an example of how bad she felt when her psychiatrist raised the issue of their unpaid balance.)

T: So did you tell her that you felt really bad?

C: Um, no. [Possible CRB1, non-assertion of feelings with therapist.]

T: So one thing I ask is that you tell me when you feel bad about something or are upset, 'cause you were reading in this rationale, one focus of our treatment is going to be on our relationship and how it connects to all your other relationships. (Therapist gives a brief version of the 'FAP rap'.) I notice you've got some other good relationships going.

        (Therapist and client spend the next few minutes exploring the client's sense of isolation and loneliness despite her good relationships.)

C: I feel emotional.
T: You feel emotional talking about your loneliness.
C: I think so, it's one thing to circle numbers on questionnaires...
        (Begins crying.) May I bother you for some tissues? [Client crying
        in first session is CRB2.]
        (Therapist naturally reinforces client with kind and attentive
        body language, and also decides not to exacerbate client's discom-
        fort by overly focusing on her crying.)
T: What's it like for you to notice what you circle?
C: For me personally I can kind of deny my miserableness on paper,
        but if I to have to talk to somebody about it, it's painful.
T: How much hope do you have that this treatment will help you?
C: I have a lot of hope actually.
T: Tell me what you feel positively about.
C: ... It feels like I've been treading water for a long time, and this
        feels like something I do need. I do need a direction, so I feel like
        this is going to be beneficial for me.
T: I'm good at giving direction and I'm good at hand holding.
C: You seem like you are. You have very kind eyes. And I'm also
        hopeful that I'll quit smoking.
T: You seem really motivated to quit smoking and I'm really moti-
        vated to help you... One of the things the form says is that therapy
        is a sacred space for you. When I'm here, I'm not thinking about
        anything else, this space is protected. I take it really seriously...
        (Therapist and client spend time discussing the handout "What
        We Will Focus on In Therapy.")
T: What are your thoughts about your session, as we are coming to
        the end of it?
C: Good, I feel encouraged.
T: What stands out to me is your perseverance. You've been depressed
        since you were 13, and there's something about you that perseveres,
        there's some incredible strength inside you that keeps you growing
        and keeps you hopeful. I'm excited because if you like to take risks,
        you and I are going to get along really well. What stands out to you?
C: I was able to cry. I don't spend a lot of time crying alone. I always
        feel a little better.
T: After you cry.
C: Yeah. I'm surprised and encouraged.
T: You're surprised you were able to cry.
C: I push it away and push it down.
T: It's also good for me to know that you feel encouraged that you
        could cry, there has to be a certain amount of trust...
C: I feel good, comfortable with you; I like you. You don't freak me
        out or anything. Obviously people don't get along with everybody.

T: It's really important to me that we matter to each other.
C: I felt encouraged that we have rapport.
T: Yes, me too.

Middle Phase of Therapy

The middle of therapy is essentially the heart of FAP. By this time, the therapeutic relationship should be well-formed. The CRBs occurring in therapy are those that probably would occur in an ongoing relationship in the client's daily life, as opposed to one in its initial stages. It is important to remember that there is no clear delineation between the beginning and middle stages of FAP. This is due, in part, to the idiographic and functional nature of the treatment. As clients vary in presenting problems and characteristics, they also vary in the rate and depth at which they form relationships.

Gradually, as a case conceptualization is collaboratively built and a relationship is formed, the therapeutic focus on trust, safety, and generalized contingent reinforcement of broad classes of such behavior sharpens to include behaviors that are more relevant to the client's goals. Therapists focus more directly on CRB1s, calling attention to them or blocking them, and promote CRB2s, including fostering relationship skills as assessed by the FIAT (refer to Chapters 3 and 4). Generalization strategies (Rule 5) also should be of greater focus in the middle of therapy. Homework assignments require clients to try out new behaviors in daily life that were effective in the therapy session, and CRB2s ideally occur every session.

Several behavioral considerations should also be mentioned at this point. Ideally, the FAP therapist should be reinforcing successive approximations to the targeted behaviors the client will acquire. At the onset of therapy the therapist reinforces a broad response class. As therapy progresses, the therapist should increase the specificity of the response required for reinforcement. This may mean what was considered a CRB2 at the beginning of therapy no longer meets the threshold[1]. In other words, the case conceptualization should be evolving as the client improves, and therapist responding to CRBs should evolve in tandem (for a primer on behavioral principles and shaping, refer to Pryor, 2002). This process is fluid in that ever more specific instances of improvement will be encouraged and reinforced by the therapist. Occasionally, the therapist may return to an earlier, broader set of reinforced client behaviors and will express appreciation for the client's willingness to come back to treatment when it is clearly difficult to do so. By reinforcing these client responses acquired earlier in treatment, the therapist is attempting to reinforce intermittently the necessary but not sufficient client behaviors required for treatment to effect change.

---

[1] This may be reminiscent of footage of Skinner shaping pigeons to turn in a circle; a 30 degree counterclockwise head movement that was initially reinforced is no longer reinforced once the pigeon has learned to turn 180 degrees.

In this stage of therapy FAP therapists also focus a great deal on the function of client and therapist behavior, the moment-to moment in-vivo processes between therapist and client, the impact of client responses on the therapist, and the impact of the therapist's behavior on the client. Forms that are assigned or referred to in this phase include "Typical FAP Questions", the "Emotional Risk Log", and the "Mid-Therapy Questionnaire" (see Appendices E, N, G). These forms can help therapists evoke client thoughts and feelings about the therapeutic relationship.

Focus on Avoidance

A typical focus within FAP is avoidance and the central role it may play in client difficulties. Avoidance may appear in-vivo when clients are not in contact with features of the therapist-client relationship that reflect their outside life relationships. For example, a client may work very hard to view the therapist as a professional, rather than a real person who cares about him or her. A caring statement may be reinterpreted as, "Something you have to say because I am paying you." In this situation the therapist may wonder aloud if the client also has reasons for why others in his or her life may not be telling the truth about how they feel. More importantly, the therapist can gently block this avoidance by repeating the caring statement, which will function as exposure and hopefully prompt CRB2s.

Avoidance may also appear in the therapy room in a much more basic sense. Specifically, a client may work to avoid truly feeling whatever there is to feel in a given therapy moment. This is an interesting FAP situation because the CRB1 of avoidance may not be particularly interpersonal in that the client may avoid the experience of true emotion even when alone; on its surface this does not appear to be an interpersonal repertoire that can be shaped by a FAP therapist with reinforcement. For many clients who have difficulty experiencing emotions, however, this difficulty parlays into problems with intimacy, trust, and empathy. How can one truly understand and accept the experience of another if one cannot do so with oneself? For example, in the case of Alicia, avoidance at first appeared simple—she had not allowed herself to cry about her beloved dog's death. But for her, grieving about one loss led to contacting the pain from other losses in her life, such as relationship break-ups that were heart-breaking for her. Letting herself cry was associated with a loss of control that most likely had been punished by those close to her in the past.

Thus, although the CRB1 of emotional avoidance may not be interpersonal, the CRB2—experiencing the emotion fully and without defense—can be extremely powerful when shared with another human being. FAP therapists therefore work a great deal with the CRB1 of avoidance and promoting the CRB2 of contact with experience for both intrapersonal and interpersonal reasons, and deep emotional contact almost always strengthens the therapeutic relationship.

In FAP the key to promoting and responding to deep emotional contact is often to focus on the direct visceral experience. Clients may be encouraged to experience their avoidance fully by describing what they are feeling in their bodies, and as emotions surface, to stay in contact with the visceral experience. Reinforcing this contact may be quite simple but profound by accepting clients' experiences and pain, letting them feel one's support, and amplifying one's own closeness that is felt in response.

Several other considerations are also important in situations where there is a great deal of fear of contacting what is being avoided. As in all good exposure therapy, it is important to allow clients to be in charge of their own pacing, and to feel fully their choice to stay where they are. It may also be helpful to explore what it means to avoid versus to move forward, and to validate all that they are already doing in the service of their growth. It may be easy for a therapist to underestimate the tremendous difficulty of contacting the pain of grief and loss. Needless to say, therapists have to be fully committed to facing their own avoidance issues in order to be effective in reducing their clients' avoidance.

A Typical Ideal FAP Interaction

During the middle phase of therapy therapists pay attention to opportunities to create 'ideal' FAP interactions. A typical FAP interaction often begins with discussion of a problem a client is having in the outside world. For example, consider the transcript between JWK and a depressed young adult woman, 'Nathalie,' presented below. The transcript has been slightly modified for the present purposes to enhance clarity.

During the session Nathalie was describing her fear of being genuine with a man, Ryan, she had been attracted to at a social event. JWK asked Nathalie if she ever felt a similar fear with him. Such out-to-in parallels (see Chapter 4) can shift the focus to CRBs. Nathalie responded that she did feel such fear with JWK, and that she was feeling it "right now." JWK asked how she knew she was feeling it in the moment and she responded, "Because I am working very hard at not crying, at not showing any emotion to you right now."

Often, especially earlier in therapy, the first CRB to occur in a session is a CRB1. This was the case with Nathalie. JWK observed that Nathalie's response was a CRB1 (Rule 1), specifically emotional avoidance, and attempted to evoke a CRB2 (Rule 2) by saying, "What can you do right now to be more genuine, more real with me?" Over the next several minutes, Nathalie continued to avoid being more genuine, and JWK gently continued to encourage her. This also is not uncommon, as CRB repertoires can be quite persistent. Eventually she began to cry a little and asked, "What does it mean to you, that I am sitting over here feeling so much?"

JWK recognized this as a CRB2 and amplified his feelings to her in an attempt to be naturally reinforcing. He said, "When you cry like this, it pulls at my empathy, it warms me up to you, I feel a sense of caring for you when I see you like this and I just think, this is the honest truth, I just think I really like this person and I hope I can help her on this. I see you're struggling, and it feels a little sad for me—just because you're sad, and I like you, and so it makes me a little sad."

JWK's response was quite evocative for Nathalie and she began to cry a great deal, continuing for several minutes. This was, in fact, the first time Nathalie had truly cried in therapy. JWK recognized this as unusual and a significant CRB2. He continued to offer support but said very little. When Nathalie had stopped crying naturally, he asked her, "How do you feel right now?" (Rule 4).

Nathalie responded, "Relieved. Exhausted. A little nervous still but intense." After some discussion of this, JWK provided a summary of what happened (Rule 5) by saying, "You started out feeling emotional, showing that a little bit, and having some fears about it, and you checked it out with me. Once you heard what I was really thinking, it kind of opened up a lot for you and you came all out, and now you feel relieved, a little safer, but still some nerves; it didn't all go away obviously. Am I getting that about accurately?" Nathalie agreed. "Okay. So you feel safer... by not avoiding." After some discussion, JWK ended the interaction with an in-to-out parallel (Rule 5) to assist in generalization of this CRB2, "Well, if I had reacted differently, you wouldn't feel safer. And so the question is, how are people out in the world going to react? Right? You know how your mom and dad will react but the question is what do you do with the rest of the world, like Ryan?"

In summary, the ideal FAP interaction begins with an out-to-in parallel based on therapist observation of a similarity between an outside problem and a CRB1 (Rule 1). This is followed by attempts to evoke (Rule 2) and, when they occur, naturally reinforce CRB2 (Rule 3). The therapist then checks the reinforcing value of his/her response (Rule 4) and provides a series of generalization strategies (Rule 5), including a functional description of what just occurred, an in-to-out parallel, and a homework assignment in which the client is encouraged to take the CRB2 'on the road.'

Another transcript is presented below to help increase clarity. While most therapeutic communications are not this succinct, additional talking has been excluded to highlight the ideal interaction and application of the five rules in sequence.

Client: [Description of an outside problem.] Every time my wife criticizes my behavior, I get defensive.

Therapist: [Thinking about a potential CRB earlier in-session (Rule 1) and draws an out-to-in parallel.] Is it possible that this occurred between us earlier in-session?

C: [CRB1.] No, it's completely different here. Why would you ask that?

T: [Rules 2 and 3: Notices and responds contingently to CRB1 and evokes a CRB2, not necessarily in the same statement.] Well I asked because it seemed like you were a little defensive then and you seem a little defensive now. What could you try right now that would appear less defensive?

C:	[CRB2.] I guess I feel like when I receive criticism, my mood changes very quickly and I feel kind of like my esteem has deflated.
T:	[Rule 3: Responds contingently to CRB2.] You know, hearing you say that makes me feel so much more connected to you than getting a defensive response.
T:	[Rule 4: Checks on reinforcing value of response to CRB2.] How was it for you to hear me say that I feel closer to you? [or] After hearing that from me are you more or less ready to talk about what happened earlier in-session?
T:	[Rule 5: Describe functional relations involved in in-session behavior.] So what I just saw happen was: I said something that deflated you and you told me how it felt for you, your sharing that made me feel closer to you and I told you so, which allowed us to have a difficult discussion.
T:	[Rule 5: Draws parallel to outside relationships.] So it sounds like this situation is very similar to what goes on between you and your wife.
T:	[Rule 5: Gives homework.] Do you think that you could try this same thing with your wife over the course of the week?

The Middle of Therapy with 'Alicia'

In this transcript from the middle phase of therapy (Session 10) with Alicia, MT is focusing on Alicia's progress in 'loving' herself, behaviorally defined as being less harsh and more loving in her self-talk, engaging in self-care such as exercising and eating more healthily, and letting herself believe MT's high positive regard of her. As you read this transcript try to identify components of the ideal FAP interaction.

Therapist:	Let's both take a breath and be with each other here... I'm reading on your Session Bridging form that you are starting to love yourself. That's so exciting for me to hear; it's so huge.
Client:	It is, and maybe this is what I really need to drive home, that you help me be better for myself... This is the tool that I've never learned.
T:	Loving yourself?
C:	Yeah. I wrote it down and put it in my special locket that I got from my grandmother. I play with my locket every once in a while and when I touch it, I think "Oh I know what's in there." It says, "Of all the people in the world I deserve my love the most. You, yourself as much as anybody in the universe, deserve your love and affection."
T:	What does this commitment feel like, that this is the tool that was missing?

C: Exciting, but nebulous. I'm still kind of in training. I'm figuring it out.

T: So we're in the middle of me responding to how you're changing, and you're so engaged in this process. I feel every bit as engaged. The ways that you're thinking about things and writing about them, it's really, really exciting to me. I find myself trying to contain myself, because you're probably not used to it.

C: And I probably wouldn't believe you. I can understand how it would be exciting though, to have somebody working with you, who's going with the flow.

T: So you don't believe me?

C: No. I mean I do, but, it's just ... I guess if I let it sink in I would believe you.

T: How would you let sink in, in this moment? That I'm excited about the ways you're changing.

C: If I think about it in the third person ... like, I have a friend who's a therapist and she has a really engaged client who's willing to really try. Then I realize that that would make me pretty psyched. Especially because this is your work, it's what you're interested in, I mean, it's huge and this could help a lot of people.

T: Yes, it could help a lot of people.

C: I also think I'm not used to people expressing their feelings either, I mean you express your feelings and I'm not used to that ... I really value honest relationships; that's so important to me. I guess I have to trust the person, in order to believe what they're telling me. It's just hard because ... at work my supervisor ... doesn't give me concrete support.

T: So you wish she would give you back more concrete feedback. And when I do it here ...

C: I believe you.

T: When I was telling you earlier that I was excited about all the ways you've changed, you said 'I don't believe you.' But now you're saying you do believe me?

C: 'Cause I think I've processed and now that I thought about it, it makes sense. I just need to do that for a while. I have a reflex that throws up a wall, "No I don't believe you. Why would I?"

T: And then you processed it and ...

C: Once I soften it, yeah.

T: What does it feel like physically?

C: When you first said it there wasn't even a physical feeling.

T: Just like a wall?

C: Yeah, and now I feel like I've let it in my body, it's in my body and it feels good.

T: I haven't even started telling you all the reasons I'm excited. Well, I started . . . by saying, that's just awesome that you showed me this locket that's more than 60 years old, with the message that there's no one more important to love than you. And that hits me hard, in the stomach, I feel it. I actually feel a little teary. [T2, MT is expressing strong feelings; Rule 2, evoke CRB; Rule 3, naturally reinforcing client's progress.]

C: That's nice. The funny thing was that when I did it I thought I was just doing it as a tool to help myself remember. Now I realize I was doing it because it meant so much more to me.

T: Yeah and I really get it that this means so much to you and you're really committed to this process of loving yourself.

C: Yeah. It's a tool. It's not even a tool; it's a part of life that I miss out on. And I really want to do it.

T: This feels like a turning point. [Rule 3, natural reinforcement.]

C: This week felt really important. . . I have so much sympathy, I mean I work in a hospital and I want to be a caregiver. And I can't do any of those things if I can't do them for myself. I won't be all there, there'll be part of me missing.

T: . . . Can you tell that I'm emotional about what we're talking about? [Rule 2, evoke CRB.]

C: Yeah.

T: How does that affect you? [Rule 2, evoke CRB; Rule 4, assess impact.]

C: I don't know, it's kind of weird, but I'm comfortable with it. It doesn't bother me.

T: I'm kind of surprised at how I'm reacting. I think I really get how big this is and that's what I'm reacting to. [Rule 3, natural reinforcement.]

C: Yeah, I kinda got hit psychically, by a two-by-four. Which I needed, and it took a long time. I don't know, I never realized, whenever I've tried to take care of myself or have self-love for myself. . . In my relationships with my boyfriends, it was always about my sacrifice, always.

T: . . . And in this moment what does loving yourself mean, in this process with me? [Rule 2, evoke CRB, bringing her feelings and behavior into the moment.]

C: I just have so much fear involved. I'm so afraid of connecting with myself because I've hated myself for so long. So I'm just completely convinced that part of me is just so awful and ugly, and so pitiful. And how could I possibly love that. But I was thinking about things that I could say to myself, and actually today I was really pissed off 'cause I have this huge zit on my chin. . . But you know I just got up and looked in the mirror and said "this will pass."

T: ...And part of loving yourself more is being able to do these things, being open to the experience of the present moment. It seems like you've been doing that with me in sessions. Really being here. [Client gave MT an example of how she was being more loving to herself, but not an in-vivo example as asked for. MT suggests that the client is being more open to herself by being truly present in the moment with her.]

C: ...I mean you say you're so excited and everything, but I just can't imagine having to sit across from me, and listen to me...

T: ...I feel so much compassion for you.

C: But, I don't know how you could...

T: Do you want me to go into it, why I feel compassion?

C: Yeah. I mean that's the part I don't get. [CRB2, asking for what she wants, even though the information may be uncomfortable for her to hear.]

T: Okay... Be open to what I have to say. When you were born, first of all you had this really difficult labor and you started having all these physical illnesses, asthma, the infections, it's not your fault. Your mother was depressed, and it sounds like she was self-focused, you've used the word narcissistic. You said you felt emotionally abused, and abandoned. So how else could you be when you haven't had the kind of support that's rightfully yours? It leads to feeling depressed and hopeless. You've had all these obstacles and suffered so much, and here you are trying your best and making all these changes. And I could tell that from our first session, that you're not a quitter, that you persevere, that you wanted to try and that you have these ideals for yourself, about your goals and dreams, you want to do acupuncture and develop a relationship again, to be healthy, to commit to not smoking. So that's mainly what I'm aware of... [Rule 3, naturally reinforcing her commitment to therapy; rule 2, evoke CRB of having a hard time believing positive feedback.] How are you doing with my feedback right now?

C: Good.

T: Good, 'cause I started by saying I really want you to be in your body and listen to me, that this is why I feel compassion, and you took it in?

C: It makes me feel better, I feel kinda psyched.

T: Yeah? How does that feel?

C: It's the times when I actually believe somebody's compliments.

T: It's not a compliment, unless that's just a shorthand way of saying something that's positive about you. But it feels like the truth.

C: Yeah.

T: It's how I see and experience you.

C: Yeah and compliments aren't necessarily honest. I guess that's the difference.

This interaction is an example of MT giving Alicia a great deal of genuine and positive feedback in terms of her personal reactions, and working with Alicia's CRB1 of not believing and facilitating her CRB2 of letting in MT's positive regard. This type of therapist feedback, an authentic and positive personal reaction to the client, may be both evocative (Rule 2) and naturally reinforcing (Rule 3), and thus is an important component of FAP.

End Phase of Therapy

As at the beginning of therapy, the end phase of therapy in FAP has unique CRBs. Termination of therapy is likely to be difficult for both the client and the therapist, especially if a strong relationship has been formed. Therefore, termination should be discussed early, so that both participants can have a number of sessions to discuss the ending of therapy. This process may vary depending on the length of treatment. For example, in short-term or time-limited therapy, the client and therapist may know at the outset that treatment only will consist of 20 sessions or a given number of months. In long-term treatment, termination may occur once the client and therapist agree that goals have been met or that sufficient progress has been made. To reiterate, as FAP is an idiographic treatment, there is no set length of time for treatment and no set number of sessions needed to process termination.

Termination should be viewed as an opportunity to help the client build a new repertoire for loss and endings. Often, relationships in the outside world do not end well. Sometimes they end cordially, sometimes angrily, and on some occasions the individuals just gradually slip apart without ever saying goodbye. But rarely is the ending (except perhaps when a death is imminent and is being prepared for) seen as an opportunity to truly explore its meaning and to feel it fully. FAP therapists strive for such meaningful endings. The therapist may initiate a conversation about termination by saying something such as, "Endings and loss are a part of life and relationships, and therapy and the therapeutic relationship allow for a unique opportunity to end an important relationship thoughtfully by acknowledging the impact we have had on each other."

The "End of Therapy Tools" (see Appendix K) can help the process of consolidating gains and saying a meaningful goodbye. One question on the form that can be explored in great detail is, "For many clients, the end of therapy brings up feelings and memories of previous transitions and losses. What thoughts and feelings do endings in general bring up for you? What thoughts and feelings are you having about the ending of this therapy relationship?" Given that the therapist will now have a well-formed and evolved case conceptualization of the client, he/she should then determine if the client's responses are CRB1s or CRB2s and then respond appropriately.

FAP therapists also may choose to write an end-of-therapy letter—such a letter can be an important component of the parting process. The letter may include a description of progress made, what the therapist appreciates about the client, any interactions that were moving to the therapist or stood out during therapy, what the therapist will remember or take away from therapy, what the therapist wants the client to take away, hopes and wishes for the client, and parting advice. These are also types of issues the client and therapist should discuss when talking about termination. Providing clients with a closing letter gives them something tangible to take away from therapy and a concrete reminder of their progress and the relationship. Here is an example of one such letter written by MT to Alicia, and read aloud to her in the final session.

Our life is an apprenticeship to the truth that around every circle another can be drawn; that there is no end in nature, but every end is a beginning... Ralph Waldo Emerson (n.d.)

Dear Alicia,

This letter signifies a graduation with honors on your part. Looking at the list of lofty goals we set for you, it's absolutely amazing how you have either attained or made significant progress towards all of them: establish a therapeutic alliance, clarify your values, take steps in valued directions, be more social, be smoke free, increase self-acceptance, increase mindfulness, increase empowered thinking, be with and process avoided feelings, process losses, decrease depression, increase health, learn from our therapy relationship as a microcosm of daily life relationships. Although we may be seeing each other again, we have completed a major symphony in our work together. It's been said that "Great is the art of beginning, but greater is the art of ending" (Lazurus Long, n.d.). How can I adequately summarize in a letter the highlights of this important and meaningful journey we've undertaken? I am grateful that our paths intersected, that the universe brought us together for this span of time. In your work, there's been much pain, but many glimpses of the happiness that percolates underneath, awaiting liberation. There's been much struggle, but so much more triumph.

I've really, really enjoyed working with you. The purpose of this therapy is to involve our clients in life-changing work, and you are well on your way. You quit smoking on March 24th, a feat that was awesome and inspiring for me to witness. I will never forget the determination you showed, the suffering you endured, the urges you tolerated, nor the 6am phone calls I made so that you wouldn't smoke that first cigarette of the day. If you have the determination and guts to quit smoking given how excruciating difficult that was for you, *you can do anything* you commit to do.

A turning point in our work was when I took on the role of your critical voice and reflected it for you. That was the beginning of a deep recognition on your part of the importance of being more caring towards yourself. I will never forget a few weeks later, after completing the book *Loving Yourself* by Kingma (2004), how you told me you were starting to love yourself, that you hugged yourself goodnight and said, "Alicia, I love you," and that you had put Kingma's quote in the locket that your grandmother gave you: "Of all the people in the world I deserve my love the most."

What I am most thrilled about, in addition to your quitting smoking and finding/acting on your self-love, is that you reclaimed your inner poet and writer. Your eloquence in expressing yourself in writing is a special gift—you have the power to make me (and others) laugh, cry, reflect, and be inspired by your words. It is a talent I hope you will use frequently in the future.

Before you participated in this therapy, you had been depressed much of your life. Now that much of your depression has been alleviated, it is normal for periods of darkness to come and go, to intensify and to ebb. If you regularly incorporate the skills you've acquired from our work together, feelings of depression will be less tenacious, and you will be in touch more consistently with your core inner voice that is so full of light:

1) *Mindfulness*. This is a skill that people often spend a lifetime working on. It involves the ability to observe your inner processes, your thoughts and feelings, without being overtaken by them. It is a powerful tool to be able to use your cue word 'breathe', to describe to yourself your visceral sensations, to observe your thoughts and not be persuaded by ones that are not helpful, such as those of your critical voice. When thoughts happen that you don't want to buy into, you can say to yourself, "Oh well, that's just a thought."

2) *Behavioral Activation*. Remember that behavioral activation is really helpful for you. You filled out many activity commitment charts for me (e.g., on walking, doing bills), and the pattern was typically that your depression would decrease, your willingness would increase, and your sense of struggle would decrease when you engaged in productive activity.

3) *Moving into your avoidance*. You made huge breakthroughs into dealing with an almost universal tendency, that of avoiding what is painful. We focused on how our ability to validate feelings of grief and loss opens the gateway to joy. Avoiding grief can lead to a numb depression, a superficiality to life where we feel the gnawing ache of something missing. You shared a lot of grief with me that I held tenderly; there is much more to feel when you are ready. On the interpersonal front, we discussed how when someone has made a commitment to you, in this case, me, it can make you want to pull away. Remember the best thing to do is what you did with me, to talk about it in a thoughtful way.

4) *Self Care*. Quitting smoking is one of the hugest self care accomplishments one can do. You've also been eating more healthily and exercising more and thus have dropped over 10 lbs, on your way to fully reclaiming your health and vivacity. You wrote on a session bridging form how important it was for you to directly share problems and issues that

you are having, to honor "How I do things for *myself*". Honoring yourself is an ultimate form of self care.

I have been in practice for over 25 years, and you are one of my most unforgettable clients. I have been so inspired by your drive, your commitment to heal yourself. When I have moments of weakness, like when tempted by junk food, I think about how you were able to resist cigarettes, and I am able to pass on what's not good for me. I will always remember and be inspired by your ability to resist your monumental urges to smoke.

You brought me a very symbolic gift after you quit smoking—a dragonfly decoration with a Shakespeare quote, "All that glitters is not gold. All who wander are not lost." These words are very apropos for you since they epitomize to me your inner knowing. I witnessed how powerful your intuition is, how you know at a deep level what you want and what is right for you. You listen to your own inner drummer, have your own pacing, rhythm and timing in terms of how you want to live your life. The dragonfly itself also symbolizes who you are. With its shimmering wings and delicate form, it is a magical creature. Dragonflies symbolize transformation. You are in the process of major transformation, Alicia. As you keep in tune with your inner voice, you will know when to initiate the changes you know are necessary, and which ones you may be avoiding.

I totally believe in you, Alicia, your ability to attain your dreams, and the vibrance you bring to those whose lives you touch. If you need a tune-up session, I am only a phone call or an email away. Until I see you again, I wish you continued success on your chosen path and the full expression of your wondrous true self.

In conclusion, the final phase of FAP is a time to consolidate gains, and to ensure that the positive interactions that have taken place in the therapeutic relationship have generalized to the clients' outside lives. It is a chance to model how a relationship can end positively, with meaning and feeling. Clients should have a clear sense of the ways in which they are special, and clarity about what they have to contribute to the relationships in their lives, their communities, and perhaps the world.

References

Callaghan, G. M., Gregg, J. A., Marx, B., Kohlenberg, B. S., & Gifford, E. (2004). FACT: The utility of an integration of Functional Analytic Psychotherapy and Acceptance and Commitment Therapy to alleviate human suffering. *Psychotherapy: Theory, Research, Practice, Training, 41*, 195–207.

Emerson, R. W. (n.d.). Retrieved August 1, 2007, from http://www.cccircles.com/

Follette, W. C., Naugle, A. E., & Callaghan, G. M. (1996). A radical behavioral understanding of the therapeutic relationship in effecting change. *Behavior Therapy, 27*, 623–641.

Holman, G. I., Sanders, C., Kohlenberg, R. J., Bolling, M. Y., & Tsai, M. (2006). *Pilot study of a behavior analytically informed integrated treatment for depression and smoking cessation*. Poster session presented at 40th Annual Convention of the Association for Behavior Analysis, San Diego, CA.

Kanter , J. W., Manos, R. C., Busch, A. M., & Rusch, L. C. (in press). Making Behavioral Activation more behavioral. *Behavior Modification.*

Kanter, J. W., Tsai, M., & Kohlenberg, R. J. (Eds.). (in press). *The practice of Functional Analytic Psychotherapy.* New York: Springer.

Kingma, D. R. (2004). *Loving yourself: Four steps to a happier you.* Boston, MA: Conari Press.

Kohlenberg, R. J., Kanter, J. W., Bolling, M. Y., Parker, C., & Tsai, M. (2002). Enhancing cognitive therapy for depression with functional analytic psychotherapy: Treatment guidelines and empirical findings. *Cognitive and Behavioral Practice, 9*(3), 213–229.

Long, L. (n.d.). Retrieved August 1, 2007, from http://www.wisdomquotes.com/cat_beginning.html

Pryor, K. (2002). *Don't Shoot the Dog!* Lydney, Gloucestershire: Ringpress Books Ltd.

Rogers, C. R. (1957). The necessary and sufficient conditions of therapeutic personality change. *Journal of Consulting and Clinical Psychology, 21,* 95–103.

Chapter 8
Supervision and Therapist Self-Development

Mavis Tsai, Glenn M. Callaghan, Robert J. Kohlenberg, William C. Follette, and Sabrina M. Darrow

> *The type of FAP supervision I have received has been about moving radically in the direction of interpersonal intimacy and profound trust. I have come to trust my FAP supervisors not because they operate predictably in the domain of emotional comfort and interpersonal distance, but because they have shown me consistently that they want to interact with me as a whole person. They want to take the risk of emotional discomfort – to venture into unknown territory because they value me unconditionally. Working together as whole people, and bringing our personal histories into our supervisory relationship, has created a profound trust that I find imperative to this work. And learning, by experience, that we are willing to stay committed to the relationship, to shape and be shaped by each other, to endure the potential unpleasantness of natural contingencies in the service of connecting with the relationship and the other person in the present, rather than artificially curtailing it given the punishment we've experienced in the past. Because I can tolerate so much more discomfort, I can venture to create this sort of relationship with my own clients, and I have never developed more powerful alliances with my clients. I am more willing to go to the uncomfortable places with them because I have a sense – from my own personal experience – that our therapeutic relationship can tolerate it, and that the deep trust and intimacy we're forming becomes the core reliable foundation upon which we can experiment with new behaviors. As I am more willing to take risks and be vulnerable in the therapeutic relationship, my clients take more risks and exhibit deep vulnerabilities as well.*
>
> (FAP supervisee MP)

Supervision is integral to the development of therapeutic skills (Armstrong & Freeston, 2006), and thus this chapter delineates a conceptual framework that facilitates an understanding of the FAP supervision process (Callaghan, 2006a;

M. Tsai (✉)
3245 Fairview Avenue East, Suite 301, Seattle, WA 98102, USA
e-mail: mavis@u.washington.edu

M. Tsai et al., *A Guide to Functional Analytic Psychotherapy*,
DOI 10.1007/978-0-387-09787-9_8, © Springer Science+Business Media, LLC 2009

Kohlenberg & Tsai, 1991). Successful FAP supervision produces the profound experience and improved therapeutic skills described in the above quote. As experiential as it is didactic, FAP supervision emphasizes the self-development of the therapist, and supervisees have been almost uniformly positive in their evaluations of the training process. In this chapter we will discuss: (1) the two kinds of knowing that are the goals of FAP supervision; (2) individual FAP supervision methods; and (3) additional training modalities, including group supervision and practicum courses. The chapter concludes with a discussion of ethics and precautions involved in FAP supervision.

Goals of FAP Supervision

Consistent with supervision across all theoretical orientations, the first goal of FAP supervision is to increase the supervisee's knowledge base, or 'intellectual knowing' inherent in the development of critical and conceptual thinking skills of scientist/practitioners. Accomplished via the modeling of competence, specific instructions (including reading assignments), goal setting, and feedback on performance (Milne & James, 2000), this type of knowing can be termed 'knowing that.' It consists of a verbal repertoire for describing the important features of the therapeutic process (Hineline, 1983). For example, FAP supervisees learn to *know that* it is important to: (1) develop a case conceptualization in order to understand which client behaviors may be CRB1s and CRB2s; (2) evoke and naturally reinforce CRB2s; and (3) conduct a functional analysis of T1s (therapist problem behaviors) and T2s (therapist target behaviors) occurring during treatment and supervision. The describing process that constitutes 'knowing that' guides the therapist during treatment by evoking the general class of self rule-governed behavior (see Chapter 2). 'Knowing that' essentially refers to a basic knowledge base of what is important in FAP to help alleviate client suffering. This knowledge base is provided in part to teach the therapist essential skills, such as knowing when and how to respond to client problem behavior and provide responses to clinical improvements in-session. The rules that the therapist follows can help him or her remember to watch for, respond to, and evoke those clinical improvements that occur in-session. A key goal of FAP training is to develop flexibility, such that therapists can watch the impact of their own responses on clients and then adjust their style, strategy or repertoire as required. All of the above need to be undertaken in the context of remaining genuine in the delivery of a response, and depends on therapists noticing their own feelings as they occur toward the client—leading to the second goal of training.

The second goal of FAP supervision is to increase the 'emotional knowing' that plays a central role in noticing, evoking and strengthening CRBs. This type of knowing, 'knowing how,' is essentially what the therapist *does*. 'Knowing how' tends to correspond with contingency-shaped behavior and can occur outside of awareness. It is described in everyday language as 'deep,' 'emotional' and 'intuitive' (Skinner, 1974). Consistent with the distinction between contingency-shaped and rule-governed behavior (see Chapter 2), 'knowing how' is learned through direct exposure to an intense interpersonal relationship with the supervisor, in which emitting and noticing important emotional responding occurs. This exposure is the experiential component of FAP supervision. The contrast between intellectual knowing ('knowing that') versus emotional knowing ('knowing how') is aptly described by a supervisee in the following quote.

> Many other supervisors tried to teach me to be emotionally present with my clients. But I am finding that going there is something I do heart-first. To do this task, I needed more than hearing it in supervision, reading it in an article, or watching it on a video. I needed to experience it myself, in-vivo, within the supervisory relationship. That, for me, is the core of FAP and FAP supervision that is transforming me and my work.

Although FAP involves both 'knowing how' and 'knowing that,' and both types of knowing inform each other, one concern is that strict rule following can interfere with attending to what is actually occurring during the session and responding to the contingencies as they change (Follette & Callaghan, 1995). Safran and Muran (2001) similarly suggest that in supervision, as in therapy, all interactions take place within a relational context. They contend that supervision should include in-vivo experiential opportunities because learning primarily at a conceptual level is insufficient.

Consider clients who have difficulties that are evoked in the context of close interpersonal relationships. These broadly can be referred to as intimacy problems, and they tend to occur to a greater or lesser extent in nearly all clients as well as in ourselves as therapists and supervisors. FAP is very difficult to conduct if therapists have similar intimacy problems to those held by their clients, and this dilemma worsens if they have little awareness of how their interpersonal limitations emerge in their role as therapists. When supervisees participate in a supervisory environment that both evokes intimacy CRB1s and gently shapes and reinforces intimacy CRB2s, they acquire the emotionally tinged pure contingency-shaped responding that better positions them to do the same with their clients. In other words, experiential training during the supervisory session helps to nurture and evoke supervisees' best selves (defined as emitting CRB2s) as authentic human beings, hence allowing them to help their clients do the same.

There is a note of intellectual tension in this process that is worth acknowledging with supervisees. It is important to 'know that' one must watch for the contingencies to occur or even shift in the therapy session. Simultaneously, the therapist should not be bound by rules that require a particular response, regardless of context. For example, a client may engage in an emotionally connecting behavior (e.g., disclosing an often unshared fear) that the therapist recognizes as a CRB2. This is 'knowing that' a CRB2 has occurred. Similarly, the therapist will need to respond to the client's behavior. Again, the therapist 'knows that' a response is warranted to the client's behavior. The style of that response, its impact, and the ability of the therapist to notice that impact and then adjust his or her behavior is all part of 'knowing how' to respond. This requires a different skill compared to the intellectual knowledge of noticing that a response is required. It necessitates the therapist being in touch with his or her feelings in-session and being sensitive to his or her impact on the client.

More generally, good FAP is facilitated when supervisees apply FAP rules not only as therapists, but also as human beings in their daily life relationships. As stated in Chapter 4, the first four rules translate into common language as being aware (Rules 1, 4), being courageous (Rule 2) and being loving (Rule 3). These critical skills or response classes were delineated in the FASIT (Functional Assessment of Skills for Interpersonal Therapists) by Callaghan (2006b) for therapists, and parallel the response classes clients address (Callaghan, 2006c). Thus the training modalities, assignments and exercises used during the supervisory process are intended to help supervisees further develop those qualities. Table 8.1 lists the optimal therapist repertoires we seek to foster in training.

Table 8.1 Optimal therapist repertoires

Therapist Interpersonal Skills	Daily Life	In-Vivo
Assertion of needs	To identify and authentically assert one's thoughts, feelings and needs. To speak truths compassionately and to take risks appropriately.	To identify and authentically assert one's thoughts, feelings and needs in the moment, to ask client or supervisor to respond in different ways, to speak truths compassionately and to take risks appropriately that are in service of client growth in therapy or personal/professional growth in supervision.
Bi-directional impact	Ability to discriminate one's impact on others and vice versa.	Ability to discriminate one's impact on client or supervisor, and vice versa.
Handling conflict	Engaging in healthy conflict and conflict resolution effectively with others	Not avoiding interpersonal tension; resolving conflict effectively with client or supervisor.
Disclosure and interpersonal closeness	Appropriately engaging in disclosure and interpersonal closeness with others. To be interpersonally intimate and effective. To create close relationships, to give and receive love.	Disclosing one's feelings in the service of client growth in therapy or personal/professional growth in supervision. To be therapeutically intimate and effective. To create a close and caring relationship with the individual in the room.
Emotional experience and expression	To discriminate, experience and express one's feelings with others.	To discriminate, experience and express one's own feelings in the service of client growth in therapy or personal/professional growth in supervision.

FAP Individual Supervision Methods

The supervision methods described below delineate a range of methods whereby supervisors can create powerful relationships with their supervisees. Such relationships aim to facilitate emotional knowing ('knowing how') with respect to FAP.

Create a 'Sacred' Space for Supervision

Just as FAP therapists create a sacred therapeutic space for their clients, FAP supervisors create a similar sacred space for their supervisees. As stated in Chapter 4, a 'sacred' space is exclusively dedicated to some person or special purpose, protected by sanction from incursion. Whether or not it is labeled in this way, the key proposal is that FAP supervisors provide an environment in which supervisees can feel safe and cared for as they learn how to implement FAP. This is achieved by minimizing the presence of aversive discriminative stimuli and maximizing positive reinforcement. Supervisors need to be authentic in describing their thoughts and feelings, and see, evoke, value and reinforce their supervisees' best qualities. At its best, supervision evokes descriptions from supervisees such as, "It's like there is no one else in the world but me, you are totally present and tuned into me. You mirror back to me the best of who I am, and you see the best of who I am capable of becoming." But keep in mind that the supervision described above represents an endpoint in the development of FAP supervisory skills; any improvement that moves the supervision in this direction constitutes progress. Functionally, the more sacred the space, the more likely the supervisee will take risks, leading to major repertoire changes that can be transforming.

The following is a transcript excerpt of an interaction between MT and her supervisee RN that captures the essence of sacred space. They are processing the ending of an intense four-year supervisory relationship characterized by a great deal of mutual vulnerability, caring, and respect. The bracketed notes provide a description of the FAP rules implemented by MT at different points.

Supervisor: I feel tears just underneath the surface. I don't quite know how to describe it 'cause I've never described it before. It has to do with my connection with you and my connection with my advisor Ned. I first felt it when I was thinking about saying goodbye to you. I would feel these words come up "I can't do this without you" (MT is referring to RN acting as her teaching assistant for the graduate student FAP course). I know I can do this without you, but I think there's something about the way he mentored me and the way I mentored you, there's a pretty strong connection there. [Rule 2, Evoke CRBs.]

Therapist: I don't know what to say. I have this I can do it. You taught me how to do it without you, and I'm going to go out and *do it*. I think this letter (good-bye letters were written by MT and RN) feels really celebratory to me, like we stated stuff.

S: Maybe I was able to give you what he didn't finish with me (Ned died at the end of MT's second year as a graduate student).

T: I'm still going to call you for supervision. I'll be seeing some really stubborn kid (on internship)...

S: You're having a hard time with my sadness [Rule 1, Awareness of CRBs; Rule 2, MT's sadness is evocative.]

T: Yeah. I don't want you to be sad. Of course you can do it without me... Yeah, I have this whole heap of historical context stuff. I don't want you to be sad. I don't want to be the cause of your sadness. I don't want you to wish that I would stay. I don't want you to worry about things in your life.

S: I don't. I'm fine with not being fine. And it's okay for me to be sad.

T: I don't like it.

S: So what's it been like, this process of you making more room for me? (referring to RN learning to take MT off a pedestal and seeing her a genuine person with emotions) [Rule 2, Evoke CRBs—MT's vulnerability is evocative.]

T: Um, it hasn't just been making room for you, it's been making room for you and us and me...

S: So I feel fine being sad. Why is it so hard on you when I'm sad?

T: Because if you were my dad you would kill yourself.

S: It's really good that we are talking about this... [Rule 3, Reinforce CRB2s.]

T: I was all set to go, and he was all proud and happy for me, then all of a sudden "Don't go, oh shit, don't go. You can't leave me like this. I can't do it without you." I don't know if he said any of that directly. But you know I was accepted to go to Haverford in the fall, and he started talking about the local community college.

S: I actually think this is the perfect experience for us to be having, because I can have those feelings (of I can't do it without you), and I *can* do it without you and you can do it without me. I'm so happy you are growing and expanding and soaring. You are leaving with my blessings. I am so proud of you. So I don't have this, "Oh how can you leave me, I'm not going to survive." It's nothing like that. It's sadness we're not going to have this. And what it triggers from the past is what I told you. I feel a ton of pride and joy. [Rule 3, Reinforce CRB2s; Rule 5, Generalization.]

T: And you're not going to suicide in any way, and you're going to keep supervising and running classes?

S: Of course I'm going to do the FAP class.

T: I want you to miss me and be okay. [CRB2, Assertion of need.]

S: I'm going to miss you terribly and I'm going to be fine. I don't get suicidal. [Rule 3, Reinforce CRB2s.]

T: I know. We've had this whole conversation.

S:	I loved our whole conversation just now. [Rule 3, Reinforce CRB2s.]
T:	Why?
S:	'Cause I think it was a really important conversation for us to have in terms of a corrective emotional experience for you, and I had enough of it that it really triggered your dad stuff.
T:	I wasn't expecting it, I wasn't expecting to be so clearly thrown back 13 years.
S:	Isn't that great, that you can be thrown back 13 years and we can process it?

In this example of a sacred space interaction, MT was authentic and vulnerable when describing her tremendous sadness at saying goodbye to RN and her feelings of not being able to teach without her. These statements in turn evoked RN's feelings of guilt from her past experience of leaving her father. This was an important learning experience for RN, such that she viscerally understood that someone truly can be sad about her leaving, can miss her greatly, and still feel joy and say goodbye with pride and blessings. This interaction is exemplary of countless supervisory interactions in which MT modeled for and shaped RN to be a more aware, courageous and naturally reinforcing FAP therapist, and RN in turn had an equally powerful influence in shaping MT to be a more impactful supervisor.

Focus on In-Vivo Work When Appropriate

While it is necessary to spend time increasing the supervisee's intellectual knowledge (e.g., discussing what to say to a client and how to implement a treatment plan), it is important to focus on in-vivo work that is relevant to the supervisee's growth as a therapist whenever possible. Applicable methods include contextual modeling, contingent natural reinforcement and parallel process work, all of which center on the real relationship between the supervisor and the supervisee.

Contextual modeling. When using contextual modeling the supervisor models for the supervisee the process of implementing FAP rules (being aware of CRBs, evoking CRBs, naturally reinforcing CRB2s, being aware of one's impact, and provision of functional analytic interpretations to facilitate generalization) within their relationship. The response classes called for by the FASIT are also contextually modeled (assertion of needs, awareness of impact, resolution of conflict, disclosure and interpersonal closeness, emotional expression). This is referred to as 'contextual' modeling because it is based on what is happening in the moment in the relationship. This is more powerful than typical non-contextual modeling because the supervisee participates in the interaction and is not only an observer. As a participant, he or she experiences the emotional knowing that is an important component of learning FAP.

In fact, research has indicated that non-contextual modeling or skills training, such as role playing and social skills training, have limited effectiveness (e.g., John, 2006; Scott, Himadi, & Keane, 1983). An example of non-contextualized modeling would entail the supervisor saying, "Watch me act like I really care and am concerned about the client," and then stating, "you do the same thing."

As we discuss in more detail towards the end of this chapter, while FAP supervision may at times overlap with therapeutic interaction, it is qualitatively different from therapy because the goal of supervision is to increase the supervisee's strengths as a therapist. For example, in FAP being therapeutically loving is equated with being naturally reinforcing (Rule 3). Being therapeutically loving is a broad class of therapy behaviors that supervisors can model contextually, and such training is likely to be relevant to the supervisee's therapeutic work. Being therapeutically loving towards supervisees (and clients) means that supervisors operate in their supervisees' best interests and are reinforced by their improvements and successes. This can be considered a generally applicable class of therapist behaviors as most therapists can benefit from being more therapeutically loving (T2). One way the supervisor can model this is by taking the risks needed to engage in therapeutically intimate relating in the service of evoking and reinforcing improvements (Rules 2 & 3). That is, the supervisor takes the risks needed to evoke therapeutically intimate relating. Supervisors should be aware of their own 1s (limitations) and 2s (target behaviors) in intimate relating in order to effectively detect when the supervisee is improving.

Evoke and naturally reinforce supervisee target behaviors. Evoking and naturally reinforcing supervisee target behaviors that apply to FAP (e.g., being aware, being courageous, being therapeutically loving) goes hand in hand with contextually modeling these behaviors. Decreasing avoidance or being courageous is one such broad class of behaviors (a focus of Rule 2, evoke CRBs) that is reinforced in-vivo as well as contextually modeled. Decreased avoidance by therapists involves taking risks, having and expressing feelings (such as caring, sadness, anger), being vulnerable, asking someone in pain to do difficult things, facing one's own fear and asking others do the same, and welcoming silence, criticism and conflict or disagreement. Decreased avoidance facilitates application of the five rules. Table 8.2 lists evocative questions that help decrease avoidance and increase awareness regarding supervisees' relationships with their clients, their relationship with their supervisor, and the supervisors' own feelings regarding their supervisees. This progression of focusing on questions regarding the supervisees' thoughts and feelings toward the client, and then bringing these questions to bear on the supervision dyad, can help supervisors evoke their supervisees' avoidances, concentrate on what is happening right here right now, and bring up target behaviors which can then be naturally reinforced, thus capitalizing on the power of in-vivo learning.

Table 8.2 FAP questions for supervisors

Supervisee toward client	Supervisee toward supervisor	Supervisor toward supervisee
What feelings/thoughts do your client bring up in you?	What feelings/thoughts do I bring up in you?	What feelings and thoughts do my supervisee bring up in me?
Which feelings/thoughts accurately reflect how others would respond to your client?	Which feelings/thoughts accurately reflect how others might also respond to me?	Which feelings and thoughts accurately reflect how others might also respond to him/her?
Which feelings/thoughts reflect your personal triggers from unresolved hurts?	Which feelings/thoughts reflect your personal triggers from unresolved hurts?	Which feelings and thoughts reflect my personal triggers from resolved hurts?
What feelings do you tend to avoid letting yourself get in contact with towards your client?	What feelings do you tend to avoid letting yourself get in contact with towards me?	What feelings do I avoid getting in touch with towards my supervisee?
What do you identify with in your client?	Is there anything you identify with in me?	What do I identify with in my supervisee?
Does your client act with you in ways that also come up with others in his/her daily life? (CRBs)	Is there any parallel process happening, a dynamic between you and your client that's also happening between you and me?	Is there a dynamic with my supervisee that also occurs with other people in my life?
What are you avoiding addressing with your client?	What are you avoiding addressing with me?	What am I avoiding addressing with my supervisee?
What would feel risky for you to say to your client? Would this be helpful? Why or why not?	What would feel risky for you to say to me?	What would feel risky for me to say to my supervisee? Would this be helpful?
What feelings do you have in-session with your client? (If there is a recording of session, isolate supervisee's feelings at key moments)	What are you feeling right now as you tell me this? What are you feeling right now as you hear this from me?	What am I feeling right now?
What are your client's CRB1s and 2s? What are your T1s and T2s with this client?	What are your 1s and 2s in supervision with me?	What are my 1s and 2s with this supervisee?
How can you mirror for your client the best aspects of who he/she is?	[Notice if your supervisee brings out the best in you; if not, why not?]	How can I mirror for my supervisee the best aspects of who he/she is?
What self-disclosures might be helpful to make to your client? Why might this be a good idea? Why not?	What self-disclosures might be helpful with me?	What self-disclosures might be helpful with my supervisee?

Table 8.2 (continued)

Supervisee toward client	Supervisee toward supervisor	Supervisor toward supervisee
How can you evoke CRBs for your client?	How can you evoke supervisor relevant behaviors in you?	How can I evoke my supervisee's T1s and T2s?
How can you be more naturally reinforcing of your client's improvements?	How can you be more naturally reinforcing of what you want in me?	How can I be more naturally reinforcing of my supervisee?

Case example. The following transcript excerpts involve interactions between MT and her supervisee CT, and between CT and her client. They illustrate the concepts of sacred space, contextual modeling, and natural reinforcement. CT's client, Leslie, is a 20 year-old female who attends college part-time and also works at an advertising agency. Her presenting problems included depression, grief over recent-break-up with a boyfriend, difficulty in establishing intimate relationships entailing not allowing others to care for her, difficulty trusting others (e.g., taking interpersonal risks) and showing and expressing emotions. CT wants to become a more effective source of positive reinforcement (referred to as salient reinforcer in the transcript) for her client.

Supervisor: How have I become a more salient reinforcer to you? Is it because of the things that you said – I think all that is a foundation: being caring, being nonjudgmental. But what makes me different from other people, other supervisors, other mentors? [MT is suggesting that CT look at the supervisory relationship for answers.]

Therapist: You are overwhelmingly positive about the stuff I do. That is just really different from most people in my life. You notice when I do good things, and you let me know what I did right. And then if there are things I didn't do well, it's not like "you did it badly, or poorly", just that this is something to work on. That makes it more salient because then there aren't aversive contingencies operating. Not like I have to come see Mavis because she's my supervisor and I have an ethical obligation. It's because I know when I come in here I won't be punished for trying new things, for being myself. I think that's what makes you a salient reinforcer, it's very different. [These are the properties of a sacred space.]

S: And that has everything to do with who I am. So what I'm trying to pull out of you, is what's distinctively you, because I think that all decent therapists, all good therapists are reinforcing, nonjudgmental, and I think that there's something that's uniquely you that nobody else can offer her. As my feelings for you grow, and they've been growing by leaps and bounds, it's because of the things that are distinctly you. [MT is contextually modeling taking risks by 'being open' and expressing her caring for CT.]

T: Can you tell me what those are, 'cause I don't know honestly. [CT is asking directly for what she wants, a 2.]

S: That you are so committed to learning, to working on yourself, and overcoming your barriers, 'cause you've been so wounded, and you just keep working at it. Here you choose to excel at FAP, which will force you to directly deal with everything you want to avoid. You have so much courage, and you struggle with me every step of the way. I know I've pissed you off many times and you keep coming and working it out with me. And you keep saying, no I'm not going to do this, (FAP experiential exercises), no forget it, and then you come back to it. I just see this phenomenal growth in you, such strength and courage, and it means so much to me. It separates you from anybody else because it's so meaningful that you keep working at it and struggling with what's difficult. [MT naturally reinforces the direct request and contextually models for CT the behavior of valuing someone by expressing what she sees and appreciates about CT.]

T: It's interesting 'cause I guess for myself I don't see that as unique. I know that I struggle and that I go to battle a lot over about certain exercises that we have to do. And it feels like particularly in class, the people struggle, but maybe it's just because I'm biased towards myself, but I feel like, they struggle, but they do it, and maybe it's not as difficult for them. But then I feel weak 'cause I have to struggle so much with it.

S: I think you are stronger because you struggle so much, because the reason you struggle so much is that you were wounded that much more... So how do you put yourself in the room more with Leslie? How do you feel about her. 'Cause you know how I told you my reactions to you. I'm really touched by our interaction, we're both engaged and emotional about it, and obviously our relationship has developed over a long period of time. And you are at the beginning of your relationship with her. But you are already having very positive feelings about her... So tell me what you feel about her?

T: I identify a lot with her, a lot of her struggles, and the way she reacts to them, very similar to how I react to things. So there's this strong connection with her because I can identify with her struggles. And she's very sweet; trying so hard, and wants to struggle with these big issues, that I'm also struggling with, very similar issues with her. I feel an instant and strong connection with her. I enjoy seeing her, I enjoy being in the room with her.

S: Do you think she has any idea you feel that way? How would she know unless she read your mind? If I were her, and you said I just feel so connected to you, I'm so happy I'm working with you, I would be really touched.

The following transcript segment is an excerpt from CT's session with Leslie subsequent to the above supervision session.

Therapist: I know that part of the reason I'm bringing this up is that oftentimes people are kind of unaware of how they impact people; both in good ways and in bad ways. I was thinking about the impact that you've had on me, even in the short amount of time we've been working together. Just starting to think about I wonder if Leslie knows how she affects people. I know for myself, that even though we've only been working together for five sessions, and today is our fifth session, that I feel really warm towards you, I really enjoy working with you, and I just have this sense of hope for our work together that we'll be able to get a lot done. My sense of you is that you're a really warm, caring and passionate person. I see you struggling to make sense of this passionate part of your personality, the crying and the feeling like that's (her emotions) almost too much...
[CT is taking risks in expressing her warm feelings for her client, as was contextually modeled by MT in their supervisory relationship.]

Client: Yeah.

T: ...you don't want to do that. But then there's a part of you too that you've talked about in here, I get the sense that, also kind of likes that part, in some ways accepts that part of you, and even likes that part of you and kind of wants to integrate those two parts.

C: Um-hmm (tears come to her eyes).

T: What's going on for you right now? I notice you starting to tear up.

C: Umm, it's always moving when people reflect back to you what you are. It's so rare that even your friends or family tell what kind of impact you have. I don't know... I'm moved. [Client acknowledges the positive impact of the therapist's comments.]

T: Say a bit more.

C: Umm, I'm sure that my mother would say things similar to what you're saying. But in general life, we don't talk about those things. I don't tell her how she affects me and she doesn't tell me how I affect her. So, I'm sure I'd have the same, and have had the same reaction when she tells me like... I can't think of anything now. Sometimes she'll just say what I mean to her and what kind of person I am and I'm like "oh." I get kinda emotional. [Client is learning an important component of intimate relating.]

(Five minutes later.)

C: Um-hmm. You're not just like an expert, I guess.

T: So then... obviously I am the therapist (laugh) and that's what you're coming here for (for help from a therapist), but it sounds like when I shared that with you it kind of took away some of that "I'm in my own bubble surrounded with scholarly journals, here to make diagnoses, and things like that. Now I'm more of a real person."

C: Yeah. You couldn't have learned what you just said in class, you know? It's personal about me. It's not like what you would say to every client you have.

T: What is that like?

C: Um, it makes me feel like I'm being cared for in the therapeutic setting.

T: So you feel like I care about you and I value our relationship.

C: Um-hmm. I'm just thinking about what kind of impact this type of interaction could have on my relationships outside of here. If I went through this kind of thing with my mom, or dad, or J (client's ex-boyfriend), what that would be like. [This is a CRB3 as the client is drawing parallels between the session and daily life that can aid in transfer from therapy to daily life.]

In sum, CT had a powerful and intimate interaction which increased her valence as a salient reinforcer for her client. This interaction originated with the contextual modeling and natural reinforcement that she experienced in her supervision session prior to the therapy session.

Focus on parallel process. Use of the parallel process hypothesis is another method that can help facilitate awareness of supervisee problem behaviors (1s) and naturally reinforce target behaviors (2s). Although the term 'parallel process' is a psychoanalytic concept, FAP supervisors can use this concept (without having to 'buy into' the underlying psychodynamic theory) to increase in-vivo learning opportunities. Parallel process stems from the concepts of transference and counter-transference (McNeill & Worthen, 1989), and occurs when therapists consciously or unconsciously recreate the presenting problems and emotions of the therapeutic relationship within the supervisory relationship (Ladany, Friedlander, & Nelson, 2005). Imagine a client presents as frustrated, confused, indecisive and helpless. The therapist works hard to help the client but to little avail. The therapist then enters supervision feeling frustrated, confused, indecisive, and helpless, and unknowingly encourages the supervisor to completely take charge by problem solving. Hence the process in supervision parallels the process in therapy. Resolution of the issue in supervision (involving use of contextual modeling and natural reinforcement) also resolves the issue in therapy. That is, the process is reversed and the therapist adopts the attitudes and behaviors of the supervisor when relating to the client. Awareness of this parallel process where it exists can shift the focus of the supervisory session to more productive content. When there is conflict in the supervisory dyad, the parallel process hypothesis can be applied as a way to understand and reduce the conflict.

The following transcript is an excerpt from a supervisory session in which the therapist/supervisee FM is seeking help with a very difficult client who is not improving. The supervisor, RJK, has suggested a number of FAP-informed empirically supported treatment-based interventions.

Supervisor: I wonder if there is anything that's happening between you and me that parallels what is happening between you and your client. The parallel process hypothesis is that the issues that exist between you and your client also come up in here between you and me. So I'm wondering if there are any issues that possibly are coming up in here that are similar to the issues that come up between you and your client.

Therapist: I think there is an issue of me letting her down and I think that comes up in here too, as well, that I am not being a good therapist and letting my client down, and with you, I am not being a good supervisee and letting you down (becomes tearful).

S: I understand how hard this is for you. Let's switch the focus a bit, rather than you being deficient, what about me not being a good supervisor?

T: It doesn't work that way (both laugh).

S: It's like you're not being a good enough therapist for her and the parallel process hypothesis would suggest that I'm not being a good enough supervisor for you.

T: No, it's me.

S: So it's not that I'm letting you down—it's like you take full responsibility—you are both being a bad therapist and a bad supervisee?

T: Yeah. [FM assumes responsibility and does not explore other possibilities. Specifically FM does not examine what could be different, what he needs in the supervisory session that would help his therapeutic work. Although an important issue, this is not parallel process.]

S: From my perspective, I do wonder if I am being a good enough supervisor. I know this has been a difficult case for you, and I felt what I needed to do in part was to be there to offer you support and guidance. [Pushing for parallel process material.]

T: I felt confused about what we were doing and I was trying to figure it out. I wish that it would have been clearer what to do with her; I've never worked with a client this difficult before.

S: Okay, so you are left with not knowing what to do after our supervisory session. My understanding is that is her (the client's) feeling too? Is that right? She doesn't know what she is supposed to be doing after your sessions with her?

T: Yeah, well that is something she brought out she wasn't sure what she was supposed to be doing, and I really wasn't certain what you (the supervisor) were going for at that point. So I kind of worked on clarifying the goals and talked about strategies to get to those goals. So, I think that was helpful for her.

S: So are you saying that that problem has been taken care of?

T: Not really. The last time I saw her, she again wanted to know what to do and what our goals were. We discussed it.

S: So you didn't have a sense of where you are going with these goals? That's what you're saying?

T: No, I had a sense in the therapy session but then I find out she didn't have a sense.

S: And you're saying that with me, you don't have a sense of where we're going with her treatment, of what my idea was about what the goals are. And I am in exactly the same position you are, I thought we had a very clear idea of what our goals were and where we were going. This is very parallel process. I then thought you didn't stick with them (the goals arrived at during supervision) and I wondered where you were going. I think that what is happening between you and her is almost exactly what's happening to us. So if we can solve this problem between you and I....

T: Then... I think I can solve it between her and me (both are laughing).

   [It was then discovered that one major issue was that RJK had not adequately explained the underlying behavioral theory that provided the coherence that FM needed. FM, in turn, did not directly ask for explanations when needed. This was remedied in future supervisory sessions. Correspondingly, FM was more methodical in explaining goals to his client and encouraged the client to ask for clarifications when needed.

As illustrated in this transcript, parallel process does occur and, at least in this instance, was useful in helping the supervisee deal with a difficult client. Needless to say, for many supervisors it may be risky to say to a supervisee, "You seem to be acting just like your client and I am having the same difficulties and frustration that you seem to have when you are doing therapy. Perhaps if I can figure what to do with you, then you could do the same thing with your client." Thus, when a supervisee acts like his or her client, and interacts with the supervisor as if he or she were a therapist, the resolution can occur via contextual modeling by the supervisor. Another explanation as to how this process works is based not on behaviorism, but instead on recent research into the mirror neuron system. This research suggests that there are neural mechanisms (mirror neurons) that allow us to directly understand the meaning of the actions and emotions of others by internally replicating them, without any explicit reflective mediation (Gallese, Keysers, & Rizzolatti, 2004).

It is unclear how often parallel process occurs in general, but when it does, resolving it with a supervisee typically leads to similar resolution in the therapist-client relationship. While it can be useful and instructive to identify to the therapist in training that a parallel process has occurred, it is essential that the supervisee refrain from making rigid rules about how to respond to current and future clients. This again illustrates the importance of the therapist knowing 'how' to respond. The therapist can do this by creating and maintaining a coherent case conceptualization, noticing his or her feelings toward the client on a moment-to-moment basis, and being aware of how he or she impacts the client's behaviors with respect to targeted treatment goals.

Group Training Modalities

FAP is designed primarily to enhance interpersonal effectiveness and functioning, hence resulting in more satisfactory life interactions. The way one therapist becomes meaningful and influences clients to take risks for their ultimate benefit can be quite different from how another therapist accomplishes the same goal. That is, there are many ways to 'know how.' Part of supervision is to help therapists find their own path to becoming meaningful to clients. One useful means to highlight this point is to make opportunities to observe how other therapists develop repertoires to support change in clients. It is also enlightening for therapists who are in supervisory roles, as they can find different ways to impact the therapists whom they supervise. Just as with clients, not all therapists hear helpful messages the way the speaker intended.

Besides the obvious pragmatic advantages of group training, there are benefits for therapists that can occur more easily in groups than in individual supervision. Over the years we have developed methods of providing FAP supervision in groups at both the University of Nevada and the University of Washington that we will describe below.

Group Supervision Model (University of Nevada, Reno)

FAP supervision at the University of Nevada, Reno, is conducted on multiple levels. Each week students meet with their supervisor and all other students learning FAP in a large group. In addition, each case is supervised by a peer and other therapists-in-training in mini-teams of three to five students. The final level of supervision is provided through individual consultation with the supervisor. Students are encouraged to consult with their supervisor at any time for feedback related to their case or on aspects of their own repertoires. In this way, students have many different contexts in which to explore their roles as therapists, supervisees, and peer supervisors. Although the structure of supervision has evolved, this particular arrangement has served students learning FAP quite well. This section will cover the process and the benefits that we have found to be associated with group supervision.

Therapist case conceptualization. The first step towards participating in group supervision is the development of a case conceptualization of therapist issues to which the group should be especially attentive. As with client case conceptualizations, these are functional and evolving. Students are encouraged to disclose what they think are their strengths and areas needing improvement with respect to practicing FAP, giving and receiving supervision, and how these interact with particular situations (in supervision and in therapy). As with all steps of the group supervision process, other students and the supervisor offer relevant observations based on their interactions with the student, and attempt to contingently respond to them. Importantly, these case conceptualizations are initially limited to those parts of a student's repertoire that are relevant to therapy and supervision, and do not involve commenting on aspects of the student's personal/social life outside of learning FAP (see ethical section for discussion). It can be the case, however, that therapists themselves will make links between their own therapy repertoires and areas of outside interpersonal functioning. Many response classes that appear on student case conceptualizations will be relevant both for providing therapy and for giving and receiving supervision.

Several common therapist problem behaviors (TIs) are worth noting. Not having a repertoire for addressing client problems (CRB1s) and only reinforcing improvements is a common T1. Addressing interpersonal problems is an important component of any therapist's repertoire for building effective relationships. Finding a means to address CRB1s directly (versus only reinforcing CRB2s or behaviors we like) is a more expedient way to proceed.. In therapy, addressing CRB1s directly can expedite the change process when certain behaviors interfere with building intimacy. Without this repertoire improvement can be very slow to emerge.

Consider the following interaction with a therapist seeing his first FAP client.

Therapist:	And then I got confused about what was going on in the session.
Supervisor:	Was this an instance where it was difficult to recognize that this might have been another way for the client to control the session, rather than understand how you were feeling? [S is trying help the therapist discriminate a different behavior as being part of a functional class in client's case conceptualization.]
T:	Yes...well, maybe. I'm not really sure. [On both the mini-teams and the next couple of larger supervision sessions the therapist exhibits difficulty explaining what he thought was happening in the sessions in spite of many attempts to define the case conceptualization.]
T:	It seems like the client just doesn't pay any attention to what I'm saying, and I'm not sure what to do.
S:	What exactly were you noticing about how you were responding in that moment? [Referring to an interaction the group was observing on tape.]

T: Well, I didn't want the client to get angry. . . I didn't know what
                to do. It may have been that he just doesn't like me. . . Wait, I'm
                confused.
S: On several occasions over the last few weeks you have said "I'm
                confused" in a way that makes it hard to know how to be
                helpful. [This is intended to decrease that response, a T1, since
                it interferes with further discussion.] I'm wondering if it might
                not be the case that it seems scary to risk stating your hypothesis
                and then being wrong?
T: It's embarrassing to be wrong. Everyone in here seems so smart.
Group   I know that I remember feeling that way when I first started out
   member A: on the team in spite of people saying it's okay to make mistakes.
Group
   member B: That's (the experience) so familiar.
S: It's our job to find ways to be helpful. I don't want to put you on
                the spot, but I was just guessing that 'confused' wasn't exactly
                what you were feeling. Since you've shown plenty of under-
                standing about some pretty complicated issues, I was just gues-
                sing that there was more going on.
T: You're right.
S: So what can we do to make it easier to say that this is scary?
T: Everyone has already said that before. It's just different when
                it's me and my first client. I appreciate what that's like now.
S: It's probably scary for your client, too. I wonder if that could be
                related to why he controls the session?
T: It might be.
S: Or he could be confused (all laugh).

Thus, although the application of aversive stimuli is circumscribed in FAP,
'punishment' (i.e., a therapist response that weakens a client CRB1 such as
withdrawing reinforcement) in the context of a strong therapeutic relationship
may be used to address problem behaviors. Again, even punishment is used
from a place of caring. We often tell therapists not to be overly cautious about
evoking negative reactions in the client; if a strong relationship exists, it should
be able to be repaired. In fact, this is modeling an important repertoire as well
(the ability to repair ruptures in the relationship), and it is also something that
can help therapists and clients build a better understanding of each other.

    Another common T1 is a lack of affect, which also can be understood as a
lack of a repertoire for giving natural reinforcement that will then hinder the
therapist in establishing oneself as a meaningful person to the client. This can
emerge in the therapy room as being overly focused on problem solving and
failing to respond as another human trying to relate to the client. This sets the
scene for arbitrary rather than natural reinforcement. In the following example,
the therapist becomes aware of how he can be more naturally reinforcing to his
client by showing more affect and caring before focusing on problem solving.

Therapist:	(Stops tape) I felt so badly for the client.
Supervisor:	What did you say to her?
T:	I told her that what he did was terrible and then we spent the rest of the session talking about a safety plan (the team then watches next segment of tape).
Group member A:	Wow, that must have been so scary for your client.
Group member B:	God, I'd have felt so alone.
T:	Yeah, I felt really terrible for her.
S:	Let's watch the first few seconds of the tape again. I'd like you to watch as if you are your client and tell me what you, the therapist, are feeling (the tape is reviewed).
T:	Oh, no. It doesn't even look like I care. It just looks like I'm sitting there thinking about what to do next.
GMA:	The safety plan was a good thing to do, but I couldn't tell how much compassion you were feeling at the time.
T:	I felt so sorry for her, but there's no way she would have been able to tell.
GMB:	Sometimes in group it's hard to tell how you are feeling.
T:	When I see my friends in trouble, I think I just want to fix their problems right away. I don't like to sit there and feel bad.
S:	Does that happen in here?
T:	I think so. When someone is having a hard time, I want to just tell them what to do next.
S:	And?
T:	And what?
GMB:	And sometimes I'd just like to know that you know what I'm going through.
T:	I don't know why I skip over that part.
S:	What can we do to point out those times when it might be useful to hear how you are feeling before jumping to a solution?

As discussed in Chapter 1, a very important issue to address in FAP is a therapist's ability to notice function, and not just topography of behaviors. Surprisingly enough, we can find no established procedure for teaching this skill by direct instruction. This recognition has to be shaped. For example, a therapist may mistake an expression of negative emotion at face value and not recognize it as an attempt to escape a difficult conversation. Of course this same topography (negative emotional expression) can function differently in different contexts. If this T1 is not addressed, the therapist is in jeopardy of reinforcing CRB1s and missing CRB2s—in other words, not using FAP. This part of a therapist's repertoire will be further addressed below, as group supervision seems to be particularly advantageous in addressing this class of behaviors.

As therapists and supervisors we need to be able to respond to problematic behaviors in ways that decrease them if they interfere with the progression of development. As behavior analysts, we expect behavior change to occur over time as part of the shaping process. A common problem in therapists' repertoires is an inability to discriminate subtle improvements in another's behavior. This discrimination is necessary for the shaping process as therapists strive to reinforce each improvement while raising the bar with each step, requiring the other person to work a little harder and improve incrementally before reinforcing these successive approximations.

The final T1 to be discussed is an almost universal problem, namely doing too much work for others. As therapists become accustomed to interacting with a given individual, they become tolerant of their deficits because there are many other features they value. This can lead to missed opportunities to help clients develop a repertoire that will function better across various contexts and with people who are not as well acquainted with them. Making up for others' deficits can build complementary relationships. This process, however, can hinder the ability to encourage each other to grow and to build more sophisticated repertoires.

Consider the following example.

Therapist:	This session went much better. The client was making much better eye contact and really seemed to be paying attention. I told him how much better I understood him.
Supervisor:	You've done a great job of making him feel comfortable in sessions. He seems very committed to therapy. He obviously values your relationship.
T:	Thanks. I really do care about him.
Group member A:	I know that you and the mini-team see him all the time, but I have to say, if I were interacting with him in a new relationship, I can't imagine that I'd find him at all interesting. He just seems off in his own world.
T:	Therapy seems much more comfortable for us.
GMA:	On our team people have been pointing out how much work I do for my client. I fill in sentences for her, and I overlook vocabulary mistakes and laugh at jokes that aren't very funny.
T:	But I really like this client.
S:	The question is would anyone else work as hard as you have to get to know this person? After twenty sessions, you now find him fun to work with, or at least you look forward to seeing him.
T:	But if you're asking would anyone else, my guess is no.
S:	I find that I bump into this very issue in here. I like working with you guys so much, and I appreciate how hard you work, it's sometimes difficult to step back and ask each of you to take the next step.
Group member B:	I think sometimes on the mini-teams we conspire to not push each other.

S: That's easy to understand, but it's a little bit of a different issue. Once we have a strong relationship with someone, we get into roles where we accept each other's deficits because we're so familiar with them we find simple work-arounds. You guys do that with me as well. I can let humor interrupt an important moment, but you hang in there. In the long run, it doesn't serve us well. How do we express our compassion and appreciation for our clients and each other and still ask for changes?

There are also certain common problems (TIs) regarding giving and receiving feedback. The program described above incorporates a social network in which many students establish friendships with other students. Due to the interactions inherent in these multiple roles, it can be difficult to negotiate such situations. One common problem is individuals feeling uncomfortable giving negative feedback because of worry about ramifications for other aspects of their relationships. It is important to establish a supervision context where feedback is expected and does not affect the social side of a relationship.

On a related note, students often neglect one of the most central tenets of FAP when in the supervision setting: building a relationship. It is often assumed that being in supervision is equivalent to being ready and willing to hear all feedback. Students over-generalize the academic context, being as critical of therapy sessions as they would a research article. This bypasses the essential step, however, of establishing oneself as a source of social reinforcement. Students learn to build a supervisory relationship where they meet the other students where they are in their stage of development as a therapist. On many occasions, difficulties in receiving or providing feedback occur. When this takes place it is best to draw a comparison with therapy, where the aim is to create an environment in which everyone's words can be heard and actions understood as being caring and in the interest of helping one another. When students are having difficulty hearing what others are saying, it can be highlighted how hard it is for a client to hear and make changes.

The TIs described above are by no means an exhaustive list, but rather some important problems to assess. As mentioned earlier, case conceptualizations are functional and evolving. Initially, a therapist case conceptualization can be simply to increase the quantity of participation (i.e., emitting behavior to be shaped), but as time goes on it may evolve to include many different TIs. Some of the TIs might be circumscribed to certain cases or particular peer supervisors. The following sections will describe the advantages of the group supervision process with respect to addressing these different TIs.

Addressing key TIs: Advantages of group supervision. One of the key advantages of group supervision lies in the number of people that participate in the process. Incorporating more people ensures it is easier to establish the emphasis on function that is necessary to conduct FAP well. Every individual participating in supervision is likely to emit topographically different behaviors while trying to achieve the same function—namely being a competent therapist and supervisor. By interacting with and viewing multiple therapists, students are provided with diverse models of responding. This process makes salient the concept that many topographically distinct and dissimilar responses can be involved in a single response class. Not only does this reinforce the idea that different topographies have the same function, it also helps students build more flexible repertoires. This modeling of behavior can provide therapists with a range of options as to how they can vary their responding in order to accomplish a given function. Such flexibility also is necessary when working with different clients who have various repertoires of their own. Therapist flexibility is essential both in terms of establishing themselves as sources of social reinforcement for their clients and in responding in ways to provide natural reinforcement.

One emphasis in the supervision process is natural over arbitrary reinforcement. As mentioned earlier, natural reinforcement is the broad reinforcement individuals encounter in their natural environment that benefits them. Conversely, arbitrary reinforcement is that which is encountered in circumscribed conditions (e.g., only in therapy) and does not sustain behavior in other conditions. Arbitrary reinforcement is particularly problematic, as the behavior producing the reinforcement is subject to extinction. A high rate of arbitrary responding is a typical T1, especially for those learning FAP subsequent to practicing other types of therapy. As therapists, individuals often develop arbitrary ways of reinforcing others or even encourage idiosyncratic ways of talking to others. It thus can be easy for a therapist to lose track of contingencies that function for him or her, but not for the majority of the population. This is one way in which group supervision is particularly beneficial. Because the group is composed of individuals with various backgrounds and experiences with different settings and people, it provides a check on this arbitrary kind of responding. For example, a common therapeutic response to a client expressing anger at the therapist, "Thank you for sharing" might function well in therapy to increase a client's emotional responding. It is unlikely, however, that clients will encounter this type of response in their natural environment; thus it will be more helpful for therapists instead to address the source of the anger.

In light of the above, those involved in the FAP supervision process are constantly assessing whether or not a therapist is providing responses that are likely to be encountered outside of therapy. Note that not all arbitrary responding is disallowed. Indeed, it might be highly important to the shaping process. A therapist has to be able to acknowledge and reinforce improvements (CRB2s) that are successive approximations. These responses are not likely to effectively produce natural reinforcement from the therapist or others, but it is necessary for the therapist to reinforce these responses. Thus arbitrary responses might be necessary to sustain behavior until the client develops a more sophisticated repertoire. A group format can help prevent students from developing idiosyncratic ways of helping clients generalize behavior change.

Greek Chorus. One of the most important functions that differentiates group supervision from individual supervision is what we refer to as the Greek Chorus function. Clients have very diverse backgrounds. The group helps keep students from responding under the control of their own history. Consider an individual whose background includes a tightly knit family where humor is used to express caring. This history thus has established humorous responding in a functional class with other expressions of caring. So when a therapist uses humor in a way that has been established in his or her history to show caring, the Greek Chorus steps in to help the therapist discriminate whether or not this is functioning in the same way (i.e., whether or not he or she is having the impact intended). Thus, the Greek Chorus function refers to the group's ability to point out how different topographical responding functions for the majority of the group (i.e., across contexts). Although this function can be accomplished in individual or smaller group supervision, it is limited by the range of histories of the individuals involved.

The Greek Chorus function also is important in the shaping process for the client. Members of the group can help a therapist respond to the client in a way that is more similar to the client's peer group, rather than the therapist's peer group. For example, a client from a particular religious or ethnic background might well be more comfortable with confrontation than a therapist from a different background. If the client's social community is different from the therapist's, the Greek Chorus can enable the therapist to recognize that behaviors the therapist finds aversive may be quite functional in the client's culture.

The ultimate purpose of the Greek Chorus is to help create flexible repertoires that will function under many different setting conditions. Thus, a supervisor should never attempt to extinguish a therapist's use of humor if it can be shaped to promote caring and understanding. The goal is to help the therapist discriminate under which conditions it will function in this way. The Greek Chorus function specifically refers to attempts to approximate a normative response. This might seem contradictory to the individual focus of the functional analytic rubric of FAP. The goal, however, is not to limit a repertoire to one that will work just with the majority of people, but to expand an individual's repertoire such that he or she can be flexible in diverse situations. Emphasizing the normative response is an attempt to build discrimination skills and provide awareness as to what strengths and weaknesses an individual brings to different situations. In other words, the ultimate goal is to help therapists understand their own stimulus functions across different situations. This includes understanding their stimulus properties, learning how to effectively consequate behavior and how to work around deficits or build a more sophisticated repertoire.

Broad outcomes. An important consequence of participating in the group supervision process is an increased understanding of the change process. Younger therapists can observe the change process that others experience. Individuals see how it happens for others and for themselves, learn the important ingredients of a useful interaction, and observe how the process occurs over time.

Finally, it is worth mentioning the impact this process can have on therapists' relationships outside of therapy. Beyond enhancing therapist and supervisory repertoires, this process can impact meaningfully therapists' personal lives. As will be mentioned below in the section examining ethics, this is not the goal of supervision. Supervisors should be careful in maintaining appropriate relationships and avoid creating dual roles (i.e., engaging in therapy with the supervisee). Supervision targets those parts of a therapist's repertoire that impede therapy. Due to the nature of FAP, however, these repertoires are likely to function in similar ways outside of therapy. Therapists learn to look for function, and it cannot be helped that this will affect their outside lives. Individuals participating in the group supervision process learn that their values and goals in therapy can be coherent with how they live across different contexts. They come to understand the way in which behavioral psychology makes sense as a world view. It sets the stage for accepting people at their stage of evolvement while being able to ask for change.

FAP Practicum Model (University of Washington)

This unique and emotionally challenging class facilitates substantial personal growth. In this course students learn about FAP both didactically ('intellectual knowing' through lectures, the viewing and discussion of instructor client tapes as well as their own) and experientially ('emotional knowing' through exercises where students personally experience any method used with a client, and through participating in the creation of a close intentional community). The vision for this practicum is for participants to create: (1) an intellectually stimulating learning atmosphere where creativity, diversity, collaboration, questions and contributions are valued; (2) an intentional community where students feel the support, acceptance and compassion of mighty companions in their outward journeys as doctoral students and in their private journeys of personal exploration and growth; (3) a place with no pretenses, where they can be seen and heard as who they are, where they express their true voice, where their wounds are validated and their gifts are nurtured; (4) an environment where they are reinforced as powerful thinkers and agents of change, not only in the therapy room, but in their daily lives; and (5) a haven from the typical demands and stresses of graduate school, where they can laugh and have fun, celebrate their uniqueness, quirks and accomplishments. The experiential learning process in this practicum focuses on the three following components.

Increasing emotional risk-taking and decreasing experiential avoidance. A description of the class states the following.

> In our interactions, you will be asked to be more open, vulnerable, aware and present. Attention may be paid to what we are experiencing at the moment in terms of issues of connection, power, conflict, avoidance, trust, and whatever else is difficult to discuss. Please try for a level of openness and emotional risk taking that feels like a CRB2 for you. Challenge yourself to be outside of your comfort zone, to go deeper than you are typically comfortable into learning, thinking, feeling, being and expressing. At the same time, we all know the difference between the form and function of a behavior; so for one person, just being in this class may feel very risky, whereas for another, his or her task may be to work on much deeper disclosure. You are the only one who can gauge what is best for you; adjust your behavior accordingly.

Although risk-taking is facilitated, it is emphasized that student therapists should tailor all experiential and disclosure exercises to their level of risk tolerance. The rationale for these exercises is that they will help students: (a) increase empathy for clients; (b) notice how and what they tend to avoid so they can be more aware of their clients' avoidance behaviors; (c) build in their own repertoires what their clients may want in their target repertoires (e.g., so they can model and reinforce intimacy skills, such as vulnerability when appropriate); (d) personally experience exercises and homework that may be useful with clients and see if it evokes their own clinically relevant behaviors; (e) highlight their values, biases and hidden assumptions so that they do not inadvertently push their clients in those directions. As Callaghan (2006a) so aptly stated, "It is ultimately the goal of supervision to help the supervisee deliver FAP effectively while keeping in mind not only the ongoing client case conceptualization but the therapist's own conceptualization of his or her problems as well" (p. 422).

The list provided below describes examples of exercises which bring students into contact with what they may be avoiding.

1) Telling their life stories in class, focusing on major self-defining memories.
2) Focusing on the important people and events that have shaped who they are.
3) Sending weekly emails to other class members that build closeness through the sharing of emotional risks, challenges, CRB1s and 2s, potent personal experiences, etc.
4) Taking turns leading a meditation at the beginning of class to facilitate connection with oneself and with others in the class.
5) Sharing one's own personal case conceptualization with the class, including one's own CRB1s and 2s in the classroom setting.
6) Sharing one's own FASIT results with the class.
7) Expressing difficult feelings and asking for what one needs.
8) Telling secrets and letting go of guilt and shame.
9) Engaging in a behavior change project.
10) Using a loss inventory (see Appendix I).
11) Preparing a mission statement (see Chapter 9).

Developing accurate empathic reflection. The above exercises assist student therapists in developing empathy by taking them beyond their comfort zones, and enabling them to experience feelings similar to their clients. In addition, the course seeks to facilitate the development of accurate empathic reflection through students repeatedly providing feedback to other class members regarding their disclosures. The functions of such feedback are to take the recipient deeper into his or her experience, to see things in a new way or observe a facet of self previously not conscious of, to feel seen, heard or otherwise reinforced for having shared, and/or to feel more connected to the person doing the reflecting. Students practice: (1) conveying compassion; (2) identifying themes (e.g., difficulty in self-care, sensitivity to rejection) to make connections between seemingly disparate topics; (3) self-disclosing reactions, thoughts, insights or similar feelings or experiences in response to what was shared; (4) linking what was shared with the individual's past sharing experiences.

Becoming more trustworthy. Trust is an essential element in the establishment of a strong therapeutic alliance. We focus on developing and practicing behaviors that foster trust. These behaviors include speaking one's truth, keeping one's word or being accountable, being consistent and predictable, recognizing another's expectations and correcting them if not accurate or explaining why they will not be met, remembering the important things someone says (regarding people, events, memories, etc.), taking responsibility for mistakes and for repairing ruptures, seeing what's in someone's best interest and not taking advantage of them or hurting them, admitting when one doesn't know the answer, and willingness to match another's vulnerability.

Willingness to take emotional risks, development of accurate empathy, and becoming more trustworthy are all behaviors that will increase therapists' value as social reinforcers for their clients, and hence will impact on the effectiveness of therapeutic interactions. The student comments provided below eloquently capture how this practicum has impacted them.

> One theme I want to appreciate is how privileged I feel to work in a context that supports and encourages my dissolving the border between my personal and professional life in ways that enrich both. FAP class is the best example of that privilege. What an honor to do this work with you all... I notice a process in myself where, as I become more accepting, I become more unguarded and consequently the behaviors that emerge are my genuine CRBs (the kind of blind spots and misjudgments that emerge unconsciously when I am not so focused on self-presentation)...
>
> (FAP class student, male)

> ...Each time I interact with FAP I am changed... I have taken risks that have helped me become a more trusting and open person... I feel a sense of possibility and hope with each interaction that I have with each of the students in the class...
>
> (FAP class Teaching Assistant, female)

> FAP... helped me find and build the concept of connection. Connected to human beings on a broader level, connected to those in the group, and connected to myself. I feel more connected to basic human suffering and emotions, to my own life story, and to the threads that run parallel in all our lives... I love the meditations we open class with and that we have the opportunity to lead these ourselves. This entire process has helped me learn how to come into my own body, to the present moment, and to self-awareness... Those moments we take to look at each of the class members in the eye, to welcome them with open arms and an open heart, are an extremely validating and loving experience. It fosters connection. I feel like for those two hours, when we sit in our group of nine, something magical happens, and the reverberations follow me throughout the week and beyond it. I am truly loving every minute of this—the growth, challenges, and connection.
>
> (FAP class student, female)

Ethics and Precautions in FAP Supervision

FAP is Difficult to Do

Being present, open, and reducing emotional avoidance is not easy. In the following transcript from a supervisory session, supervisee SB vividly describes and struggles with this difficulty. Every FAP therapist must deal with these issues, and it is important to keep in mind the notion of T1s and T2s. One therapist's T1s are another's T2s, and what is important is improvement and not meeting any absolute standard of what 'good' is. Essentially, good FAP involves exhibiting T2s.

In the following case example, SB's client Belinda is depressed and anxious, avoids close relationships, has difficulty expressing her feelings, struggles with job seeking, and feels worthless. SB has not yet told her client what she values about her even though she knows it would evoke CRBs, model openness and the expression of feelings, and MT has contextually modeled such expression in the supervisory relationship. SB, in describing why it is difficult for her to do FAP, understands at a gut level the importance of groundedness in the therapist's personal life.

Therapist: ...Mavis, I'm not doing FAP. I've been in FAP class for a year and a half and I'm not doing FAP... there's a way that doing FAP necessitates my being transparent and open, and less protected, which for me means I need to be stronger, not like I got my shit together stronger, but in a real way, that's where I feel I have to go on some retreats and do some work and get my life in order, get a lot less stressed out, not feel I have to be really vigilant about getting myself together in order to be able to do this. Otherwise I'd feel like, okay I could maybe make myself go through the motions of this, but to really be that present and that open and to be able to use myself in that way as a reflection for her, that openly, I need to be in a different place. So it's just safer, it's more protected, it's more comfortable not to do it.

Supervisor: I think the analogy is when people question whether they can be adequate parents, whether they can bring a child into this world and give him or her adequate nurturing, and they question all that is wrong with this world, then there are people who blindly go ahead and have babies. I think there are people who are gung ho about FAP and rush in there thinking, "I can do this," and you with all these reservations and who cares so much, I would trust you so much more to do what is best... so let's look at the very specific interaction about valuing her... how does everything you just said relate to you not being able to tell her how much you value her?

T: There's a way that it opens up a different level of engagement. It's no longer like, you're sitting over there, I'm sitting over here, you're talking and I'm doing some things, and it's helpful, and great, I'll see you next week. It becomes, it sinks down a level, it introduces much more of an interpersonal factor, I know that's the point, it becomes a different relationship. It feels somehow unsafe to me, like I'm not sure I can sustain it. Like I need to be consistent. where if I imagine how I want to tell her that, in a way that feels clean, like 'I'm telling you this because I trust it's going to be helpful in some way, and because it's the truth.' When I imagine that, there's a place that I would need to be in. I also could just do it and it feels just a little off. [SB is describing her feelings that, in turn, suggest variables that account for her reluctance to do FAP—the beginnings of a functional analysis.]

S: This is really valuable, what we're going through. [Natural reinforcement.]

T: So I'm just kind of getting this, Mavis, why I've been so resistant to this. The times I have seen and felt FAP, when I get it, when I think of that, and where would I need to be and feel, with that kind of energy, that kind of intent and interaction. I can get like almost an embodied sense, what kind of place I would need to be in for that to be a clean reflection, and not about being compliant, or not about trying to do something strategic, but in a way that's open, not like, I'm going to do this because Mavis said so... it's like my whole life would have to change. I'd have to find some peace and some time and I'd have to live in a way that's congruent with, I can't walk into a session and be this other person, and relate in this other way, turn it on... I have to *be* a different way, my whole being has to actually *be* congruent with that.

S: I think that's the ideal, but I think there are approximations to the ideal. When we look at our relationship, what's it like for you to be yourself in here? [Rule 2, Evoke CRBs.]

T: It's totally different though. In this context it's okay. I guess I don't understand where you're going.

S: Okay, there's a similar process, because what's been happening here is that you are experiencing what it's like to be yourself and you don't have your mask on, and you can be just as engaged, whereas in the rest of the world you have your persona. So you're telling me that you have a certain persona with Belinda, and I'm saying you can experiment with this process, can you be more open with her without being this completely whole grounded clear person? Before your therapy ends, it's important so she doesn't go away without knowing how much you value her. You see her in a way no one else does, so don't go away without sharing that with her. You just get her in such deep ways.

T: Yeah, I never thought about that. I don't think there's anyone else who sees her that way. I feel really sad.

S: I love how you're engaging with me on this.

T: Good, me too, it feels good 'cause I'm just getting part of why I'm so resistant.

After this supervision session, SB was able to take more risks with her client, and their relationship deepened. In turn, her client responded by also taking more emotional risks in-session and in her daily life.

Boundary Issues (Supervision Versus Therapy)

Supervisory and therapeutic relationships have important aspects in common, such as a collaborative mindset, the importance of goal setting and measuring progress, the sensitive handling of power imbalances, and an atmosphere of encouragement and hope. Supervisory and therapeutic relationships have distinct differences, however, in that supervision focuses on treatment of the client (not the supervisee), multiple supervisors are more beneficial in training than are multiple therapists in treatment, and there is flexibility for supervisory relationships to evolve into collegial or personal relationships (Newman, 1998).

In interpersonally deep interactions, the risk of supervision treading on therapeutic territory becomes more likely. Because supervision focuses on treatment of the client, even though supervisees or supervisors may raise topics that overlap with what is covered in personal therapy, the emphasis is on the development of supervisee clinical skills. There is not a sustained focus on supervisees' personal issues, but rather an exploration of how these personal issues impact their work. Supervisees are encouraged to pursue their own individual therapy in order to work through personal issues that arise.

Power Differential

Within the power differential in therapy and supervisory relationships exists the possibility for exploitation, and it is imperative this potential be guarded against (Falender & Shafranske, 2004; Holloway, 1999). In order to prevent an abuse of power, it is crucial that the supervisee provide informed consent for the type of interpersonally intense supervision he or she will be receiving (Callaghan, 2006a). Specifically, the supervisee should be informed that: (1) due to the in-vivo focus in FAP supervision, intense feelings that often come up in therapy relationships may arise in the supervisory relationship (e.g., hurt, anger, sadness, fear, dependence, attachment, attraction); (2) the openness and vulnerability that are valued and evaluated highly in FAP supervision may at times be antithetical to the supervisee's need to appear composed and competent; (3) personal issues that require a sustained focus need to be addressed in individual therapy elsewhere; and (4) the supervisor will also meet the supervisee from a place of authenticity and vulnerability, and is prepared to address variables that affect the power structure, including evaluative authority, gender, age, race, sexual orientation and cultural differences.

Creating a Therapist Case Conceptualization

One of the ways to maintain the focus on the therapist's goals with the client is for supervisors to ask themselves consistently, "Am I trying to change the supervisee or help him or her become a better therapist?" The broader agenda of creating sweeping behavior change in a supervisee is akin to the goal of psychotherapy. The other goal of training or of creating more effective therapist skills, remains the purpose of supervision. One means of achieving this is to create a supervisee case conceptualization, as described above. Each therapist has his or her own T1s and T2s. These, however, are limited to those behaviors relevant to becoming an effective FAP therapist. While the therapist behaviors described in the FASIT system (Callaghan, 2006b) parallel those of the client, there are important differences. One such point of difference lies in the scope of the interpersonal repertoire. The FAP supervisor has the responsibility to limit his or her intervention and skill development with respect to the therapist behaviors of interest to those areas that directly impact the treatment of the client being supervised.

It is assumed that therapists are in the business of doing therapy because they want to help. Wanting to help a supervisee with life problems thus makes a great deal of sense, but there are ethical prohibitions against this for good reason. As the supervisor begins to develop a dual role with the therapist in training, his or her capacity to serve as trainer and ultimately evaluator of the therapist's skills may become compromised. To remain an effective FAP supervisor, he or she must continue to be present, compassionate, thoughtful, flexible and consistent—all in the service of helping the supervisee develop better skills as a FAP therapist.

Many FAP therapists become more effective, honest, open and even more loving people as an effect of learning FAP. Part of this is accomplished by 'living FAP' in their own lives and acting consistently with FAP training. We would note that although this is a wonderful outcome of learning FAP, it is not required nor can it be the necessary goal of FAP supervision. If, empirically, it were determined that good FAP therapists must do these things in their lives to be effective in treatment with a client, then we may move toward that recommendation. Until then, the supervisee-supervisor relationship remains the professional interaction of training with the agenda of improved therapist skills. This training can appear intense, uncomfortable, compassionate and powerful at any one time, just as in therapy. The goals of supervision, however, remain more circumscribed.

There are a variety of supervision styles and approaches. The goal of each must be to train effective and ethical therapists. Regardless of age and sophistication, supervisees will be influenced by their mentors. It is up to the mentors to discharge this responsibility with care and regard for their influence.

Having listed these cautions and constraints, it is difficult for anyone learning FAP not to see the broad implications of understanding and influencing behavior change. We caution our students to become intensely meaningful to clients without creating debilitating dependency. The same is true for the supervisory relationship.

Learning to be a psychologist is a choice. This choice is influenced by experiences and personal values. The 'choice' to become a FAP therapist should not be taken lightly because 'informed consent' is an ideal rather than a reality. At the beginning of FAP training, although we tell students that FAP training is not intended to be therapy, it is difficult to conceive how this training will not cause them to examine their own interpersonal repertoires, values and goals. On one occasion, after several sessions of struggling to be present in the room with a client, a young therapist said, "I understand what I need to do to become good at this, but I don't want to make those changes in myself. My life works well for me, and I don't want to do anything that would jeopardize that. I know how to do other empirically supported treatments, and I think I'll stick with that." That was a healthy decision that gives us reason to think that one can examine the possibilities of FAP while maintaining autonomy. This is a good thing.

Conclusion

We began this chapter with a student's description of the training experience, and we conclude with a reflection by MT to her supervisees on what an equally profound experience it was to work with each of them.

> I'm sad that this is my final e-post, that our class is coming to an end, and that we won't ever be this close as a group again after our retreat. In writing my appreciations and your student evaluations, I spent many hours reflecting on the ways you are uniquely special. It's been such a privilege to be privy to all of your lives in a profound way, to be aware of the depths of your struggles and joys, private feelings and events that are meant only for those closest to you to know. In addition to being more facile with FAP in a visceral way, one of the lessons that I'd like you to take away from our class is that intimacy is a choice. Due to the weekly writing assignments and to all the sharing that was prompted by class and small group, we communicated at a deep level regularly whether we were happy or sad, stressed or relaxed, overwhelmed or in charge, whether we felt like talking or not. Through that consistency, we created an atmosphere of intimacy and trust with risk-taking, self-disclosure, acceptance and compassion. I'm chagrined to say that because I communicated with you more, I actually feel closer to you guys than to some of my dear friends who I did not connect with as regularly. Coming back to us, we have built a foundation of closeness and trust that is solid. Any one of you can come to me at any time if you need input or help from me. I hope you will email the entire group when you want to share something significant in your lives, but even if I never hear from you again, know that what we have shared is unforgettable, and that you will always have a place in my heart.

References

Armstrong, P. V., & Freeston, M. H. (2006). Conceptualising and formulating cognitive therapy supervision. In N. Tarrier (Ed.), *Case formulation in cognitive behavior therapy: The treatment of challenging and complex cases* (pp. 349–371). New York: Routledge/ Taylor & Francis Group.

Callaghan, G. M. (2006a). Functional analytic psychotherapy and supervision. *International Journal of Behavioral and Consultation Therapy, 2,* 416–431.

Callaghan, G. M. (2006b). Functional assessment of skills for interpersonal therapists: The FASIT system: For the assessment of therapist behavior for interpersonally-based interventions including Functional Analytic Psychotherapy (FAP) or FAP-enhanced treatments. *The Behavior Analyst Today, 7,* 399–433.

Callaghan, G. M. (2006c). The Functional Idiographic Assessment Template (FIAT) system. *The Behavior Analyst Today, 7,* 357–398.

Falender, C. A., & Shafranske, E. P. (2004). *Clinical supervision: A competency-based approach.* Washington, DC: American Psychological Association.

Follette, W. C., & Callaghan, G. M. (1995). Do as I do, not as I say: A behavior-analytic approach to supervision. *Professional Psychology: Research & Practice, 26,* 413–421.

Gallese, V., Keysers, C., & Rizzolatti, G. (2004). A unifying view of the basis of social cognition. *Trends in Cognitive Sciences, 8,* 396–403.

Hineline, P. N. (1983). When we speak of knowing. *The Behavior Analyst, 6,* 183–186.

Holloway, E. (1999). A framework for supervision training. In E. Holloway & M. Carroll (Eds.), *Training counseling supervisors* (pp. 8–43). Thousand Oaks, CA: Sage.

John, W. M. (2006). Social skills training for students with emotional and behavioral disorders: A review of reviews. *Behavioral Disorders, 32,* 4–18.

Kohlenberg, R. J., & Tsai, M. (1991). *Functional analytic psychotherapy: Creating intense and curative therapeutic relationships.* New York: Plenum Press.

Ladany, N., Friedlander, M., & Nelson, M. L. (2005). *Critical events in psychotherapy supervision: An interpersonal approach.* Washington DC: American Psychological Association.

McNeill, B. W., & Worthen, V. (1989). The parallel process in psychotherapy supervision. *Professional Psychology: Research and Practice, 20,* 329–333.

Milne, D., & James, I. (2000). A systematic review of effective cognitive-behavioral supervision. *British Journal of Clinical Psychology, 39,* 111–127.

Newman, C. F. (1998). Therapeutic and supervisory relationships in cognitive-behavioral therapies: Similarities and differences. *Journal of Cognitive Psychotherapy, 12,* 95–108.

Safran, J. D., & Muran, J. C. (2001). A relational approach to training and supervision in cognitive psychotherapy. *Journal of Cognitive Psychotherapy, 15,* 3–15.

Scott, R., Himadi, W., & Keane, T. (1983). Generalization of social skills. In M. Hersen, R. Eisler, & P. Miller (Eds.), *Progress in behavior modification* (pp. 113–172). New York: Academic Press.

Skinner, B. F. (1974). *About behaviorism.* New York: Knopf

Chapter 9
Values in Therapy and Green FAP

Mavis Tsai, Robert J. Kohlenberg, Madelon Y. Bolling, and Christeine Terry

> *We realize the huge calling of history at this time. We have been called to a collective genius, and each of us is being prepared to play our part. Our world needs spiritual giants, and it takes not ego but humility to sign up for the effort. Many of our problems arose because we chose to play small, thinking there we would find safety. But we were born with wings, and we are meant to spread them.*
>
> (Williamson, 2004, p. 250)

Traditionally, FAP has been conceptualized as a relatively value-free therapy. FAP aims to help the client have a productive, meaningful and fulfilling life, but it is left to the client to specify what is personally productive, meaningful and fulfilling. As discussed in Chapter 3, the therapist's job is to help clarify his or her client's personal goals and provide guidance in how to achieve them. With the exception of the behavior analytic goal of maximizing long term positive reinforcement and minimizing aversive control, the therapist is expected to refrain from imposing his or her personal values on the process. Over recent years, however, as global problems have intensified, we have proposed a variant of FAP that we term 'Green' FAP. Green FAP is thus named because it encourages the overt introduction into treatment of personal therapist values that are consistent with ideals of the 'Green' movement (Green politics, n.d.). Green FAP incorporates a socially conscious ideology that places a high importance on ecological, environmental, social justice and nonviolence goals. Specifically, Green FAP values call for caring and helping of others, social consciousness and responsibility, and using one's talents and passions to contribute to the world.

Given the central role of 'values' in this chapter, it is appropriate to describe what is meant by this term in the current context. In its broadest sense, values are verbal statements specifying reinforcers and the activities that produce them

M. Tsai (✉)
3245 Fairview Avenue East, Suite 301, Seattle, WA 98102, USA
e-mail: mavis@u.washington.edu

M. Tsai et al., *A Guide to Functional Analytic Psychotherapy*,
DOI 10.1007/978-0-387-09787-9_9, © Springer Science+Business Media, LLC 2009

(Baum, 2005; Skinner, 1971). Given our focus on values relevant to psychotherapy, we are interested in clarifying the nature of value statements made by therapists.

Three types of value statements potentially can be asserted by therapists. The first loosely can be referred to as therapeutic 'facts.' These facts predict reinforcers based on scientific data. An example is advising depressed clients of research suggesting that improved interpersonal functioning increases resistance to recurrence of depression, and hence noting that it should be a goal of treatment. The second type we refer to as therapeutic 'ethics,' and include ethical standards of practice that ostensibly improve the welfare of clients. Therapeutic ethics are more or less universally adopted and sanctioned by the larger professional group of which the therapist is a member. Clients reasonably might expect their therapists to issue therapeutic fact- and ethics-based value statements. The third type of value statement we refer to as 'personal' therapeutic values. Such personal values are not universally associated with the larger professional group. Clients thus may not expect their therapist to state their personal values. Before exploring how Green FAP is implemented, we will address briefly why we believe therapists' explicitly stated personal values can have a place in therapy.

The Role of Therapists' Personal Values in Psychotherapy

We propose that it is time to introduce the personal values of Green FAP into therapy because we believe the world is at a crossroads. As implied by Williamson's quote above, we are members of a generation that holds the fate of civilization in our hands. We are concerned with a number of key issues: (1) large-scale deprivation (3.7 billion people live in poverty on $2 a day or less; 24,000 people die every day from hunger; 30,000 children under five die every day from preventable causes; 2.4 billion people live without decent sanitation; and 4 billion people are without wastewater disposal) (Planet facts, n.d.); (2) the perils of global warming; (3) the devastation of our natural environment; (4) political violence/war, extreme deprivation, and/or unbearable living conditions across the globe (e.g., Myanmar (Burma), Middle East, Darfur (Sudan), Congo Chechnya, Northeast India, Somalia, Colombia, Uganda, Ivory Coast); (5) severe world health crises (e.g., 2.9 million AIDS deaths/year, one every 10 seconds; 1.7 million tuberculosis deaths per year, one every 20 seconds) (Top 10 most underreported humanitarian stories, 2007); and (6) the atrocities of terrorism.

We recognize that the identification and prioritizing of world problems is somewhat arbitrary and will vary from person to person depending on the type and nature of the data they encounter. Nonetheless, as socially conscious therapists we question whether it is enough simply to help clients alleviate distress, change self-defeating behaviors, or pursue purely personal goals. Green FAP is based on the proposition that social consciousness has a crucial role in treatment that can serve both the well-being of clients and the world. We are not suggesting that therapists abandon the process of addressing their clients' presenting problems and goals. Rather we are urging that therapists also pursue, whenever possible, the development of client repertoires incorporating Green FAP values.

Some will argue that therapists' personal values have no place in their professional roles, and that therapists should limit themselves to the task of discovering what their clients' values and goals are, and helping them achieve those goals. On closer examination, however, this view does not preclude the use of personal values based on the caveat that therapists must be willing to help a client work towards a specific goal. Take the example of a client whose goal is to reduce guilt and increase wealth ensuing from a legal exploitation of employees who do not have realistic options for finding work elsewhere. In this context the therapist's personal values will influence how they proceed. Similarly, consider 'willingness' in the situation where a client cannot pay for services, but such payments support the therapist's valued standard of living, leisure time with friends and family, and commitment to give to charity. All of these influences are values that may affect who therapists decide to treat.

Furthermore, whether or not therapists explicitly state their personal values, we are all influenced by them in treatment. For example, Bilgrave and Deluty (2002) found that most of the therapists in their sample tended to identify themselves as politically liberal Democrats, and about half believed that their political beliefs influence their practice of psychotherapy. Gartner, Harmatz, Hohmann, Larson, and Gartner (1990) determined that ideological match affected the degree to which clinicians empathized with and liked their patients. Politically liberal clinicians tended to have a negative personal response to politically conservative patients and conservative clinicians had an even stronger negative response to liberal patients. Further, the clinicians' assessments and personal responses to patients were influenced by the degree of ideological congruence between themselves and their patients. Gartner and colleagues referred to this congruence as 'ideological transference.' From a FAP viewpoint a mismatch would be counter-therapeutic if the therapist's ability to naturally reinforce CRB2s was compromised. Conversely, a mismatch might be evocative of CRBs that are related to the client's presenting problems, and thus might offer opportunities for therapeutic interventions.

Under conditions where a mismatch of values leads to a lack of empathy and a therapeutic rupture occurs, clients may blame themselves for the failure if they are not aware of their therapists' values. In contrast, a Green FAP therapist, who would be more forthcoming with his or her values, is better positioned to take responsibility for ruptures. If values are presented in the initial phone call or the first session, clients who do not agree with these values have the option of choosing another therapist. For example, MT states to potential clients, "In addition to working on individual problems and goals in therapy, I am also interested in helping my clients get in touch with their unique talents and passions that can address the larger problems in our community and the world. Is this something that you would be interested in?" If a client holds similar values, the stage has been set for a productive therapeutic environment.

A good alliance also can occur even if clients have not yet identified their own values but are curious about and are attracted to Green FAP values.

Implementing Green FAP Values

In the following discussion we explore how Green FAP values can be implemented during therapy. Some methods are fairly easy to put into action and probably occur regardless of the therapist's awareness of the process. Others are more risky, require courage, and need to be tailored to fit the particular therapist and client involved.

Naturally Occurring Implementation of Green FAP during FAP

In FAP, clients are nurtured to experience the therapeutic relationship as a safe place in which previously punished behavior is encouraged, even though it may be frightening. Over time the operants of being 'present' (see Chapter 5 on Self and Mindfulness), courageous and taking interpersonal risks are strengthened and avoidance is reduced. The therapist also encourages and can use ACT (Acceptance and Commitment Therapy) interventions (Hayes, Strosahl & Wilson, 2002; Kohlenberg & Callaghan, in press) in the service of helping clients stay present with personal discomfort, overcome emotional avoidance and act in more courageous and caring ways. All these behaviors depend on the availability of natural reinforcement that is intrinsic to a therapeutic relationship in which a genuine and mutual caring develops. With successful treatment, these same behaviors then transfer to daily life and clients eventually are reinforced by achieving the goals that brought them into treatment. Thus FAP incorporates the potential to reduce experiential avoidance, to increase attachment and intimacy repertoires (see Chapter 6 on Intimacy), to give and accept caring, and to increase a stable sense of self. These repertoires in turn, have benefits that apply to an individual's relationship with the world, as touched on briefly in each section below.

   Reducing experiential avoidance. A recent review of the literature generated the conclusion that most clinical problems stem from unhealthy efforts to escape and avoid emotions, and that these difficulties are ameliorated through reduced experiential avoidance (Hayes, Wilson, Gifford, & Follette, 1996). A recent study also documented the role that experiential avoidance plays in the relationship between materialism and diminished well-being (Kashdan & Breen, 2007). Reducing materialism is consistent with Green FAP values and holds promise for improving meaningful connections with other people and promoting the welfare of others.

   Improving attachment repertoires. FAP specifically has been identified as having potential for improving attachment repertoires (Meyer & Pilkonis,

2001). Secure attachment has been shown to increase toleration of inter-group diversity and the humane and compassionate regard of others (Ginsberg et al., 1997). Mikulincer and Shaver (2007) suggest that interventions aimed at improving attachment repertoires would allow humans to be better able to create a kinder and more tolerant, harmonious and peaceful society.

Giving and accepting care. The FAP environment encourages mutual caring, concern and compassion. Although the focus of FAP is on the therapeutic relationship and the transfer of its gains to other interpersonal relationships, once established it is possible that these repertoires will generalize to larger communities, thereby enabling Green FAP values.

Increasing a stable sense of self. Features of a stable sense of self, which is a possible target of FAP, include the ability to be assertive with others and to be less subject to adopting the values of the immediate interpersonal environment (Kernis, Cornell, Sun, Berry, & Harlow, 1993; Kohlenberg & Tsai, 1991). If a client is inclined toward Green FAP values, improved stability of self will lead to actions consistent with these values.

Case Example. The following case example illustrates the process through which a client of RJK's treated with FAP became more socially conscious and politically active, values consistent with Green FAP. Initially the client sought treatment for depression and anxiety. The therapy resulted in CRB2s of taking interpersonal risks, reducing interpersonal experiential avoidance and improving intimacy and attachment repertoires. Towards the end of therapy she wrote the following note to RJK.

> After the years of graying elders – experienced leaders, leaders of good will and intention—my country and heart have been broken. The politics of 'vast conspiracies' and special interests, right or left, are tearing us apart, I dropped out of political and social activism. To me, the need to believe is worth me taking the risk of being involved in this election. As I've learned so well in your office, 'we are all special,' 'I can risk, lose, and live through it,' and 'without hope there is no wholeness.'

As this correspondence illustrates, the client became more willing to re-engage in political and social activism as a result of FAP, without Green FAP strategies directly being implemented. Therapists who want to assist their clients in more actively pursuing ways to help alleviate community or world problems can use the Green FAP strategies discussed below.

Direct Implementation of Green FAP

In our first book (Kohlenberg & Tsai, 1991), we discussed how our culture isolates us from the deeper contingencies of eating meat. The key points are: the amount of grain used to produce one meal of meat can be used to make ten vegetarian meals; the energy used in raising animals for meat is depleting natural resources and contributing to pollution; rain forests are being cut down to create grazing land for cattle, with dire effects on the environment (Robbins,

1987). We are similarly estranged from other, deeper contingencies. For example, we are shielded from the homeless and the hungry, the elderly in nursing homes, people dying, the complex process of obtaining of drinking water, the cutting of trees to make paper, and processes of garbage and sewage disposal. People generally avoid contact with these situations because positive reinforcement for dealing with them is remote or delayed, and the immediate consequences are quite aversive. From a Green FAP standpoint, we believe that contacting these contingencies will improve the world and benefit those (including ourselves) who live in it. In this section we address ways to increase staying present and in contact with these 'hidden' contingencies and the aversive private experiences they may evoke, and how each of us can use our unique talents, inclinations, interests and/or passions to play a role in addressing larger social problems.

Being more altruistic. Compelling data suggest that altruistic behavior, or unselfish concern for others and the doing of good deeds for them, leads to improvements in well being and alleviates depression (Seligman, Steen, Park, & Peterson, 2005). There is also growing evidence of an evolutionary basis for altruism (Haidt, 2007; Wilson, Van Vugt, & O'Gorman, 2008; Wilson & Wilson, 2007). In behavioral terms, altruistic behaviors are naturally reinforcing.

In a plea for altruism, Australian ethicist Peter Singer (1999) enables readers to get in touch with the fact that average American families spend almost one-third of their incomes on unnecessary luxuries, such as going out to nice restaurants, buying new clothes because the old ones are no longer stylish, and vacationing at beach resorts. The income that is spent on things not essential to the preservation of our lives and health, if donated to a charitable agency, could mean the difference between the life and death of children in need. Singer describes a case given by philosopher Peter Unger in his book entitled *Living High and Letting Die*, such that a $200 donation to an organization like UNICEF (800-367-5437) or Oxfam America (800-693-2687) would help a sickly 2-year-old Third World child transform into a healthy 6-year-old, offering safe passage through childhood's most dangerous years. Singer donates one-fifth of his income to famine relief agencies and urges everyone else to do the same.

After reading the above, are you inclined make a donation? If you do donate, you still may be unconvinced of its efficacy and have slightly less money—both aversive consequences. We and others, however, have donated in spite of these short-term effects. The research on altruism cited above indicates possible positive reinforcement to account for this behavior. If your history has inadvertently kept you from donating, you may be missing an opportunity for positive experiences. Our suggestion is to try giving money or time, or some other more personally appealing altruistic act that you typically would not engage in, and see what happens. Here is another contingency—if you do it, let us know (mavis@u.washington.edu), and we will respond.

Here is another idea that may enable you to take an altruistic action you may have been delaying—by trying to contact your own mortality. In his book, *Naked Buddhism*, Deida (2001) reminds us of the following.

> No matter how much money or love you have made, one day your legs will become cold and numb, your heart will stop, your breath will cease, and all will disappear. In some now-moment as real as this present one, your life will end. Are you ready for your death? Are you ready for the death of your children, your parents, and your friends? Have you loved fully and given your deepest gifts? A life lived well embraces death by feeling open, from heart to all, in every moment. Wide open you can offer without holding back, you can receive without pushing away... (pp.1–2).

Although the technique of contacting our own mortality may feel aversive at first, the ultimate goal is to contact the positive reinforcers that come from altruism and making a difference in the lives of others.

Developing a sense of universal responsibility. All human beings seek happiness, security, comfort and peace. Yet as individuals and members of groups we identify with (e.g., couples, families, communities, nations), we value our own individual or group happiness over others'. The evolutionary basis of altruism suggests that we are inclined to identify with a group (e.g., kin, colony) that in turn determines the scope of our responsibility.

The writings of the Dalai Lama seem intended to influence our perception of group membership. Buddhism teaches that the erroneous perception of a dualistic split between self (and our group) and others is the root of personal and collective suffering. The solution proposed by the Dalai Lama (2006) is for each individual to cultivate a sense of universal responsibility, such that we become aware of the basic humanity that binds us as a single human family, and hence have a deep concern for all, irrespective of creed, color, gender or nationality. The premise of universal responsibility is that all life is interrelated, and that the happiness of one person or group should not be sought at the expense of others—that we are "caught in an escapable network of mutuality, tied in a single garment of destiny." (Martin Luther King, Jr., cited by Johnson, 2006, p. 30). The experiential exercise in Chapter 1 is intended to convey a similar sense of interconnectedness.

Acknowledgment of our interdependence and interconnectedness with one another will help us experience a sense of universal responsibility and evoke actions to overcome the dangers to our very existence. The wiser course is to think of others when pursuing our own happiness. The more we can move beyond national boundaries and embrace the international community at large, the less likely people in poorer countries will be denied adequate reinforcement density. From our Green FAP standpoint, nations have no choice but to be concerned about the welfare of others because it is in the mutual and long term interest of all concerned.

Cultivating an open heart. The heart metaphor is discussed in Chapter 6 on intimacy. Cultivating an open heart can help create a sense of connection in all relationships, including the therapeutic one. All relationships involve questions of power and conflicting interests. Whether it is intimate affairs or international affairs, human relationships all operate on the same basic principles: love, forgiveness, awareness, kindness and selflessness lead to peace; hatred and violence produce misery. Given the world conflicts we face, we have much to gain by opening our hearts.

The development of an open and kind heart—love and compassion for others, a true sense of community, and a feeling of closeness with all human beings—is related to altruism, the common goal of moral precepts laid down by the great teachers of humanity. The goal is an altruism that enables a spontaneous compassion for all sentient beings. It ultimately benefits the giver as much as, if not more than, the receiver. Individual happiness ceases to be a conscious self-seeking effort and instead becomes an automatic and far superior by-product of the whole process of loving and serving others.

Working to change our communities begins with a feeling of connection with all other beings. This feeling, however, cannot be selective, "for we are one with both our friends and our enemies, with those who suffer and those who cause suffering" (Hanh, 2006, p. 38). In order to end war and suffering, and to bring about peace, we must each live mindfully in the present moment. "We must simply stop the endless wars that rage within. . . imagine, if everyone stopped the war in themselves—there would be no seeds from which war could grow." (Johnson, 2006, p. 37).

Advancing a sense of purpose and personal mission. We believe that people experience a high level of fulfillment when they contact the passion, talent, or sense of purpose that enables them to be of service and to help better the world. This can be facilitated in Green FAP by asking clients to craft a personal mission statement, a systematic values statement that plays an important role in taking charge of one's life. Mission statements can help us focus on what is most important—the principles that anchor our life, who we want to be, what we want to accomplish, what we want to dedicate our time to, and the legacy we want to leave. They can be a compass, a strong source of guidance amid the stormy seas and pressing, pulling currents of life (Covey, 2004).

Behaviorally speaking, the mission statement is a set of rules involving predictions about what events will be reinforcing and what behavior will be reinforced. Explanations of apparently purposive action and self reports of felt purpose rely on present circumstances coupled with past reinforcement in similar circumstances. In other words, all intentional statements, although they appear to refer to the future, actually refer to past reinforcement. Words such as intend, want, try, expect and propose can be paraphrased by, "In circumstances like these in the past, my behavior was reinforced."

The following tools can help in the crafting of a mission statement.

1) Borrow freely from whatever values speak to you in "Living a fulfilled life" (Table 9.1). This table describes a series of values or ways of being that we believe will lead to a fulfilled and evolved life. Some of them may be more important to you than others. Some may already be ingrained in your life; others will require persistent attention. Some will constitute the work of a

Table 9.1 Values for fulfillment

Values	Description
Health	I feel good physically. I take care of my body by feeding it healthy food, exercising regularly, and giving myself enough rest. I understand the importance of balance in all that I do.
Spirituality	I integrate a spiritual path with my daily activities. I am aware of my connection to all living things, and feel a sense of wonder for the miracle that is life. I am conscious of the fragility and transience of life. I live with gratitude, grace, and value simplicity. I am aware that I have a mission, that my life has a purpose. I am in touch with my inner voice of wisdom, my higher self.
Love and Intimacy	I feel an abundance of love in my life. I nurture and feel nurtured by people I love. I am vulnerable and reveal myself to those I trust. I act with honesty and integrity, and am able to make commitments that I honor. I understand that conflicts are inevitable in close relationships, and work to resolve conflicts and learn from them.
Meaningful Work	My work brings me a deep sense of personal satisfaction. It challenges, stimulates me, and I know I am using my talents.
Beautiful Space	I surround myself with beauty, and create living and work space that bring me peace, inspiration and joy. There is a place for everything, and everything is in its place.
Mindfulness/ Insight/Awareness	I can focus awareness on the present moment and go beyond old mechanical patterns and compulsions. I am interested in the meaning and causes of my (and others' behavior), in what causes me to act, think, or feel a certain way. I understand how my family of origin, and other salient people and experiences impact me today. I examine my behavior for maladaptive patterns and work to change them.
Compassionate Communication/ Reinforcing Others	I communicate in a way that brings harmony to my relationships. I can diffuse conflict with empathy, and motivate with compassion rather than with fear, guilt or shame. I see the best in other people. For every criticism or negative judgment, I am aware of five positives. I catch others in the act of doing well or being good. Positive reinforcement is especially important when it comes to raising children.
Sexuality	Erotic energy is a source of life energy. I feel good about my body and am able to give and receive sexual pleasure.
Social Consciousness/ Activism/ Altruism	A purely personal life lacks a sense of connection and purpose. I have a community to which I belong. I see what is wrong with the world and act on my convictions in working for social change.
Emotional Awareness	I am in touch with my feelings, am accepting of them, and allow myself to feel a wide range of feelings. I grieve losses fully. I know that when pain is blocked, so is joy.

Table 9.1 (continued)

Values	Description
Authentic Expression of Core Self	"It takes courage to grow up and be who you really are." I relate to others with truth and authenticity, and I can speak my mind without creating resistance or hostility. I feel comfortable expressing my true thoughts and feelings to others when appropriate.
Creative and Artistic Expression	I cultivate artistic expression through music, art, writing, or other channels which foster my creativity.
Problems as Opportunities	I see problems as challenges and as opportunities for learning and growth. I focus on my role in the problem, or how I've contributed to the problem rather than what is wrong with the other person. Thus I can feel my power in solving the problem.
Wonder	I experience wonder on a daily basis, and feel a sense of appreciation for children, animals, nature, art, music, literature, and the arts in general.
Discipline	I am able to set realistic goals and follow through on achieving them. I do what I say I am going to do, so that others can rely on my word.
Cognitive Flexibility	Other people and events don't cause my feelings; I can impact greatly my own feelings and reactions by how I interpret events. I am able to recognize and challenge distortions in my thinking which lead to negative feelings. I am able to come up with creative solutions to my daily life problems.
Activities that Bring Pleasure	I regularly engage in activities or hobbies that give me pleasure. I am in touch with my inner child and can be spontaneous and playful in my pursuits.
Finances	I feel good about my finances. I have enough money, am able to spend money on things I need and want. I am generous with others. I save, invest and plan for the future.
Courage	I face and deal with my fears directly. I don't let my anxieties and fears curtail my life. I take risks in going after what is important to me.
Lifelong Learning	I take classes or read books to learn about topics that interest me. I stimulate my mind with new information.

lifetime. Please select the values that are important to you and use them to create your own vision for how you would like to live your life.

2) Answer the Seligman Values in Action Signature Strengths survey (short version) to identify your top five values. It takes about 20 minutes to complete the survey online (VIA Signature Strengths Questionnaire, n.d.)

3) Answer these questions:

a) What do you stand for? What principle, cause, value or purpose would you be willing to defend to the death or devote your life to?

b) What are your happiest moments, experiences or greatest achievements? Describe how you were 'being' in those moments. What traits or qualities were present?

c) What are ten things that bring you great joy?

d) What excites you in or about the world?

e) What do you long for?

f) What would you do if you had the courage?

g) What would you do if you had the resources?

h) What would you do if you believed it were possible?

i) What motto do you try to live by?

j) What five things do you want to be remembered for when you die?

4) Feel free to take from the examples below whatever moves you or speaks to you. They include our personal mission statements and ones created by our clients, supervisees and colleagues.

As we stand at the cusp of planetary survival, my mission is to dare to be powerful and visible in using my gifts for the greater good of humanity. I want to live and to teach broadly the core principles of FAP which are awareness, courage and love. With an open heart, I give that which is most mine to give—I mirror for others their best selves as I help them heal, awaken spiritually and honor their callings. I speak my truth compassionately, and I aspire to cultivate sacredness and beauty in every moment and in every interaction. I want to connect with my divine guidance daily, to nurture my creative spirit, and to surrender to life's mysteries and wonders. I am committed to helping create peace for future generations. MT

My mission is to engage as fully and deeply as I can with the world—including interpersonal, cultural and physical realms. This includes: (1) striving to love ever more deeply and increasing the scope and intensity of my attachment to, caring for and benefiting others; (2) increasing my concern and involvement with solving sociopolitical problems; (3) passionately playing with ideas that foster creativity and intellectually challenging myself and stimulating others to do the same; and (4) learning about, deepening my understanding, and having hands-on involvement and connection to the physical and technological features of the world in which I live. RJK

My mission is to turn against the current:
to live and act from my deepest experiences;
to bear witness to the mystery of each ordinary thing;
to step through assumptions of duality
and pull others from the swamp of despair;
to be open to life and death as our wholeness;
to practice complete simplicity;
to trust, refusing hurry;
to re-enter the wild Heart continually:
to celebrate our essential belonging. MYB

I strive to be:
- able to have my fear and not have it control my life.
- fully connected with others with an open heart.
- open and to use my talent of creative expression every day.
- a person who takes a stand against those who preach inequality and intolerance.

- a person who never gives up.
- able to cultivate and live in a space where problems are unrealized opportunities.
- able to recognize my strength and to use it to help others.
- able to view my weaknesses as areas of continued growth.
- able to give and receive compassion.
- a person who lets herself take risks, even if this means that I may look like a 'fool' sometimes.
- in full contact with life's experiences and opportunities, with the knowledge that this will inevitably lead me to experience great pain and great joy. CT

Other inspiring mission statements written by our clients and colleagues include:

"My mission is to teach love, inspire hope and create healing in others and myself."
"My mission is to bring a child into my life, share my love and insights, and create an environment for this child to know what it's like to love himself/herself."
"With mortality as paradoxical liberator, my mission is to, quite frankly, 'go for it.' To stop flying below the radar, frightened of illusions and ancient dictums. My vow is to live a life of full integrity. To ROAR when noise is needed, to console when consolation is called for, to shine brightly when illumination is the order. And, to help others, and myself, awaken to the truth—you are, quite simply, splendid!"
"Ad astra per aspera
To the stars through difficulties.
I aspire to...
- have the courage to fail in order to be great.
- work for equality and dignity of those less fortunate.
- educate and inspire others.
- find spiritual enlightenment.
- be thrilled by the stars at night.
- speak my mind, even when my voice quakes.
- beware of those who invite me to be less than who I am and stay close to those who dare me to be more than I ever imagined.
- live and love gracefully."
"My mission is
To be of use.
To understand and surrender, more and more deeply.
To move with power and grace.
To embody lovingkindness.
True gold does not fear fire."

We think it is an important exercise for therapists to write their own mission statements in order to understand how inspiring and significant this task is before giving the assignment to their clients. Mission statements are considered to be blueprints or drafts that can be revised as one changes and grows, but continue to remain inspiring and powerful throughout their iterations.

Engaging in a daily practice. While some people use a daily meditation practice to increase their mindfulness, others find it difficult to incorporate such an activity on a regular basis for a number of reasons, including lack of time or proclivity. What we advocate is a daily practice of some kind, not necessarily meditation, that will enliven you with regard to one or more of the above categories—altruism, universal responsibility, open heart, or personal mission. What type of practice can you engage in daily that takes you away from the hectic and distracting demands of living and returns you to your core voice, creates poetry in action, and brings out your best and most wise self? One can choose the same daily practice, or engage in a different one each day. Examples include journal writing, reading books that motivate, taking a bubble bath, going out into nature, working in the garden, taking a walk, creating art, writing poetry, spending time with one's children or elders, doing volunteer work, working out or exercising, listening to or creating music, making love, cooking healthy meals, refraining from eating a meal, capturing timeless moments with photography or videography, and/or connecting with others. To continue developing ourselves, it is essential to engage in a daily practice that opens us to what is truly important. Johnson (2006), a Buddhist, spoke like a behaviorist with his quote, "I cannot think myself into a new way of living, I have to live myself into a new way of thinking" (p. 36).

Conclusion

Green FAP is a model for understanding the relationship between the avoidance of contact, the personal development of clients and therapists, a concern for larger cultural issues, and a plea to be in touch with what is possible. Green FAP urges us to: (1) claim a world where every life is precious:

> "We are all just human beings who experience sorrow, need, sickness, loss and other kinds of suffering, and who rely on relationships to help deal with adversity and to maintain well-being; whether these relationships are with one another, the animal world, the spiritual realm, or the earth" (British Museum, 2006).

(2) love in a way we've never loved before; and (3) take our sense of personal agency (capacity of exerting power to achieve an end) to its highest level, applying our passions and gifts to personal, interpersonal and global transformation.

> "Thou shalt not be a victim.
> Thou shalt not be a perpetrator. Above all, thou shalt not be a bystander."
> (Holocaust Museum)

References

Baum, W. M. (2005). *Understanding behaviorism: Behavior, culture, and evolution.* Malden, MA: Blackwell Publishing.

Bilgrave, D. P., & Deluty, R. H. (2002). Religious beliefs and political ideologies as predictors of psychotherapeutic orientations of clinical and counseling psychologists. *Psychotherapy, 39*(3), 245–260.

British Museum (2007, Viewed July 27). *Living and Dying.* Exhibit in Room 24, London: British Museum.

Covey, S. R. (2004). *The 8th habit: From effectiveness to greatness.* New York: Free Press.

Dalai Lama (2006). A new approach to global problems. In M. McLeod (Ed.), *Mindful politics: A Buddhist guide to making the world a better place.* (pp. 17–27). Boston, MA: Wisdom Publications.

Deida, D. (2001). *Naked Buddhism: 39 ways to free your heart and awaken to now.* Austin, TX: Plexus.

Gartner, J., Harmatz, M., Hohmann, A., Larson, D., & Gartner, A. F. (1990). The effect of patient and clinician ideology on clinical judgment: A study of ideological countertransference. *Psychotherapy: Theory, Research, Practice, Training, 27*(1), 98–106.

Ginsberg, J. P., Klesges, R. C., Johnson, K. C., Eck, L. H., Meyers, A. W., & Winders, S. A. (1997). The relationship between a history of depression and adherence to a multicomponent smoking-cessation program. *Addictive Behaviors, 22*(6), 783–787.

Green Politics. (n.d.). Retrieved March 15, 2008, from http://en.wikipedia.org/wiki/Green_movement.

Haidt, J. (2007). The new synthesis in moral psychology. *Science, 316*(5827), 998–1002.

Hanh, T. N. (2006). Call me by my true names. In M. McLeod (Ed.), *Mindful politics: A Buddhist guide to making the world a better place* (pp. 39–43). Boston, MA: Wisdom Publications.

Hayes, S. C., Strosahl, K. D., & Wilson, K. G. (2002). Acceptance and commitment therapy: An experiential approach to behavior change. *Cognitive and Behavioral Practice, 9*(2), 164–166.

Hayes, S. C., Wilson, K. G., Gifford, E. V., & Follette, V. M. (1996). Experiential avoidance and behavioral disorders: A functional dimensional approach to diagnosis and treatment. *Journal of Consulting and Clinical Psychology, 64*(6), 1152–1168.

Holocaust Museum (2008, Viewed February 17). Washington, DC.

Johnson, C. R. (2006). Be peace embodied. In M. McLeod (Ed.), *Mindful politics: A Buddhist guide to making the world a better place* (pp. 29–37). Boston, MA: Wisdom Publications.

Kashdan, T. B., & Breen, W. L. (2007). Materialism and diminished well-being: Experiential avoidance as a mediating mechanism. *Journal of Social and Clinical Psychology, 26*(5), 521–539.

Kernis, M. H., Cornell, D. P., Sun, C.R., Berry, A., & Harlow, T. (1993). There's more to self-esteem than whether it is high or low: The importance of stability of self-esteem. *Journal of Personality and Social Psychology December, 65*(6), 1190–1204.

Kohlenberg, B., & Callaghan, G. (in press). FAP and Acceptance and Commitment Therapy: Similarities, divergence and integration. In J. Kanter, M. Tsai, & R. J. Kohlenberg (Eds.), *The practice of FAP*. New York: Springer.

Kohlenberg, R. J., & Tsai, M. (1991). *Functional analytic psychotherapy: Creating intense and curative therapeutic relationships*. New York: Plenum Press.

Meyer, B., & Pilkonis, P. A. (2001). Attachment style. *Psychotherapy, 38*(4), 466–472.

Mikulincer, M., & Shaver, P. R. (2007). Boosting attachment security to promote mental health, prosocial values, and inter-group tolerance. *Psychological Inquiry, 18*(3), 139–156.

Planet Facts. (n.d.). Retrieved March 15, 2008, from http://planetinperil.org/category/planet-facts/

Robbins, J. (1987). *Diet for a new America*. Walpole, NH: Stillpoint Publishing.

Seligman, M. E. P., Steen, T. A., Park, N., & Peterson, C. (2005). Positive psychology progress: Empirical validation of interventions. *American Psychologist, 60*(5), 410–421.

Singer, P. (1999, September 5) The Singer solution to world poverty. *New York Times Magazine*. Retrieved February 12, 2008, from http://people.brandeis.edu/~teuber/singer-mag.html

Skinner, B. F. (1971). *Beyond freedom and dignity*. New York: Knopf.

Top 10 most underreported humanitarian stories. (2007). Retrieved March 15, 2008, from http://www.doctorswithoutborders.org/publications/ reports/topten/

VIA Signature Strengths Questionnaire. (n.d.). Retrieved March 15, 2008, from http://www.authentichappiness.org/

Williamson, M. (2004). *The gift of change*. New York: HarperCollins Publishers.

Wilson, D. S., & Wilson, E. O. (2007). Rethinking the theoretical foundation of sociobiology. *Quarterly Review of Biology, 82*(4), 327–348.

Wilson, D. S., Van Vugt, M., & O'Gorman, R. (2008). Multilevel selection theory and major evolutionary transitions: Implications for psychological science. *Current Directions in Psychological Science, 17*(1), 6–9.

Appendices

Appendix A: Case Conceptualization Form

FAP Conceptualization and Treatment Plan for Client:
Therapist: Date:

Relevant History:
O1s – Daily Life Problems:
  – Can include problematic thoughts for FAP Enhanced Cognitive Therapy
  – Can include socio-political problems (SP1s)

Variables Maintaining Problems:
Assets and Strengths:
CRB1s: In-Session Problems:
CRB2s: In-Session Target Improvements:
O2s – Daily Life Goals:
  – Can include improved thoughts for FAP Enhanced Cognitive Therapy
  – Can include socio-political improvements (SP2s)
Planned Interventions:
T1s (Therapist in-session problems) & T2s (Therapist in-session target behaviors):

Appendix B: FAP Preliminary Client Information Questionnaire

Please try to complete as much of this as you can and bring to the first session.

Name: Date:

1. Life Events Summary: Summarizing the main aspects of your life history will save us time in therapy. On a separate sheet of paper, reflect on your life from birth to present in terms of the highlights, challenges, celebrations, relationships, enduring circumstances, turning points, accomplishments, losses, adventures, and the peaks and valleys that have shaped who you are as a person. You can do this in chart form or narrative form, or both. If you

do draw a chart, divide it into 5–10 year periods, where the middle of the paper is the neutral zone. Mark each significant memory in a way that reflects the variance from neutral of your experiences. Write a few words next to each event or relationship to indicate their significance. Put a star by the events you want to talk about in therapy.

2. If possible, please list some of your strengths, assets, or things you are proud of about yourself.

3. What are your goals for this therapy?

4. Is there anything else that is important for me as your therapist to know about that will help me in working with you?

Appendix C: FAP Life Snapshot

Name:	Date:									
1 = not at all satisfied; 5 = average; 10 = extremely satisfied										
Satisfaction with life	1	2	3	4	5	6	7	8	9	10
Self care	1	2	3	4	5	6	7	8	9	10
Time management/discipline	1	2	3	4	5	6	7	8	9	10
Meaningful work	1	2	3	4	5	6	7	8	9	10
Love and intimacy	1	2	3	4	5	6	7	8	9	10
Sexuality	1	2	3	4	5	6	7	8	9	10
Health and nutrition	1	2	3	4	5	6	7	8	9	10
Exercise	1	2	3	4	5	6	7	8	9	10
Home management/uplifting home environment	1	2	3	4	5	6	7	8	9	10
Life purpose	1	2	3	4	5	6	7	8	9	10
Friendships and social support	1	2	3	4	5	6	7	8	9	10
Family relationships (parents/siblings/kids)	1	2	3	4	5	6	7	8	9	10
Finances	1	2	3	4	5	6	7	8	9	10
Courage/ability to take risks	1	2	3	4	5	6	7	8	9	10
Spiritual life	1	2	3	4	5	6	7	8	9	10
Contribution to community/activism/altruism	1	2	3	4	5	6	7	8	9	10
Emotional insight/cognitive flexibility	1	2	3	4	5	6	7	8	9	10
Mindfulness	1	2	3	4	5	6	7	8	9	10
Authentic expression/speaking your inner voice	1	2	3	4	5	6	7	8	9	10
Creative and artistic expression	1	2	3	4	5	6	7	8	9	10
Problems as opportunities	1	2	3	4	5	6	7	8	9	10
Sense of gratitude	1	2	3	4	5	6	7	8	9	10
Activities that bring pleasure	1	2	3	4	5	6	7	8	9	10
Lifelong learning	1	2	3	4	5	6	7	8	9	10
Other values/target behaviors, list:	1	2	3	4	5	6	7	8	9	10
	1	2	3	4	5	6	7	8	9	10
	1	2	3	4	5	6	7	8	9	10

Appendix D: FAP Session Bridging Form

Name: Date:

<u>Part A (to be completely shortly after therapy session):</u>

1) What stands out to you about our last session? Thoughts, feelings, insights?
2) On a 10 point scale, how would you rate the following items a)—d)?

   <u>Not at all</u>   <u>A little bit</u>   <u>Moderate</u>   <u>Substantial</u>   <u>Very Substantial</u>
   1   2   3   4   5   6   7   8   9   10

   a) Helpfulness/effectiveness of session: ____ What was helpful?
                                            What was not helpful?
   b) How connected you felt to your therapist: ____
   c) How engaged/involved you felt with the topics being discussed: ____
   d) How present you were in the session: ____

3) What would have made the session more helpful or a better experience? Anything you are reluctant to say or ask for?
4) What issues came up for you in the session/with your therapist that are similar to your daily life problems?
5) What risks did you take in the session/with your therapist or what progress did you make that can translate into your outside life?

<u>Part B (to be completed just prior to next therapy session):</u>

6) What were the high and low points of your week?
7) What items, issues, challenges or positive changes do you want to put on the agenda for our next session?
8) How open were you in answering the above questions 1—7 (0-100%)?
9) Anything else you'd like to add?

Appendix E: Typical FAP Questions

Typical FAP questions are of two types: They bring the client's attention to what he or she is thinking and feeling (a) at the moment; (b) about the therapy or therapeutic relationship, preferably in the moment, but thoughts or feelings outside of the session regarding the relationship are okay too.

What are you thinking or feeling right now?
What's going through your mind right now?
What's your reaction to what I just said? To the rationale I just gave?
To being in a research study, to me as your therapist, to agenda setting, to structured therapy, to the homework assignment, to time-limited 20 session therapy?
What were you thinking/feeling on your way to therapy today?

What were you thinking/feeling while you were waiting for me out in the
   waiting room?
What are your hopes and concerns/fears as you start this therapy relation
   ship with me?
What are your behaviors that tend to bring closeness in your relation
   ships? What do you tend to do that decreases closeness in your rela-
   tionships? How would you feel about us watching for your behaviors in
   here which increase or decrease closeness?
What were your reactions to our last session?
What stood out to you regarding our last session?
What stands out to you about today's session?
What are your feelings/reactions to our session today?
What's hard for you to say to me?
How are you feeling about our therapy relationship? What's good about
   it? What needs to be improved?
What do you wish I would have done?
What do you think I'm thinking about you/ that/ what you did/ said?
How do you feel about your progress?
What do you think I'm feeling about your progress?
Are your reactions to me similar to your reactions to X? or Is that how you
   feel about me too?

Appendix F: Beginning of Therapy Questionnaire

1. In general, when I begin a new relationship or activity, I*

   – jump in quickly, ignoring any reservations I have.
   – move cautiously, taking time before I vent myself.
   – trust slowly before I make any commitment.
   – try hard to make a good impression.
   – feel shy and keep to myself until I feel comfortable.
   – am very quick to be critical of what's going on.
   – become involved and stay that way.
   – am concerned that I might get trapped.
   – start out with high hopes and then get disappointed.
   – am different depending on the situation.
   – other, describe.

2. I notice these similarities and differences between my usual style of beginning
   and how I am beginning this relationship:

---

* Adapted from Bruckner-Gordon F., Gangi, B. & Wallman, G. (1988) *Making therapy
work: Your guide to choosing, using and ending therapy.* New York: HarperCollins.

3. I will increase the likelihood of having a good experience and getting what I want from therapy if:
4. What I like about therapy so far is:
5. Therapy would work better for me if:
6. What else is important for my therapist to know that will be helpful in working with me?
7. Any other feedback—thoughts, feelings, requests?

Appendix G: The Mid-Therapy Questionnaire*

I am pleased about my progress in
I wish I had made more progress in
I'm having a hard time expressing myself about
I want you to know
It would be difficult for me to face
I am interested in changing my therapy to include
I could improve our relationship by
You could improve our relationship by
I have a hard time expressing myself about
It is hard for me to tell you about
What bothers me about you is
You are a lot like
My reactions to you remind me of
As I think about my sessions, I would like
I wish my therapy would be
We need to continue talking about
I am finding it hard to accept
I recognize I am changing because
It is getting easier for me to
I no longer feel
I saw things in a new way when
It was a powerful experience when
For the first time I
It seemed you were insensitive to me when
I felt hurt or angry when you
It is difficult for me to manage my feelings during therapy sessions when
It has been hard to cope with my feelings in between sessions when
It has been painful for me to discover
I had a dramatic, intense, or seemingly inappropriate reaction to you when

---

* Adapted fromBruckner-Gordon F., Gangi, B. & Wallman, G. (1988) *Making therapy work: Your guide to choosing, using and ending therapy.* New York: HarperCollins.

I feel closest to you when
I'm most likely to push you away when
Now that I'm in the middle of therapy, I
This is (different from) (similar to) what usually happens when I am involved
   in the middle of an activity or relationship because
Your policies are hard for me when
When the therapy session ends, I often
The beginning of a session is hard for me when
I wish you would
I am glad you

Appendix H: Grief Worksheet

I am sad/I am hurt that
I am angry that
I miss
I am relieved
I am grateful
I am sorry/ I regret
I wish I had
I wish you had
I forgive you for
Please forgive me for
My heart cries out
I never told you
You never told me
I learned from our relationship
I will always remember/ I will never forget
I want you to know
If only I could
I honor your memory/ you will always live on
Other thoughts and feelings/what else do you need to say?

Appendix I: Loss Inventory Assignment

Sometimes we stay stuck in our lives unless we look directly at the ways we've
been wounded and we grieve. This is an exercise that allows you to acknowledge what you have loved and lost, the hurts, disappointments, endings, and
betrayals you have endured. Losses are broadly defined and also include anything
wished for that did not occur. In validating our losses, we begin the grieving
process.

In writing your inventory, consider the following:

What are the losses you've endured in your life that stand out to you from earliest memory to the present? What has made you sad, what has broken your heart, what has left a gap in your life? What has been missing in your life?

What losses do you think should or could evoke a response in you now but don't? What do good-byes bring up for you?

There is no right or wrong way to do this. Just let your heart speak to you as you review the losses you have experienced. Be gentle with yourself as you complete this inventory, and contact your friends, family, or your therapist for support if needed. Below are examples from individuals who have done the loss inventory:

- One of the earliest painful memories was when I stayed with my grandmother because my mother was about to give birth and there were unexplained "complications." My dad would visit us and I can still remember seeing the red tail-lights of his care as he drove away. Longing to go with him...
- When I think of a "gap in my life" growing up, the biggest one was a sense that I never quite measured up to my dad's expectations. Envious when I would see other fathers and sons with an easy relationship.
- I moved around so much when I was little that I felt uprooted and friendless much of the time.
- My parents' divorce when I was 7.
- Loss of my wonderful mother due to lung cancer.
- Loss of my dog who our entire family loved. Felt helpless as he had multiple seizures, didn't know what was wrong.
- My sister who developed schizophrenia.
- My grandpa who died when I was 8. I remember bargaining with God to let him stay a little longer in my life and when it didn't happen, I lost my trust in God.
- Loss of my virginity at age 15 to someone who didn't care about me.
- Loss of my innocence because I was sexually abused as a child.
- Loss of my first love, loss of trust in others, loss of trust in my intuition, loss of sense of security, loss of feeling special to someone.
- Loss of belief in the inherent goodness of others after being sexually assaulted.
- My friend who committed suicide in college.
- Two of my closest friends getting married.

Appendix J: Crying Out in Your Poetry*

Give yourself permission to cry out in raw pain on the page and in actuality. Avoiding what is bewildering and painful may exact a far greater toll on you physically and mentally than expressing what is gnawing at your soul. Attempts

---

* Adapted from Fox, J. (1997). *Poetic medicine: The healing art of poem-making.* New York: Jeremy P. Tarcher/Putnam.

to explain or discuss or analyze your painful experience may not be enough to free the energy and insight you need to heal and move forward.

A more visceral, spontaneous language, originating within you, may open the gateway to greater intuition, insight and energy for dealing with your problems. Your poetry can mark the steps and resting places of your journey, the twists and turns of your life.

Don't try to intellectualize or soothe. Let words jangle and burn on the page, catch our attention and draw us into the poignancy of loneliness and pain. Poetry is a way to see the truth, and in that process, healing becomes possible. Use words that are stark, strong, and vibrant, words that bite, words that leave the roots and dirt on. Use magnetic words that stir attention and feeling. The potent energy contained within such words ignites the authentic development of your poem. Choose words that interest you, that have impact, that reveal something about you and your state of mind, problem or hurt right now. Pay attention to how the sound of a word communicates the feeling of that word. Dive into these words. Some examples include: restless, jagged, wreckage, ruthless, abandon, frighten, turbulent, bruised, caress, fertile, pungent, empty, moist, ache, rotting, stormy scream, rage, shatter, odor, exhausted, thorny, cavernous, molten. Sometimes images in nature make good metaphors or analogies.

You can also complete these stem sentences to evoke or describe feelings:

I see, I hear, I taste, I smell, I touch, I feel, I sense, I yearn, I long for, I cry out.

Use images so vivid that others will have clear visual and visceral representations.

Appendix K: End of Therapy Tools

End of Therapy Questions for Clients to Consider

1. For many clients, the end of therapy brings up feelings and memories of previous transitions and losses. What thoughts and feelings do endings in general bring up for you? What thoughts and feelings are you having about the ending of this therapy relationship?
2. What have you learned, what has been helpful for you in this therapy?
3. What are you aware of about yourself that you weren't aware of before?
4. What are the skills you've learned that you want to keep implementing in your life?
5. What do you like and appreciate about yourself? What are you grateful for in your life?
6. What stands out to you most about your interactions with your therapist?

7. What do you like and appreciate about your therapist?
8. What regrets do you have about the therapy or what would you like to have gone differently?
9. What situations, thoughts or behaviors make you vulnerable to (insert disorder/ presenting problem here), and how can you deal with them to decrease the likelihood or the severity of what you were experiencing when you first came in?
10. What are the things you can do to maintain your gains in therapy and to continue to improve your life?

End of Therapy Letter to Client

Describe the following:

1. The client's goals and progress in therapy.
2. Your client's unique and special qualities, and what you appreciate about him/her.
3. Interactions you had with your client that stand out, what impacted you personally, what you enjoyed and what touched or moved you.
4. What you take away from your work with your client, what you will remember about him/her, and how you are different as a result of having worked with him/her.
5. What you want your client to take away from his/her work with you, and what's important for your client to remember.
6. Any regrets?
7. Your hopes and wishes for your client.
8. What you will miss about your client.
9. Parting advice, what to watch out for in the future, and relapse prevention ideas.

Appendix L: FAP-ECR (Experiences of Closeness in the Therapeutic Relationship)

Attachment measure modified for therapist–client relationship

Name: Date:

The following statements concern how you feel in your relationship with your therapist. Respond to each statement by indicating how much you agree or disagree with it. Write the number in the space provided, using the following rating scale:

1		2	3	4		5	6	7
Disagree Strongly				Neutral/Mixed				Agree Strongly

___ 1. I prefer not to show my therapist how I feel deep down.
___ 2. I am very comfortable being close to my therapist.
___ 3. Just when my therapist starts to get close to me I find myself pulling away.
___ 4. I get uncomfortable when my therapist wants to be very close.
___ 5. I don't feel comfortable opening up to my therapist.
___ 6. I want to get close to my therapist, but I keep pulling back.
___ 7. I am nervous when my therapist gets too close to me.
___ 8. I feel comfortable sharing my private thoughts and feelings with my therapist.
___ 9. I try to avoid getting too close to my therapist.
___ 10. I find it relatively easy to get close to my therapist.
___ 11. Sometimes I feel that I force my therapist to show more feeling, more commitment.
___ 12. I find it difficult to allow myself to depend on my therapist.
___ 13. I prefer not to be too close to my therapist.
___ 14. I tell my therapist just about everything.
___ 15. I usually discuss my problems and concerns with my therapist.
___ 16. I feel comfortable depending on my therapist.
___ 17. I don't mind asking my therapist for comfort, advice, or help.
___ 18. It helps to turn to my therapist in times of need.
___ 19. I turn to my therapist for many things, including comfort and reassurance.

Appendix M: PTSR (Patient-Therapist Session Report) on Relationships

1. Over the last week, have your relationships with others been different than they usually are?

1 They have been much worse lately. I feel I have a harder time interacting with others.

2 They have been slightly worse; I've had some difficulties with others lately.

3 I haven't noticed my relationships with others being different than they usually are.

4 They have been slightly better. My relationships seem to work better or feel better to me.

5 They have been much better, my relationships seem to work much better or feel much better to me.

2. Over the last week, if your relationships have seemed different to you: (i.e., your response to #1 was 1, 2, 4,or 5) do you think the difference is a result of this therapy?

(continued)

	1	No, the difference I've noticed in my relationships is due to other factors.

1   No, the difference I've noticed in my relationships is due to other factors.

    I don't see a connection between how my relationships are and what happens in

2   therapy.

3   I think the changes may be related to some extent.

4   The differences in my relationships is definitely a result of therapy.

3.   If your response to # 2 was 3 or 4 (the change in relationships *is a result of* this therapy), it was due to:

1   Something that happened in the last session (the session prior to today).

2   A collective or cumulative effect over many sessions

4.   Over the last week, has your symptom(s) been different than usual?

1   It has been much worse lately.

2   It has been slightly worse.

3   I haven't noticed my symptoms being different than usual.

4   It has been slightly better.

5   It has been much better.

5.   Over the last week, if your symptom (s) seemed different to you: (i.e., your response to #4 was 1, 2, 4,or 5) do you think the difference is a result of this therapy?

1   No, the difference I've noticed in my sympto (s) is due to other factors.

    I don't see a connection between how my symptom (s) is and what happens in

2   therapy.

3   I think the changes may be related to some extent.

4   The differences in my symptom(s) is definitely a result of therapy.

6.   If your response to # 5 was 3 or 4 (the change in my symptom (s) *is a result of* this therapy), it was due to:

1   Something that happened in the last session (the session prior to today).

2   A collective or cumulative effect over many sessions.

7.   Over the last week, has the way you view events or situations in your life been different than it usually is?

1   It has been much worse lately.

2   It has been slightly worse.

3   I haven't noticed my view of events or situations being different than usual.

4   It has been slightly better.

5   It has been much better.

8.   Over the last week, if your view of events or situations has seemed different to you: (i.e., your response to #7 was 1, 2, 4,or 5) do you think the difference is a result of this therapy?

1   No, the difference I've noticed in my view of events or situations is due to other factors.

2   I don't see a connection between my view of events and situations and what happens in therapy.

3   I think the changes may be related to some extent.

4   The differences in my view of events and situations is definitely a result of therapy.

9.   If your response to # 8 was 3 or 4 (the change in my view *is a result of* this therapy), it was due to:

1   Something that happened in the last session (the session prior to today).

2   A collective or cumulative effect over many sessions

224   Appendices

Appendix N: Emotional Risk Log

Creating more of what we want in our lives usually takes courage. We will have to move beyond our comfort zones and do things that feel anxiety-provoking, scary or risky. Discuss with your therapist (1) the risks you've taken in the past that led to desired outcomes, and (2) what risks you can take now that will move you towards what you value in your life, and the benefits versus costs of these risks. Try to take one risk daily; they can be small risks (e.g., rating of 1–2), or larger ones. Examples include: expressing your true feelings to someone, taking an art class, trying a new recipe. Consider things you would really like to do, but normally would not. Include risks that you can take in your interactions with your therapist.

Date	Description of Emotional Risk	Risk Rating 1-10 (10 = highest)

Index

A

Acceptance and Commitment Therapy
(ACT), 46, 113, 121, 202
Addis, M. E., 73
Allen, L. B., 38
Altruistic behavior, 204–205
Andersen, S. M., 24
Anderson, C. A., 26
Antecedents, 48
Armstrong, P. V., 167
Arrindell, W. A., 132
Asch, S. E., 110
Assessment and case conceptualization
assessment of therapist
T1s (Therapist Problem Behaviors)
and T2s (Therapist Target
Behaviors), 58
therapist role in FAP, 56–57
therapist stimulus functions, 57–58
assessment over course of therapy, 42–43
client self-monitoring during treatment,
55–56
defining and tracking of response
classes, 56
monitoring opportunities, 56
tracking of behavior outside-of-
session, 55
context of assessment, 38
overview of functional idiographic
assessment, 38–42
functional class, 41
functional identification, 41
possible roadblocks to assessment, 58–59
structured case formulation using
Functional Idiographic
Assessment Template (FIAT),
50–53
case example: identifying FIAT
classes, 54–55
tactics in practical case formulation
assessment of antecedents, behavioral
repertoires and consequences, 48–50
behavior outside of session (Os), 46
Clinically Relevant Behaviors
(CRBs), 47–48
goals and values, 45–46
life history, 44–45
Atkinson, R. C., 25
Auerbach, A., 25
Avoidance behaviors, 49
Awareness/Relaxation/Acceptance Exercise
(ARA), 121
instructions for, 122–123
rationale for, 121
Ayllon, T., 5

B

Banko, K. M., 28
Barber, J. P., 23
Barlow, D. H., 38
Barnes-Holmes, D., 66, 105, 108
Barnes-Holmes, Y., 66, 105
Baruch, D. E., 21
Baum, A. B., 24
Baum, W. M., 200
Beginning phase of therapy
creating trust and safety
importance of fostering, 147–148
trust-enhancing behaviors, 148
Beginning of Therapy Questionnaire,
218–219
Behavior
defined, 4
operant, 7
respondent, 7
See also Discriminative stimuli; Eliciting
stimuli; Operant behavior;
Reinforcing stimuli

Behavioral approach
  advantage of, 3
Behavioral assessment, 39
Behavioral cosmology
  clients experience, 16
  contingencies of reinforcement, 16
  experiential exercise, 17–18
Behavioral theory of self, 110
Behaviorism, 3, 4
Behaviors as actions
  examples of, 4
Behavior's function, 7
  defined, 39
Benson, H., 112, 121–122
Bergin, A. E., 23
Bermúdez, M. A. L., 22
Berry, A., 203
Berry, J. W., 27
Biglan, A., 4
Bilgrave, D. P., 201
Bilodeau, E. A., 25
Bolling, M. Y., 12, 30, 42, 145, 199
Borderline personality disorder (BPD), 110
Bowlby, J., 134
Breen, W. L., 202
Brennan, K. A., 138
Brown, G. W., 21
Brown, K. W., 113
Burckell, L. A., 83
Burman, B., 132
Busch, A. M., 21, 31–32, 145

C
Callaghan, G. M., 24, 30, 31, 37, 50, 55, 64,
      145, 147, 167, 169, 170, 191, 195,
      196, 202
Calvillo, M., 22
Cameron, J., 28
Carpenter, K. M., 73
Case conceptualization, 41
  purpose, 42
Case conceptualization form, 215
Castonguay, L. G., 23
Catania, A. C., 25, 30
CBT treatment for panic
  discussion of mindfulness, 111
Chen, S., 24
Choate, M. L., 38
Client improvements that occur in-session
      (CRB2s), 13–14
Client interpretations of behavior (CRB3s),
      14–15
  functional talk, 15

Client problems that occur in-session
      (CRB1s), 12–13
Client's values
  identifying and clarifying aid therapeutic
      process, 45
  methods for clarifying, 46
Clinically Relevant Behaviors (CRBs)
  CRB1s, 12–13
    clinical problems, 13
  CRB2s, 13–14
  CRB3s, 14–15
  In-to-Out Parallels, 47
  Out-to-In Parallels, 47–48
Cognitive Behavioral Therapy (CBT), 111
Cole, S. W., 24–25
Competence in conducting FAP, 99–100
  client target behavior in own repertoire, 100
  controlled by reinforcers beneficial to
      client, 100
  therapist self-awareness, 99–100
  thorough understanding of client, 99
Connolly, M. B., 23, 24, 25, 27
Consciousness, 104, 120
Contextual modeling, 173
  See also Non-contextualized modeling
Contrived or arbitrary responses, 135
Contrived reinforcers, 9
Cooley, C. H., 106, 108, 109
Cooper, M. L., 21
Cordova, J. V., 132, 133
Cornell, D. P., 203
Course of therapy
  beginning phase
    beginning therapy with 'Alicia',
        150–153
    "Beginning of Therapy
        Questionnaire", 149
    creating trust and safety, 147–148
    instilling hope, 148
    taking time to form meaningful
        relationship, 148–149
    therapy forms, 149–150
  end phase, 161–164
    behavioral activation, 163
    end-of-therapy letter, 161–163
    "End of Therapy Tools", 161
    mindfulness, 163
    moving into avoidance, 163
    self care, 163–164
  FAP techniques, 145
  middle phase
    "Emotional Risk Log", 154
    focus on avoidance, 154–155

middle of therapy with 'Alicia',
    157–161
  "Mid-Therapy Questionnaire", 154
  "Typical FAP Questions", 154
  typical ideal FAP interaction, 155–157
  prior to, 146
Covey, S. R., 206
Coyne, J. C., 133
CRBs, 70
CRB1s, see Client problems that occur in-
    session (CRB1s)
CRB2s, see Client improvements that occur
    in-session (CRB2s)
CRB3s, see Client interpretations of
    behavior (CRB3s)
Crits-Christoph, P., 23, 25
Crocker, P., 136
Crying Out in Your Poetry, 221–222
Cullinan, V., 66, 105
Cush, D. T., 30

D
Dalai Lama, 205
Davis, M. K., 23
Davison, G. C., 38
Deaver, C. M., 26
Deci, E. L., 28
Deida, D., 136, 205
Deikman, A., 104
Delay effect, 25
Deluty, R. H., 201
Demorest, A., 25
DeRubeis, R. J., 23
Dialectical Behavioral Therapy (DBT), 22
Dickinson, A., 28
Direct implementation of green FAP
  advancing sense of purpose and personal
    mission, 206–210
  altruistic behavior, 204–205
  cultivating open heart, 205–206
  developing sense of universal
    responsibility, 205
  engaging in daily practice, 210–211
Discriminative stimuli, 6–7
Dore, J., 106
Dougher, M. J., 12
Drozd, J. F., 23
DSM (Diagnostic and Statistical Manual)-
    based diagnostic assessment, 38

E
Edelstein, S., 27
Eliciting stimuli, 7

Emotional risk log, 226
End of therapy tools
  letter to client, 223
  questions for clients to consider,
    222–223
Escape responses, 49
Eubanks-Carter, C., 83
Evocative therapeutic methods,
    74–82
  classes of avoided thoughts and
    feelings, 75
  empty chair work, 76–77
  evoking client's best self, 80–82
  evoking emotion by focusing on bodily
    sensations, 77–80
  free association, 75
  writing exercises, 75–76
Experiences of Closeness in Therapeutic
    Relationship (FAP-ECR), 138
  attachment measure modified for
    therapist-client relationship,
    223–224
Experience of self, 104–105
  verbal behavior and, 108
Experience of Self Scale (EOSS), 110
Exposure and Response Prevention
    (ERP), 123
  essence of, 124
  specific treatment elements, 124

F
Falender, C. A., 195
FAP-ECR, see Experiences of Closeness in
    Therapeutic Relationship
    (FAP-ECR)
FAP-enhanced cognitive therapy (FECT),
    30, 41
"FAP Experiences of Closeness in
    Therapist-Client Relationship"
    questionnaire, 138
FAP Life Snapshot, 216
FAP practicum model, 190–192
  becoming trustworthy, 192
  developing empathic reflection
    students practice, 191–192
  increasing emotional risk-taking and
    decreasing experiential avoidance,
    190–191
  examples of exercises, 191
  rationale for exercises, 191
  vision for practicum, 190
FAP Preliminary Client Information
    Questionnaire, 215–216

FAP principles
    CRBs evoked by therapeutic context,
        24–25
    CRBs shaped through application of
        contingencies in therapeutic
        relationship, 25–27
        contingent reinforcement and
            interpersonal expectancy effects,
            28–29
        contingent reinforcement and
            'unconditional' positive regard,
            26–27
        importance of contingent
            reinforcement live, in-session
            behavior, 25
        transference interpretations differ
            from contingent responding, 27
    existing research on, 30–32
        ACT and FAP to Nicotine
            Replacement Therapy, 30–31
        determining effectiveness of FECT
            and CBT for depression, 30
        FAP mechanism, 31
        FAPRS, 31
    importance of natural reinforcement,
        27–30
        contingent, natural reinforcement
            promotes generalization, 29–30
        contingent responding undermine
            intrinsic motivation, 27–28
FAP process feedback forms and
        questionnaires
    Beginning of Therapy Questionnaire, 74,
        149, 150, 218–219
    Crying Out in Your Poetry, 74, 221–222
    End of Therapy Tools, 74, 161, 222–223
    Grief Worksheet, 74, 220
    Loss Inventory, 74, 220–221
    Mid-Therapy Questionnaire, 74, 154,
        219–220
    Session Bridging Form, 74, 149, 217
    Typical FAP Questions, 74, 154, 217–218
FAP questions for supervisors, 175–176
FAP rationale (FAP rap)
    examples, 73
    statements, 71–73
FAP rules, 61–62
FAP, see Functional Analytic
        Psychotherapy (FAP)
    and Acceptance and Commitment
        Therapy (ACT), 22
    aim, 199
    assessment, 38

case conceptualizations, 37
case studies, 22
and Dialectical Behavioral Therapy
        (DBT), 22
function of stimulus or behavior, 39
as stand alone treatment, 22, 30
topographical analysis, 39
FAP Session Bridging Form, 217
FAP supervision process
    emphasizes self-development of therapist
        and supervisees, 168
FAP techniques
    Acceptance and Commitment
        Therapy, 145
    Behavioral Activation, 145
    Cognitive Therapy, 145
FAP theory, 28
FAP verbal behavior classification system
    detecting CRB1s in verbal behavior,
        67–70
        forms and functions of client
            statements, 68
    mands, 67
    tacts, 66–67
FASIT (Functional Assessment of Skills for
        Interpersonal Therapists), 170
Ferro, C. L. B., 22
Ferro, G. R., 22
Ferro, R., 22
Ferster, C. B., 9
FIAT classes
    Class A, 51
    Class B, 51–52
    Class C, 52
    Class D, 52–53
    Class E, 53
    difficulties, 53
    identifying (case example), 54–55
FIAT-Q, 50, 139
FIAT, see Functional Idiographic
        Assessment Template (FIAT)
Fischer, N., 123
Flessner, C. A., 121
Focus on in-vivo work
    case example, 176–179
    contextual modeling, 173
    evoking and naturally reinforcing
        supervisee target behaviors
        decreasing avoidance, 174
    FAP questions for supervisors, 175–176
    focus on parallel process, 179–182
Follette, V. M., 103, 202
Follette, W. C., 24, 37, 147, 167, 169

Foreman, S., 25
Fraiberg, S., 106
Fraley, R. C., 138
Frank, J. D., 26
Freeston, M. H., 167
Freud, S., 1, 22, 134
Friedlander, M., 179
Frone, M. R., 21
Fulton, P. R., 111
Functional analysis
    behavior's function, 7
    case study, 5–8
    discriminative stimuli, 6–7
    eliciting stimuli, 7
    patient in reinforced position, 5
    reinforcing stimuli, 6
    versus topographical analysis, 6–8
Functional Analytic Psychotherapy (FAP), 1
    behavioral concepts underlying
        behavior as action, 4
        functional analysis *versus*
            topographical analysis, 5–8
        reinforcement, 8–10
    behavioral cosmology
        experiential exercise, 17–18
    behavioral view of psychotherapy, 11–12
        application of functional analysis, 11
    definition, 1
    experiences, 1–2
    therapeutic focus
        assumptions, 12
        clinically relevant behavior, 12–15
Functional Analytic Psychotherapy Rating
        Scale (FAPRS), 31
Functional assessment, 39, 40
    aim, 40
    source of information, 40
    See also Behavioral assessment
Functional class, 41
Functional identification, 41
Functional Idiographic Assessment
        Template (FIAT), 50
Furtado da Cruz, A. C., 22

G
Gable, S. L., 132
Gallese, V., 181
Garlinghouse, M. A., 26
Garske, J. P., 23
Gartner, A. F., 201
Gartner, J., 201
Gaynor, S. T., 30
Germer, C. K., 111, 113

Gifford, E. V., 30, 145, 202
Ginsberg, J. P., 203
Gladis, L., 23
Glassman, N. S., 24
Goldberg, N., 75
Goldfried, M. R., 23, 83
Gordon, K. H., 132
Gosch, C. S., 22
Greben, S. E., 101
Greek Chorus function, 189
Greenberg, L., 76
Green FAP, 199
    personal values of, 200
    therapist, 201
Greenspoon, J., 25, 26
Gregg, J. A., 105, 145
Grief Worksheet, 220
Groom, J., 46
Group supervision model, 182–190
    advantages of, 187–188
    broad outcomes, 189–190
    Greek Chorus, 188–189
    therapist case conceptualization, 183–187

H
Haidt, J., 204
Hanh, T. N., 206
Harlow, T., 203
Harmatz, M., 201
Harris, M. J., 28
Haughton, E., 5
Hayes, L. J., 3, 106
Hayes, A. M., 23
Hayes, S. C., 3, 11, 22, 29, 37, 46, 53, 61, 66,
        77, 103, 105, 106, 108, 113, 114, 202
Hays, R. D., 21
Himadi, W., 174
Hineline, P. N., 168
Hockman, C. H., 25
Hohmann, A., 201
Holloway, E., 195
Holman, G. I., 21, 145
Hooley, J. M., 21
Horvath, A. O., 23

I
Ideological transference, 201
Immediate reinforcement, 25
Implementation of green FAP during FAP
    case example, 203
    giving and accepting care, 203
    improving attachment repertoires,
        202–203

Implementation of green FAP during FAP (*cont.*)
  increasing stable sense of self, 203
  reducing experiential avoidance, 202
Interpersonal expectancy effects, 28
Interpersonal vulnerability, 132
Intimacy
  attached or connected to others, 134–135
    behavioral repertoires, classification, 134
    Bowlby's fundamental hypothesis, 134
  case example, 139–142
  clinical importance, 132–133
  definitions, 131–132
  expressing difficult and risky thoughts and feelings, 133–134
    boundary issues, 133–134
    self-disclosure as aversive stimulus, 133
  fear of, 134
  lack of, 132
  as process, 132
  social support
    response blocks, 133
  source of happiness and well-being, 132
  therapeutic implications
    discuss and assess attachment and connection, 138–139
    reinforce interpersonal vulnerable behavior, 135–136
    specific techniques, 136–138
Intimacy problems, 169
Intimate relationship, 132
  healing trauma with therapeutic, 132
In-to-out assessment process, 47
In-to-out parallels, 93
Intrinsic motivation
  defined, 28
  versus extrinsic motivation, 28

J
James, I., 168
Johnson, K. C., 205, 206, 211
John, W. M., 174
Joiner, T. E., 132
Joyce, A. S., 24
'Judging' of interest, 113

K
Kanter, J. W., 1, 8, 12, 21, 23, 30, 31, 37, 42, 61, 84, 103, 110, 145
Kashdan, T. B., 202

Keane, T., 174
Kernis, M. H., 203
Keysers, C., 181
Kingma, D. R., 163
Klein, D. N., 21
'Knowing how' and 'knowing that', 168, 169
Koestner, R., 28
Kohlenberg, B. S., 22, 24
Kohlenberg, R. J., 1, 2, 3, 4, 12, 22, 23, 24, 30, 42, 61, 63, 66, 74, 84, 103, 107, 110, 117, 123
Kohn, A., 28
Konner, M., 134
Kovacs, A. L., 131
Krasner, L., 26

L
Ladany, N., 179
Lambert, M. J., 23
Landes, S. J., 21, 37, 145
Lara, M. E., 21
Larson, D., 201
Laurenceau, J.-P., 131
Lawrence, P., 30
Leader, J., 21
Leibing, E., 27
Leichsenring, F., 27
Leigland, S., 45
Linehan, M. M., 103
Lines of evidence in support of FAP
  existing research on FAP principles, 30–32
  principles of FAP
    CRBs evoked by therapeutic context, 24–25
    CRBs shaped through application of contingencies in therapeutic relationship, 25–27
    importance of natural reinforcement, 27–30
  therapeutic alliance, 22–24
    assumptions, 24
    focus on therapeutic relationship, 23
    importance of, 23
    See also 'Quintessential integrative variable' of therapy
Lipkens, R., 106
Lipsitt, L. P., 25
"Living High and Letting Die", 204
Long, E. S., 26
López, F. J. C., 22
Loss Inventory Assignment, 220–221
"Loving Yourself", 163

Luborsky, L., 25
Luteijn, F., 132
Lyvers, M., 132

M
McAdams, D. P., 132
McCallum, M., 24
McCarthy, P. R., 83
McLellan, A. T., 25
McMain, S., 136
McNeill, B. W., 179
Mahalik, J. R., 83
Mands
    characteristics, 67
Manos, R. C., 145
Margolin, G., 132
Marlatt, G. A., 112, 113
Marques, J., 112
Martin, D. J., 23
Marx, B. P., 22, 145
'Metaphor', 68
    example, 69–70
Meyer, B., 134, 135, 202
The Mid-Therapy Questionnaire,
    219–220
Mikulincer, M., 203
Miller, I. W., 21
Milne, D., 168
Miltenberger, R. G., 26
Mindfulness
    awareness or consciousness having
        characteristics
        focus on here and now, 113
        non-judgmentalness, 113
    definition, 103, 112
    process from therapist's perspective, 112
Mindfulness
    behavioral view of, 111–113
        focus on here and now, 113
        non-judgmentalness, 113
    case example: exposure and response
        prevention, FAP and mindfulness
        for obsessive compulsive disorder,
        123–128
    clinical implications and techniques for
        promoting
        Awareness/Relaxation/Acceptance
            Exercise (ARA), 121–123
        self-observation, 119–121
    in context of FAP, 112
    Janet Surrey's description of, 112
    therapeutic mindfulness, 114
"Mindfulness in Psychotherapy", 111

Mission statement, 46, 206, 210
    crafting of, 206–210
    inspiring, 210
Moran, P., 21
Morris, S. A., 30
Mudar, P., 21
Muran, J. C., 23, 136, 169
Murray, P., 136
"Naked Buddhism", 205

N
Natural reinforcement
    vs. arbitrary reinforcement, 188
Natural reinforcers, 9
    in-session improvement, 10
Naugle, A. E., 24, 147
Negative reinforcement or avoidance, 40
Nelson, M. L., 179
Nelson, R. O., 37
Non-contextualized modeling, 174
Non-directive therapy, 26
Nonspecific behaviors, 147
Non-specific relationship factor, 22, 29

O
O'Brian, C., 25
Obsessive compulsive disorder
    ERP, FAP and mindfulness for, 123–128
O'Connor, L. E., 27
O'Gorman, R., 204
Ogrodniczuk, J. S., 24, 27
Oliveira-Nasser, K. C. F., 22
Operant behavior (voluntary behavior), 7
    See also Discriminative stimuli;
        Reinforcing stimuli
Optimal therapist repertoires, 170, 178
Orsillo, S. M., 22
Out-to-in parallels, 93
Out-to-in process, 47

P
Parallel process hypothesis, 179
Paraphrased rationale, example, 121
Parker, C. R., 12, 30, 42, 103, 110, 145
Park, N., 204
"Patient-Therapist Session Report (PTSR)
    on Relationships", 139
Paul, R. H., 22
Peck, M. S., 61
Peirce, R. S., 21
Perls, F., 76
Personal therapeutic values, 200
Perspective or locus, experience of, 108

Peters, A. N., 106
Peterson, C., 204
Pielage, S. B., 132, 135
Pierce, W. D., 28
Pilkonis, P. A., 134, 135, 202
Piper, W. E., 24
Popovic, M., 131
Possible CRBs based on FIAT-Q responses,
    64–66
Power differential
    information to supervisee, 195
Prager, K. J., 132
"Preliminary Client Information"
    questionnaire, 44
Pryor, K., 153
Psychotherapy, 61
    therapeutic relationship, 22
PTSR (Patient-Therapist Session Report) on
    relationships, 224–225

Q
Queiroz, M. A. M., 22
'Quintessential integrative variable' of
    therapy, 23

R
Radical behavioral theory, 8
Ragan, J., 21
Randall, P., 21
Rapp, J. T., 26
Raue, P. J., 23
Reese, H. W., 3
Reinforcement
    contingencies of, 16
    contingencies, 26
    delay of, 25
    immediate, 25
    natural *versus* contrived reinforcers, 8–10
    negative, 8
    positive, 15
    within-session contingencies, 10
    shaping, 10
Reinforcing stimuli, 6
Reis, H. T., 132
Relational Frame Theory (RFT), 114
Renner, K. E., 25
Respect
    defined in context of self, 117
Respondent behavior (involuntary or
    reflexive behavior), 7
    See also Eliciting stimuli
Response repertoires, 48–49
Rigotti, N. A., 30

Rivera, L. M., 131
Rizzolatti, G., 181
Robbins, J., 203
Robitschek, C. G., 83
Roche, B., 3, 66, 108
Rogerian theory, 27
Rogers, C. R., 22, 26, 29, 85, 147
Rosenfarb, I. S., 29, 30
Rosen, G. M., 38
Rosenthal, R., 28
Rotter, J. B., 110
Ruckstuhl, L. E., 31
Ruiz, M., 42
Rule-governed behavior
    vs contingency-shaped behavior, 29
Rusch, L. C., 21, 145
Russell, M., 21
Russell, R., 132
Ryan, F. J., 25
Ryan, R. M., 28, 113

S
Sacred space, 171
Safran, J. D., 23
Salovey, P., 57
Saltzman, I. J., 25
Sanders, C., 145
Sawabini, F. L., 25
Schaffer, A. R., 131
Schildcrout, J. S., 23
Scott, R. L., 132, 174
Self
    behavioral view of
        development of sense of self,
            106–110
        experience of self, 104–105
    clinical implications for problems of
        match therapeutic tasks to level of
            private control in client's
            repertoire, 116–117
        reinforce as many client 'I x'
            statements as possible,
            117–119
        reinforce talking in absence of
            specific external cues, 115–116
    defined, 104
    develops as result of language
        acquisition, 109–110
    understanding, functionally, 105
Self-awareness, 104, 120
    See also Consciousness
Self problems, clinical implications for,
    114–119

match therapeutic tasks to level of private
control in client's repertoire,
116–117
reinforce as many client 'I x' statements as
possible, 117–119
counterproductive statements,
118–119
self-maligning statements, 119
suicidal or homicidal statements, 119
reinforce talking in absence of specific
external cues, 115–116
Seligman, M. E. P., 204
Sense of Self, 104, 110
development of, 106–110
"Session Bridging" Questions, 139
Shafranske, E. P., 195
Shapiro, D. A., 23
Shaver, P. R., 203
Sherbourne, C. D., 21
Shimoff, E., 30
Siegel, R. D., 111
Simi, N. L., 83
Singer, P., 204
Single-word speech period, 106
Siqueland, L., 23
Skinner, B. F., 2, 9, 18, 25, 29, 67, 104, 105,
134, 169, 200
Socio-political behaviors (SPs), 42
Specific discriminative stimuli (Sds), 106
aversive, 114, 120
Steen, T. A., 204
Stice, E., 21
Stimulus or behavior, function of, 39
Stricker, J. M., 26
Strosahl, K. D., 22, 46, 108, 202
Structured free association, 117
Structuring evocative therapy, 71–74
creating sacred space of trust and
safety, 74
describing FAP rationale (FAP rap),
71–72
using FAP process feedback forms and
questionnaires, 74
Summers, C. J., 30, 55
Sun, C.R., 203
Supervision and therapist self-development
ethics and precautions in FAP
supervision
boundary issues, 195
creating therapist case
conceptualization, 196–197
difficulty in FAP, 192–195
power differential, 195

FAP individual supervision methods
create sacred space for supervision,
171–173
focus on in-vivo work, 173–182
goals of FAP supervision, 168–170
increase emotional knowing, 168–169
increase supervisee's knowledge base
or intellectual knowing, 168
'Knowing how' and 'knowing that',
168, 169
optimal therapist repertoires, 170
group training modalities
FAP practicum model, 190–192
group supervision model, 182–190
Surrey, J. L., 113, 123, 137
Syndromal diagnosis, 38

T
Tacting, 105
Tacts, 66–67
Tarpy, R. M., 25
Teasdale, J. D., 21
Terry, C., 42, 199
Therapeutic ethics, 200
Therapeutic facts, 200
Therapeutic goals, 14
Therapeutic implications
experiential exercises
connection exercises, 137
instructions for combined
exercises, 137
open heart meditation, 136–137
Therapeutic love, 84
Therapeutic mechanisms, 3
Therapeutic mindfulness, 112, 114
Therapeutic technique
avoid sexual exploitation
avoid non-beneficial treatment,
98–99
competence in conducting FAP,
99–100
cultural biases, 98
ethical issues and precautions, 98
evoke CRBs
structuring evocative therapy, 71–74
using evocative therapeutic methods,
74–82
using oneself as instrument of change,
82–83
functional analytically informed
interpretations and implement
generalization strategies
assigning homework, 96–97

Therapeutic technique (*cont.*)
FAP reasons, 92–93
parallels between in-session and daily life behaviors, 93–96
natural reinforcement of CRB2s
amplifying feelings to increase salience, 87–89
caring for clients, 85
clients' goal repertoires, 85–86
matching expectations with clients' current repertoires, 86–87
responding to CRB1s, 84–85
reinforce CRB2s naturally amplify one's feelings to increase salience, 84–85
reinforcing effects of therapist behavior in relation to client CRBs, 90–92
role of T1s and T2s, 92
watch for CRBs
detecting hidden meaning in verbal behavior, 66–70
identification of possible CRBs based on FIAT-Q responses, 64–66
reactions as barometer, 63–64
therapeutic situations evoke CRBs, 63
Therapist-client relationship, 3
Therapist imperfections, 133–134
Therapist's intervention, 25
Therapy experience, 14–15
Therapy forms, 149–150
beginning phase
"Beginning of Therapy Questionnaire", 150
case conceptualization, 150
"FAP Experiences of Closeness in the Therapeutic Relationship" questionnaire (FAP-ECR), 150
"PTSR (Patient-Therapist Session Report) on Relationships", 150
"Session Bridging Form", 149
end phase
"End of Therapy Tools", 161
middle phase
"Emotional Risk Log", 154
"Mid-Therapy Questionnaire", 154
"Typical FAP Questions", 154
Thinking as process, 114
Thorberg, F. A., 132
Tolle, E., 113
Transference, 24
Transference interpretation, 27

Treatment
functional, 37
Truax, C. B., 26, 85
Tsai, M., 1, 2, 3, 4, 12, 21, 22, 30, 42, 61, 63, 66, 74, 84, 103, 107, 110, 117, 131, 132, 145, 167, 199, 203
Turk, D. C., 57
Turn-by-turn methodology
advantage of, 31
Typical FAP Questions, 217–218

U
Unstructured free association, 116–117

V
Valero, L., 22
Valued Living Questionnaire (VLQ), 46
Values, 199–200
Values for fulfillment, 207–208
Value statements
personal therapeutic values, 200
therapeutic ethics, 200
therapeutic facts, 200
Values in therapy and green FAP
implementing green FAP values
direct implementation of green FAP, 203–211
implementation of green FAP during FAP, 202–203
role of therapists' personal values in psychotherapy, 200–202
therapist's personal values influence professional roles, 201
Vandenberghe, L., 22, 123
Van Orden, K., 132, 135
Van Vugt, M., 204
Verbal behavior
development, stages of, 107, 108
functional analysis of labeling stimuli, *see* Tacting
Vives, M. C., 22

W
Wachtel, P. L., 9
Wagner, A. W., 22
Waller, N. G., 138
Weeks, C. E., 37
Weidman, M., 30, 55
Weiss, J., 27
Wells, K. B., 21
Wells, P. A., 132
Wetterneck, C. T., 121
Williamson, M., 199

Wilson, D. S., 204
Wilson, K. D., 45
Wilson, K. G., 22, 45, 105, 108, 114,
    202, 204
Wingate, L. R., 132
Witkiewitz, K., 112
Wolfe, B., 23
Woods, D. W., 121

Woody, G. E., 25
Worthen, V., 179

Y
Yeater, E. A., 24, 136

Z
Zettle, R. D., 29, 61

Breinigsville, PA USA
23 June 2010
240345BV00004B/48/P